THORACIC TRAUMA

THORACIC TRAUMA

Edited by

DeWitt C. Daughtry, M.D.

Clinical Professor of Surgery,
University of Miami School of Medicine;
Attending Staff, Jackson Memorial
Hospital, Miami, Florida, Miami Heart
Institute, Miami Beach, Florida

Little, Brown and Company
Boston

Library of Congress Catalog Card No. 80-80593

ISBN 0-316-17380-0

Printed in the United States of America

HAL

To my wife Lucille

and to the many patients
who have made this volume possible

PREFACE

This book presents a comprehensive account of the management of thoracic trauma as seen primarily in civilian life but also in certain combat situations. The contributing authors are thoracic surgeons who have had vast experience in their particular areas, and thus each chapter is highly authoritative. *Thoracic Trauma* should serve as a guide for those who are involved in the treatment of thoracic injuries in well-equipped hospitals or in trauma centers.

Trauma, although largely preventable, is the fourth highest cause of death among all ages in the United States and is the leading cause of death under the age of 45 years. Thoracic injuries are becoming increasingly significant because of the large number of automobile accidents and because of the increase in various forms of violence. Twenty-five percent of automobile accident deaths are attributable to the thoracic component of the injury. When associated with other serious injuries, the thoracic component is an even greater contributing factor in disability and death. During wartime, with its attendant rise in bullet and shrapnel wounds, thoracic injuries account for a much higher mortality and morbidity.

In addition to the emphasis placed on management techniques, attention has been directed toward transportation of the injured, the communications response system, and triage at the site of the accident. Fortunately, there is emerging a new specialty devoted to emergency medical care. This should accomplish at least two things: first, better organization of emergency care for the patient in accident care centers; and second, better triage and organization of the consultation team to care for these patients. A review of autopsy material reveals that a large percentage of accident victims could have been salvaged by a better system of care.

In recent years physicians, industry, public officials, law enforcement agencies, and the federal government have become more deeply concerned with accident causation and prevention. Stimulated by the recent fuel shortage, this concern has led to manufacture of lower-horsepower cars and a lowering of speed limits. It is regrettable that the automobile manufacturing industry has been so careless in its attitude regarding safety features. However, measures have been taken to force the adoption of safer engineering principles, and this should further enhance accident prevention and decrease the severity and extent of injuries.

In addition to industry facing its responsibilities, we, as responsible citizens, should become involved and exert pressure upon organizations and individuals to face up to the major problem of accident prevention. Human carelessness causes more accidents and deaths than all other factors combined.

I wish to thank the individual co-authors for their superb contributions to this volume. I wish to express my gratitude to Minor Duggan, M.D., Head of the Department of Publications of the Miami Heart Institute, and also Mrs. Klara Soos of the same department. I would also like to express my appreciation to Mrs. Bronia Barbash, Medical Librarian, and Mr. Rand Johns, Medical Illustrator, of the Miami Heart Institute. Special thanks are due to my wife Lucille for her perseverance and to the staff of Little, Brown and Company for their fine cooperation.

D. C. D.

CONTENTS

CONTRIBUTING AUTHORS

PAUL C. ADKINS, M.D.
Professor and Chairman, Department of Surgery,
George Washington University School of Medicine
and Health Sciences, Washington, D.C.
Chapter 4

SAFUH ATTAR, M.D.
Professor of Surgery, University of Maryland School
of Medicine; Attending Surgeon, Department of
Thoracic and Cardiovascular Surgery, University of
Maryland Hospital, Baltimore, Maryland
Chapter 1

ARTHUR C. BEALL, Jr., M.D.
Professor of Surgery, Cora and Webb Mading
Department of Surgery, Baylor College of Medicine;
Attending Surgeon, Ben Taub General Hospital,
Houston, Texas
Chapter 11

WILLIAM E. BLOOMER, M.D.
Associate Clinical Professor of Surgery, University
of California, Los Angeles, School of Medicine,
Los Angeles; Chief, Section of Thoracic Surgery,
Memorial Hospital, Long Beach, California
Chapter 16

LEWIS H. BOSHER, Jr., M.D.
Professor, Department of Surgery, Virginia
Commonwealth University Medical College of
Virginia School of Medicine; Attending Surgeon,
Division of Thoracic and Cardiac Surgery, Medical
College of Virginia Hospitals and Clinics, Richmond,
Virginia
Chapters 9 and 10

LYMAN A. BREWER III, M.D., M.S.
Professor of Surgery, Loma Linda University School
of Medicine; Distinguished Physician, Jerry L. Pettis
Memorial Veterans Medical Center, Loma Linda,
California
Chapter 20

DONALD L. BRICKER, M.D.
Chief of Staff, Saint Mary of the Plains Hospital;
Attending Surgeon, Methodist Hospital, Lubbock,
Texas
Chapter 11

JAMES W. BROOKS, M.D.
Professor of Surgery, Division of Health Sciences,
Virginia Commonwealth University Medical College
of Virginia School of Medicine; Professor of
Surgery, Division of Cardiac and Thoracic Surgery,
Medical College of Virginia Hospitals and Clinics,
Richmond, Virginia
Chapters 12, 13, and 14

ROBERT E. CARR, M.D.
Consultant in Thoracic Surgery, Former Chief,
Division of Surgery, and Former Surgeon-in-Chief,
Harris Hospital, Fort Worth Medical Center, Fort
Worth, Texas
Chapter 5

J. M. CIVETTA, M.D.
Professor of Surgery, Anesthesiology, Medicine, and
Pathology, University of Miami School of Medicine;
Medical Director of the Intensive Care Unit, Jackson
Memorial Hospital, Miami
Chapter 8

PAUL J. CORSO, M.D.
Assistant Clinical Professor, George Washington
University School of Medicine and Health Sciences;
Junior Attending Surgeon, Department of Surgery,
Division of Cardiovascular and Thoracic Surgery,
The Washington Hospital Center, Washington, D.C.
Chapter 4

WILLIAM A. COX, M.D., Col. M.C., U.S.A., Ret.
Clinical Professor, Department of Cardiothoracic
Surgery, The University of Texas Medical School at
San Antonio; Chief of Staff and Attending Surgeon,
Thoracic Surgery Section, Memorial Medical Center,
Corpus Christi, Texas. Formerly Chief of
Cardiothoracic Surgery, Brooke Army Medical
Center, San Antonio, Texas, and Consultant in
Cardiothoracic Surgery, Korean Theater, 1965
Chapter 17

DE WITT C. DAUGHTRY, M.D.
Clinical Professor of Surgery, University of Miami
School of Medicine; Attending Staff, Jackson
Memorial Hospital, Miami, Florida, Miami Heart
Institute, Miami Beach, Florida
Editor; Chapters 2 and 15

JAMES DE WITT DAUGHTRY, M.D.
Urology Staff, St. Francis Hospital and Goleta
Valley Community Hospital, Santa Barbara,
California
Chapters 2 and 15

JOSEPH H. DAVIS, M.D.
Professor of Pathology, University of Miami School
of Medicine; Chief Medical Examiner, Dade County,
Miami, Florida
Chapter 21

JAMES M. FELTIS, Jr., Lt. Col. M.C.
Deputy Chief of Staff for Professional Activities,
U.S. Army Health Services Command, Fort Sam
Houston, San Antonio, Texas
Chapter 17

ROBERT J. FLEMMA, M.D.
Clinical Professor of Surgery, The Medical College
of Wisconsin; Attending Surgeon, St. Luke's
Hospital, Milwaukee, Wisconsin
Chapter 18

T. J. GALLAGHER, M.D.
Assistant Professor of Anesthesiology and Surgery,
University of Miami School of Medicine; Attending
Anesthesiologist, Departments of Anesthesiology and
Surgery, University of Miami-Jackson Memorial
Hospital Medical Center, Miami, Florida
Chapter 8

J. LAURANCE HILL, M.D.
Associate Professor of Surgery, University of
Maryland School of Medicine and The Johns
Hopkins University School of Medicine, Baltimore,
Maryland
Chapter 4

WILLIAM H. KIRBY, Jr., M.S.(Eng.), M.D.
Chief, Biophysics Laboratory, Edgewood Arsenal,
Edgewood, Maryland
Chapter 1

LUIZ C. KUNTZ, M.D.
Department of Surgery, Medical University of
South Carolina College of Medicine, Charleston,
South Carolina
Chapter 15

EUGENE L. NAGEL, M.D.
Professor and Chairman, Department of
Anesthesiology, The Johns Hopkins University
School of Medicine; Professor and Chairman,
Department of Anesthesiology, Johns Hopkins
Hospital, Baltimore, Maryland
Chapter 19

MARUF A. RAZZUK, M.D.
Clinical Associate Professor of Thoracic and
Cardiovascular Surgery, The University of Texas
Southwestern Medical School at Dallas; Attending
Surgeon, Department of Thoracic and Cardiovascular
Surgery, Baylor University Medical Center, Dallas,
Texas
Chapter 7

CHARLES F. REUBEN, M.D.
Assistant Instructor, Department of Surgery, The
Medical College of Wisconsin; Staff Surgeon,
Department of Thoracic and Cardiovascular
Surgery, St. Joseph's Hospital and Lutheran
Hospital, Milwaukee, Wisconsin
Chapter 18

PAUL C. SAMSON, M.D., M.S.
Clinical Professor Emeritus of Thoracic Surgery,
Stanford University School of Medicine, Stanford,
California; Chairman, Department of Thoracic
Surgery, Highland General Hospital; Formerly Chief
of Staff, Samuel Mcrritt Hospital, Oakland,
California
Chapters 3 and 6

RONALD SAMSON, M.D.
Assistant Professor of Anesthesiology, University
of Miami School of Medicine; Attending
Anesthesiologist, Jackson Memorial Hospital,
Miami, Florida
Chapter 19

HAWLEY H. SEILER, M.D., M.S.
Attending Thoracic Surgeon, Tampa General
Hospital, St. Joseph's Hospital, University
Community Hospital, Memorial Hospital, Brandon
Community Hospital, Centro Español Hospital,
Tampa, Florida
Chapters 12 and 14

KENNETH E. THOMAS, M.D.
Attending Surgeon and Director, Cardiac Surgery
Unit, St. Joseph's Hospital, Atlanta, Georgia
Chapter 10

RICHARD J. THURER, M.D.
Associate Professor of Surgery, Division of Thoracic
and Cardiovascular Surgery, University of Miami
School of Medicine; Attending Surgeon, Jackson
Memorial Hospital, Miami, Florida
Chapter 18

HAROLD C. URSCHEL, Jr., M.D.
Clinical Professor of Thoracic and Cardiovascular
Surgery, The University of Texas Health Science
Center; Senior Attending Surgeon, Department of
Thoracic Surgery, Baylor University Medical Center,
Dallas, Texas
Chapter 7

THORACIC TRAUMA

1. THE FORCES PRODUCING CERTAIN TYPES OF THORACIC TRAUMA

Safuh Attar
William H. Kirby, Jr.

The primary purpose of this chapter is to review briefly current information about the biophysics of trauma modalities and to relate this knowledge to clinical observations. It is intended as a contribution toward improved understanding and prevention or minimization of serious injury in the future.

Thoracic injuries may be categorized as either penetrating or nonpenetrating. While those sustained during military activities are usually of the penetrating kind and are due to fragmentation of various types of missiles, the injuries seen in civilian practice are brought about primarily by automobile crashes and comprise a wide variety from each category, both singly and combined. Often these thoracic injuries are complicated when other organs are also involved. In addition to automobile crashes, there are other causative factors such as aircraft crashes, athletic sports, accidental falls, riots (injuries caused by anti-riot weapons), accidental blasts, and criminal and personal conflicts. The common process in all cases is, of course, one of energy transfer. The outcome is dependent on a number of factors, such as the nature of the energy delivery or loading; the age, size, and shape of the recipient; the location and manner in which the energy is dissipated; the environment and accessibility to treatment; the time the accident occurs; and the diagnostic and therapeutic facilities available.

THE LOADING PROCESS

Two major difficulties prevent a comprehensive understanding of the effects of the various forms of impacting energy on the thorax and its component subsystems. In the first place, we know little about the basic mechanics of thoracic tissue, individually or as a whole. The body has often been described as a great nonlinear damping system.

Supported by the United States Public Health Service, Research Grant Nos. HE-09341-07 and HE-09341-08.

Clemedson and associates [7] have pointed out the extreme complexity of the human body, particularly from a mechanical standpoint, and have described it as a heterogeneous viscoelastic mass. The same authors have also noted that an impacting source imparts mechanical and thermal disturbances to the body, with the former the more important. This is followed by a deformation and displacement of tissues at and near the points of contact, with the development of a pressure wave or pulse that then propagates through the tissue until damped out or further transmitted out of the body.

The role of biomechanics, by applying physical engineering and mechanical principles to the study of bodily trauma, is to provide a better understanding of the cause and effects of the mechanisms and processes involved in thoracic trauma. Goldsmith [12] speaks of these principles and their application to head injuries, but they apply equally well to those of the thorax. Specifically, the principles of continuum mechanics or of the dynamics of discrete systems can be applied to mathematical models of the response of the thorax and its attachments to a given external stimulus, which in turn leads to a prediction of the history of the field parameters, such as stress, strain, displacement, acceleration, pressure for the entire domain, and the determination of the motion of specified elements. The tools of experimental mechanics can also be employed to measure physical changes produced by impact or impulsive loading in replicas of the thorax, which could be animal specimens, cadavers, or inanimate models. Tests of this type on living animals are accompanied most frequently by concurrent physiological measurement and subsequent pathological examination for the purpose of correlation. Data from such experiments serve the following purposes: to substantiate or disprove theoretical hypotheses concerning trauma mechanisms and their patterns; to establish tolerance levels and failure limits for various types of loading; to assess the efficacy of protective devices and environments; to provide statistical data; and to make available information concerning the basic mechanical properties of the components involved.

From the standpoint of mechanics, the causes of thoracic injuries may also be divided into categories on the basis of the manner of the loading application. An impact or blow upon the thorax may be due to a solid object traveling at an appreciable velocity, e.g., missiles or bullets; automobile components under crash conditions; slower moving objects such as knives; or even the intensive pressure waves caused by a blast. Each of these impacts may be further subdivided. In contrast we might consider the static or quasi-static loading produced by a relatively long-term crushing action. These situations encompass different physical phenomena, and their mathematical representations would emphasize different loading and response factors. Some of the injuries discussed later in this chapter demonstrate that clinical effects can often be distinguished according to the type of load that caused the injury.

PENETRATING THORACIC TRAUMA

Thoracic penetration by fast-moving particles such as bomb fragments or bullets is of concern to both military and civilian surgeons. Medical interest in the battle casualty includes the type and anatomical location of wounds as well as the correlated visceral damage and the causative agents, and has existed since the earliest days of organized combat. Much speculation and some observation has been devoted to the magnitude of a missile wound and its correlation with momentum, kinetic energy of the missile, or the rate with which the energy was dissipated. It has become apparent that all physical phenomena connected with wound formation are direct results of kinetic energy, meaning that the mass of a missile is not as important as the velocity with which it strikes.

Amato and associates [2] studied the events that occur within various tissues after high-velocity bullet-wounding. As tissues are struck by a missile, multiple disruptive forces combine to produce tissue destruction. The major forces consist of the velocity, the mass, and the change in shape of the bullet when it reaches the tissue. The most important force is the velocity of the missile within the tissues. The initial velocity on impact is called *striking velocity*. If the bullet leaves the tissue, the

remaining velocity is the *residual velocity*. The effective velocity of the injury is the difference between the two velocities: $(V_1 - V_2)$. The kinetic energy (KE) imparted to the tissues expressed in foot pounds can be written:

$$KE = M(V_1{}^2 - V_2{}^2)/2g$$

where M equals mass, and g equals gravity. If small amounts of energy are released within the tissue, as in the low-velocity wound, destruction will be confined to the pathway of the bullet. The energy released by high-velocity missiles forms initial shock waves with a pressure up to 100 to 200 atmospheres, imparting momentum to the tissues both forward and laterally. These tissues accelerate in an outward direction, creating a large space known as the *temporary cavity*. The tissues undulate and undergo stretching and compression. Because of the heterogeneity and varied density of the tissues, there is added mechanical damage due to the shearing effect between these tissues. The retentive forces that combat the disruptive forces vary with individual tissues. The characteristic pattern of injury is determined by the density of tissues combined with the degree of elasticity and cohesion within these tissues. Using high-speed photography and roentgenography, Amato and his colleagues [2] demonstrated experimentally the formation of temporary cavities in muscle, liver, and lung. Although previously never visualized and thought possibly nonexistent, a temporary cavity was formed within the lung tissue by a missile striking at 3000 feet per second. In angiograms a small cavity within the lung parenchyma was demonstrated by showing disruption of the blood vessels. The temporary cavity was smaller and less impressive than that in muscle or liver tissue. The elastic fibers within the spongework of lung parenchyma absorb the energy and recoil so that the missile tract is hardly perceptible.

Stab wounds and wounds caused by large objects are in a separate category. The loading process is of a much lower order and the outcome somewhat more predictable in that the damage is more closely related to the structural and functional deficits of the components directly traumatized.

NONPENETRATING THORACIC TRAUMA

These injuries may also be subcategorized according to the loading process. Essentially we are concerned with the effects of pressure waves due to blast and impulses generated by blunt objects striking the body.

Blast Injury

When an explosion occurs, a blast or shock wave develops that is similar in all fundamental respects to those produced by supersonic aircraft or by missiles. The parameters of a blast wave have been carefully studied from a biological point of view and comprise: (1) the peak over pressure and (2) the positive duration of this peak over pressure. According to DeCandole [9], one might visualize a shock wave by considering the consequences of a very brief but violent blow impinging uniformly on the side of the body. A significant part of the energy is transmitted through the tissues.

Clemedson [6] points out that an absorbed blast wave is propagated through the body as a pressure wave. The latter may be higher than in the primary wave due to so-called damping up of pressure against the body surface. The degree of injury to a tissue or an organ from a shock wave depends on their physical properties in relation to the characteristics of the wave. If the shock wave derives from a large explosive charge at a considerable distance, the destruction is related chiefly to the peak pressure. However, if the shock wave is caused by a small charge at a short distance, then the damage will depend primarily on the impulse.

Not all tissues are equally susceptible to blast injury. Most internal organs are considered virtually incompressible and subject to minimal displacement. The most vulnerable parts of the body are those containing air or gas, namely, the ear drums, lungs, and intestines. This is thought to be due essentially to a bursting or shredding effect that occurs at the interface and strikes the internal organs one by one during the succeeding millisecond or less. Thoracic structures, especially the lungs, cause a marked distortion of the pressure wave because of large differences in tissue density. The pathophysiological events following exposure of an animal to a high-compression, high-velocity shock wave are characterized by lesions appearing in various internal organs, particularly the air-containing structures, without signs of external injury. The clinical picture may be compounded by additional trauma due to flying debris and/or bodily displacement and impact. Furthermore, there may be other significant environmental influences, depending on the nature of the explosion, temperature conditions, and so on.

The question of the immediate cause of death in blast injury has been reviewed extensively. While a number of theories are proposed, the final impression is that the immediate cause of death may differ under different conditions. The various possibilities may be classified as respiratory, circulatory, cerebrospinal, and others. In severe blast injury, massive pulmonary hemorrhage with obstruction of the respiratory passages by blood and froth leads to suffocation. One view, however, is that the respiratory symptoms apparently are not the cause of death but the consequence of circulatory failure. This suggests that attention should be focused on the mechanisms associated with the onset of circulatory shock as a sequel to the various forms of blast injury. Much more work is needed to help us clarify our understanding of the pathophysiological and biophysical aspects of this form of injury.

Blunt Injury

Information on the effects of blunt trauma to the body is very scanty, especially as it applies to the thorax. Clemedson and associates [7] believe that the pathoanatomical damage to the lungs and heart may be essentially the same in the three different types of loading (penetrating, blast, or blunt), although the thresholds and injury-producing values of impact velocity and impact energy in blast exposure are not valid for the other two types. Trinkle and colleagues [35] studied the anatomical and physiological lesions of the lung produced when a .38-caliber blank cartridge was fired against the chest of anesthetized dogs. Disruption of the alveolar-capillary integrity caused a bruise of the underlying lung with hemorrhage and edema of both the alveolar and interstitial spaces. The resulting pulmonary contusion has been described in blast injuries, direct chest trauma, and recently in penetrating wounds of the chest produced by high-velocity missiles.

Deceleration Injury

Perhaps an even more difficult correlation problem occurs when the body is the moving entity and comes to a sudden halt, with or without the impaction of external objects. A great deal of work has been done, including voluntary human experiments, by Stapp [34] and other investigators regarding the effects on body structure and function of sudden stops (deceleration trauma). This kind of investigation obviously permits the gathering and assessment of data under reasonably controlled conditions.

The form of body deceleration trauma in which there is also impact with external objects presents a complex picture due to the combination of effects from tissue displacement by both blunt and penetrating forces. This kind of injury is often seen as a result of automobile accidents. Unfortunately, while we can speak of forces, velocity, acceleration, kinetic energy, and other physical factors, we are not yet in the position of relating them to types and degrees of injury. Each serious automobile accident is so different that predictions of outcome, except in a very broad sense, are impossible.

SELECTED TYPES OF INJURY

This discussion will be concerned mainly with the biomechanics of blunt trauma, which causes the majority of thoracic injuries encountered in civilian and military practice. Of 585 deaths from traffic accidents reported by Kemmerer and associates [16], the percentage of thoracic injuries was as follows: rib fractures, 39 percent; hemothorax, 28 percent; lung laceration, 10 percent; ruptured great vessel, 10 percent; lung contusion, 6 percent; lacerated diaphragm, 5 percent; sternal fractures, 5 percent; myocardial injury, 6 percent; and lacerated trachea, 1 percent. In almost 25 percent of those deaths, death could be attributed to the thoracic trauma. In 80 percent of those with rib fractures, there was an associated serious intrathoracic injury.

The thoracic skeletal system is frequently involved in direct injury. This results in rib fractures, with or without an accompanying fractured sternum, depending on the mode of injury. Children and adolescents, whose chests are more flexible, may experience greater deformations of the chest cage without rib fractures. The upper ribs are protected to some extent anteriorly by the clavicles, posteriorly by the scapulae, and laterally by the heavy musculature of the upper thorax and shoulder girdle. Rutherford [33] points out that for this reason fractures above the fifth rib imply considerable trauma, not uncommonly associated with serious intrathoracic injuries such as rupture of the tracheobronchial tree. The fifth through the ninth

ribs are the ones most frequently involved in blunt thoracic trauma. A direct blow may cause breaks at the point of impact. With crushing injuries, however, the same is seldom the case. More commonly the ribs give way at the point of maximum convexity in the region of the costal angle.

Experimental work using human cadavers has been carried out in which thoracic response and tolerance levels were reported by Patrick, Mertz, and Kroell [30]. In this research, embalmed cadavers were seated on the sled of a horizontal accelerator and driven to a specific velocity. Having reached the desired speed, the sled was stopped abruptly. During deceleration the cadavers slid forward relative to the sled and impacted their chests. A flat and padded surface 6 inches in diameter was used as the chest impactor. The corresponding displacement of the sternum relative to the thoracic vertebrae was obtained by photographically monitoring the movement of a probe attached to the sternum and passed through the thoracic cavity. Four rib fractures were observed at a sled velocity of 16.8 miles per hour (mph) and a maximum chest load of 1340 pounds, while extensive fractures resulted at 19.5 mph with a load of 1859 pounds. The maximum chest deflection was 2.25 inches at 1545 pounds. Nahum and colleagues [27] studied the interrelationships between force of chest impact, chest wall deflections, and resulting trauma in blunt sternal impact to the human cadaver with high-speed photography. The preliminary studies showed great variations in response to trauma associated with age. The younger cadaver specimens suffered virtually no skeletal damage, whereas the older specimens sustained extensive damage, in the form of rib fractures (7 to 20 rib fractures), sternal fractures, and lacerations of heart and lungs. In a similar experiment Kroell, Gadd, and Schneider [18] concluded that force per se cannot be correlated with thoracic injury. The magnitude of skeletal deflection and the time required to develop such deflections would appear to be much more directly associable with thoracic injury, both skeletal and visceral. Significant skeletal damage was found at both the 11 and 16 mph levels. The authors suggested that a skeletal deflection not exceeding 51 mm (2 inches) for midsternal blunt impact should be a reasonable criterion for the preclusion of serious thoracic trauma.

Although visceral thoracic injuries are often associated with injury to the chest wall and sternum, they are sometimes sustained without chest wall involvement and include lung contusions, ruptured bronchus, ruptured diaphragm, ruptured aorta, and cardiac injuries.

Lung contusions may result either from blast injury or blunt trauma. In military practice they are caused by nonpenetrating wounds from high-velocity missiles, high-explosive shells, and detonations. In civilian life, they are most frequently secondary to automobile accidents, although falls and industrial mishaps may also be causative. The pulmonary injury can be traced to the direct effect of blast-induced variations of the environmental pressure. The extent of the injury depends on the magnitude of the loading force, the physical characteristics of the shock wave, the medium that transmits the shock wave, and the dissipation of energy through the chest wall and pulmonary tissue. Following a blast or violent blow to the chest, much of the energy is reflected, but at least part is transmitted to the thoracic viscera. Compressibility permits displacement, and whenever tissues of different density exist side by side, the amount of displacement and its time course vary from point to point with subsequent distortion and tearing. Within the lungs, the alveolar septa are most affected and are torn so that the parenchyma shears away from the vascular structures and the alveolar epithelium is shredded. The outcome is failure of the blood-air barrier, with collection of blood in the pulmonary tissue and escape of air into the pulmonary veins.

Although extensive data have been accumulated on blast injuries, relatively scant information is available on blunt or deceleration trauma to the thorax. Since, for obvious reasons, destructive impact tests cannot be made on living human subjects, most of the facts have therefore been obtained from animal experimentation. However, the thorax of quadruped mammals is quite different in shape from that of man. This difference influences the behavior of the intact thoracic cage under impact loading, and caution should be exercised in the interpretation of findings when applied to man.

Beckman and Palmer [4] have studied the thoracic force-deflation characteristics of an impactor in the living subhuman primate as a step toward the analysis of cardiothoracic injuries. Mechanisms of injury were investigated by subjecting Rhesus monkeys seated on a stationary, freely movable sled to static and dynamic chest wall displacement. This was achieved by means of a cartridge-fired projectile equipped with a diameter impact plate that is 3 inches in diameter and an accelerometer compensated-force transducer. Forces up to only 30 pounds were developed in static pressure tests for 2-inch deflections but reached 700 pounds for the same deflection using dynamic tests. These authors postulate that the force generated on dynamic deflection of the anterior chest wall, aside from the static reaction, may have components due to: (1) the spring mass effect of the anterior chest wall, (2) the compression of air in the lungs, and (3) the viscous or viscoelastic behavior of the thoracic tissue.

Tracheal and bronchial injuries are seen with increasing frequency following blunt trauma, especially when this has occurred in an automobile accident. Rupture separation of the cervical portion of the trachea usually succeeds a direct force, tending to avulse the larynx and cricoid cartilage from the trachea. Intrathoracic rupture of the trachea seems to result from a sharply localized force applied to a relatively elastic chest wall anteriorly, leading to compression of the trachea against the rigid vertebrae posteriorly. This in turn causes the membranous part of the trachea to be torn from its cartilaginous attachment, or, by being sharply overstretched, the trachea is fractured just above the carina. This mechanism is apparently similar to that of traumatic bronchial rupture. The following mechanism is suggested by Lloyd and colleagues [21] for bronchial ruptures: when blunt trauma is applied to the anteroposterior diameter of the chest, this diameter decreases while the transverse dimension increases. The lungs, owing to their negative intrathoracic pressure, remain coapted to the chest wall and are subjected to tension at the carina. If the lateral excursion of either lung is carried beyond the point of elasticity of the bronchi, a tear results at or near the carina. These factors are augmented when the blow is administered to the chest in the anteroposterior diameter when the glottis is closed.

Another injury that is seen with increasing frequency following blunt trauma is rupture of the diaphragm. It occurs after a steering wheel injury to the lower part of the chest and upper abdomen. In mining and industrial areas, diaphragmatic hernia is more likely to result from falls of coal and rock, or from crushing by trucks and pit cages. It is seen less frequently on the right (5 to 20 percent), probably because of the protective effect of the liver on the right leaflet of the diaphragm. Although the heart, pericardium, and lungs may act as cushions to the left leaflet, they are less effective. Most ruptures of the diaphragm seem to occur in association with severe injuries to the musculoskeletal system, especially trauma to the pelvis, lumbosacral spine, and lower extremities. The patients most likely to suffer diaphragmatic rupture from increased intra-abdominal pressure are infants, young children, and pregnant women whose abdomens have been run over. In the Evans' series [11] five out of seven hernias due to nonpenetrating injury followed such accidents; four of the patients had fractures of the pelvis, none had fractured ribs, and all escaped visceral injury.

The site of rupture of the left dome of the diaphragm correlates well with the embryological point of weakness in its posterior and lateral walls. It would appear that the relatively weak diaphragmatic structure yields between the solid viscera of the abdomen and the pliant thoracic structures when a sudden force is applied to either the thoracic or abdominal wall. According to Desforges and associates [10] the direction of trauma per se is unimportant in the disruptive mechanism. Forces applied to the anterior abdomen and the flanks are transmitted equally in all directions, and since the diaphragm offers the least resistance, it fails by disruption. Another possible mechanism suggested by Desforges is that forces compressing the chest from opposite directions could rupture the diaphragm like the membrane of a drum. Under these conditions the tear would be expected to occur in the line of compression and to be centrally located. Once a rent occurs, the abdominal organs tend to herniate into the chest due to the greater intra-abdominal pressure. In Marchand's study [23], the intraperitoneal pressure after a rent varied from +2 cm to +10 cm of water during quiet breathing in the supine position, while the intrapleural pressure varied from −5 cm during expiration to −10 cm during inspiration. This gradient of 7 to 20 cm could exceed 100 cm with maximum respiratory effort. A search of the literature for an estimate of the magnitude and distribution of the forces that lead to rupture of the diaphragm was not fruitful. One can only infer that they are of the same magnitude as forces leading to fracture of the pelvis or lumbar spine.

With the advent of the automobile, high-speed deceleration impact injuries have markedly increased. Ventricular impact, abrupt transfers of kinetic forces to the victim, and sudden decelerations

of bodily viscera and blood column momentum all operate sequentially to produce cardiovascular injuries [19]. The extent and severity of these injuries is determined by several biomechanical interactions, including (1) the magnitude of deceleration, (2) the total duration of exposure to the forces of deceleration, and (3) the rate of time change of deceleration, according to Newtonian laws of dynamics: $F = MA$, or in the case of deceleration, $F = MD$, where F is the resultant of forces acting on the viscera, M is the scalar mass of the viscera involved, D is the magnitude of deceleration, V_2 and V_1 are terminal and initial velocities, respectively, and t is the time duration of velocity change.

Traumatic injuries to the cardiovascular system following blunt trauma have been well documented. Parmley and colleagues [29] reviewed 546 cases of fatal nonpenetrating cardiac trauma. They recorded a predominance of myocardial rupture—353 cases; there was also myocardial contusion and/or laceration in 129, pericardial laceration in 36, hemopericardium in 25, and single cases of valvular injury, papillary muscle rupture, and coronary artery laceration. The incidence of cardiac contusion in 507 patients with nonpenetrating chest trauma was reported by Jones, Hewitt, and Drapanas [15] to be 9.41 percent (48 patients). They were all involved in automobile accidents and had evidence of moderate to severe trauma to the thorax. Twenty-two patients had associated rib fractures and 13 had sternal fractures. The physical forces involved in the production of such injuries were summarized by Parmley and associates [29] as follows: (1) unidirectional force against the chest; (2) bidirectional or compressive force against the thorax; (3) indirect forces, i.e., compression of the abdomen and lower extremities resulting in a marked increase in intravascular pressure; (4) decelerative forces, particularly when imparting differential deceleration to the heart and great vessels; (5) blast; and (6) concussive force, usually produced by rapid motion without bringing about demonstrable pathological changes.

In order to investigate the possible mechanism of myocardial injury secondary to blunt trauma the following methods were pursued:

1. An experimental model was developed by Anderson and Doty [3] to study myocardial contusion. Isolated myocardial injury was produced

in 20 anesthetized dogs, using the impact of a captive-bolt handgun with semielliptical steel disc positioned over a point of maximum cardiac impulse. When the weapon was discharged, the bolt was propelled forward, transferring kinetic energy through the intact chest wall to the underlying heart. Nine animals died within minutes of the contusion; the other 11 recovered until they were sacrificed for pathological study. The animals that died immediately after injury showed similar severe, isolated injury to the heart. Circular areas of transmural contusion with subepicardial hematoma and subendocardial ecchymosis were present over the left ventricle, anterior septal area, and cardiac apex. Disruption of surface coronary vessels was not observed. Animals sacrificed at intervals up to 72 hours showed injuries of identical extent and distribution, with progressive resorption of hemorrhage. By three weeks, when the last animal was sacrificed, the heart appeared to have patchy areas of scarring but its appearance was otherwise normal. The outstanding physiological consequences of isolated contusing injury to the myocardium was ventricular tachyarrhythmia, which was observed in every dog at least transiently following trauma, and which often progressed to uniformly fatal ventricular fibrillation. The severity and duration of tachyarrhythmia and consequently the survival of the animal, correlated with the size of the powder charge used in relation to the size of the animal. There is a suggestion that the location of the myocardial injury may determine the type of cardiac arrhythmia. Mosley, Vernick, and Doty [26] reported conduction defects and reduction of heart rate in sinus rhythm following blunt chest injury when the injury force was applied to the right side of the chest, presumably affecting the right atrium and conduction system. This is in contrast to predominantly ventricular rhythm disturbances when the injury force was to the left side of the chest over the ventricular mass.

2. High speed radiographs were obtained at selected time intervals during controlled deceleration of beagle dogs subjected to ± Gz impact on a decelerator [14]. Preliminary data indicate that the heart undergoes considerable inertial movement during deceleration. The average displacement suggests a sine wave function with superimposed damping after one cycle. There is first an upward displacement of the heart followed by an inertial rebound in a downward direction.

Rupture of the heart may occur immediately or within the first two weeks after trauma when softening of the contused myocardial segment occurs. The immediate rupture of a cardiac chamber usually occurs in one of the following ways: the heart may be lacerated by a rib or other bony fragments when the anterior chest is driven in by an external force, or it may be ruptured by forceful compression against the vertebral column, either when it is empty and relaxed or when it is filled. Important factors in determining whether or not heart rupture will occur are the direction of chest compression, and the phase of the cardiac cycle in which the compression occurs. Life and Prince [20] impacted dogs during either ventricular diastole or systole. Of the animals struck during systole, 85 percent had ruptures of one or both ventricles, while of the animals impacted during ventricular diastole none had ventricular rupture. The velocity with which the pressure is applied and the rise of intracardiac pressure produced are also important factors in cardiac rupture.

Rupture of the aorta is among the most frequently encountered severe injuries following blunt trauma to the thorax. Automobile accidents account for 61 to 95 percent of these cases. Greendyke [13] reported 42 cases of traumatic rupture of the aorta in 1259 medicolegal autopsies. One of every six victims of fatal automobile accidents sustains aortic rupture. In about 20 percent of the cases, rupture is caused by a variety of mechanisms such as falling from a height and landing on feet or buttocks, burial under masses of earth or snow, a blow to the chest by a stone, or a blow from a piece of wood flying from a circular saw. The site of rupture is related to the mode of injury. The most common site is the descending thoracic aorta at the isthmus just beyond the origin of the left subclavian artery and is associated with crushing and horizontal injuries. Vertical deceleration trauma occurring with jumps or falls from great heights produces a rupture of the ascending aorta just above the aortic valve. Much speculation has been generated about the mechanisms and forces leading to aortic rupture; this has recently led to experimentation that might shed light on this complex problem. The vast literature on this subject contains theories that are summarized below.

1. *Deceleration mechanism.* The most widely accepted theory to explain the frequency of rupture at the aortic isthmus is based on the fact that

the aortic arch is fixed by its major branches and that the descending thoracic aorta is mobile. During deceleration, there is a continued forward movement of the descending aorta in the presence of a fixed transverse aortic arch. Whenever one part of the body is decelerated at a rate different from that of another, the connection between the two parts is placed under stress proportional to the difference in the rates of deceleration.

On the other hand, McKnight, Meyer, and Neville [24] disagree with these anatomical considerations and claim that the aortic arch is mobile while the descending aorta is relatively fixed. The latter is immobilized by the pleural reflections and the intercostal arteries, whereas the arch is actually suspended by the major branches rather than fixed. Lundevall [22] did postmortem studies of the aortas from ten bodies and found the thoracic part of the aorta to be relatively mobile, but the isthmus was attached slightly more firmly to its surroundings than the portions of the aorta above and below. The branches of the aortic arch did not particularly restrain aortic motion nor did the intercostal arteries. The heart was relatively resistant against vertical movements but was somewhat more mobile transversely and could also be rotated to some extent along its longitudinal axis.

2. *Pressure mechanism.* Increased intra-aortic pressure has been implicated in aortic rupture. This is brought about by compression of the heart between the sternum and vertebral column, leading to displacement of an intact column of blood with propagation of a pressure wave causing a waterhammer effect. Nahum and co-workers [27] attempted to reproduce this lesion by subjecting 12 cadavers to impact injury. The thoracic aorta was hydraulically pressurized with water in an attempt to simulate to some degree the in vivo blood pressure state. Vascular occlusions were established in the aorta just above the diaphragm and in the left common carotid artery near its origin. Hydraulic pressurization of the thoracic aorta was performed immediately prior to impact in all 12 cadavers. It was not possible to elevate the intra-aortic pressure heard to the desired minimum value of 90 to 100 mm Hg in 7. In no case was rupture of the aorta produced, although there was a bruise observed near the root of the ascending aorta in one, and hemorrhages into the adventitia of the descending aorta in another. Moritz [25] found that pressures of 800 to 1000 mm Hg applied to the aorta of living rats caused rupture of the portal

veins or its branches, but the aorta did not rupture. Oppenheim [28] was able to produce intimal ruptures in cadaver aortas above the aortic valve and just below the attachment of the ligamentum arteriosum. Such lesions were produced by injecting fluid at pressures of 3000 mm Hg. Klotz and Simpson [17], on the other hand, were unable to produce lesions with intravascular pressures in the neighborhood of 1000 mm Hg. Zehnder [38] tested the tensile strength and elasticity of strips of the aorta and found a bursting tolerance equivalent to an internal pressure of 2500 mm Hg. Roberts and Beckman [31] have rejected this mechanism of increased pressure as the sole phenomenon responsible for the injury. They based this contention on the fact that aortic tears are always transverse to the vessel axis rather than longitudinal, as might be expected from the results of stress due to internal pressure and the fact that the circumferential stresses are always at least twice the magnitude of those exerted in a longitudinal plane. Furthermore, Roberts has demonstrated that a comparable lesion occurs in dogs whose blood volume has been reduced by five-sixths of the total.

3. *Displacement mechanism.* Significant displacements of the heart and aorta caused by blunt trauma have been shown to be implicated in aortic rupture. According to Cammack and associates [5], during the time of deceleration, when the chest is compressed in the anteroposterior diameter, the heart and mediastinal structures are displaced into the left chest posteriorly, causing rotation of aorta and an increase in the tortuosity of its course. Three stresses are involved in this displacement: a torsion stress tangential to the surface; a shearing stress, which is radial in direction; and a bending stress directed along the longitudinal axis of the aorta. Cammack and his co-workers [5] state that the bending stress may be ignored since the aorta is very inelastic. The torsion stresses are greater at the base of the heart, whereas those with a shearing action predominate in the descending aorta where the ruptures occur. The torsion stress gives rise to a pressure wave of blood that is transmitted through the aorta. A maximum internal pressure is produced at the point of greatest stability of the aorta, causing a concentrated shearing stress in this area.

Roberts and Beckman [31] have studied the displacement of the heart by means of high-speed flash roentgenograms taken during an actual im-

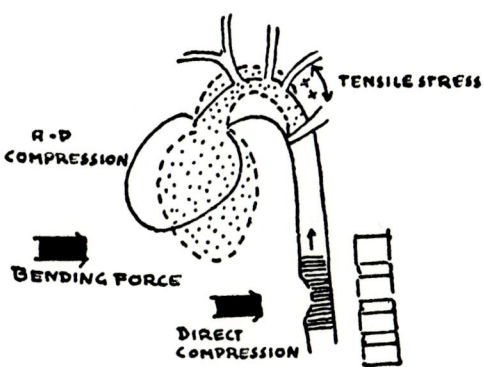

Fig 1-1. *Illustration shows the displacement of the heart and aorta upon impact.* (From V. L. Roberts and D. L. Beckman, Impact Injury and Crash Protection, 1970, Charles C Thomas, Publisher. Used by permission.)

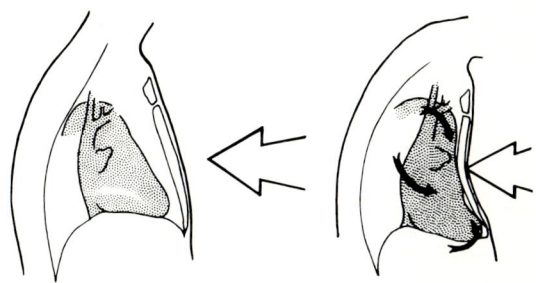

Fig 1-2. *Scheme of aortic rupture by shoveling effect* (From G. E. Voigt in Hefte Zur Unfallhei Kunde 96:115, 1968.)

pact to the thorax in dogs. They found the base of the heart to be forced anteriorly and downward while the apex moved posteriorly and downward (Fig 1-1). There was also a tendency for movement into the left chest, although this was not extreme. The great vessels were stretched and distorted, and the aorta presented a rippled appearance on its posterior surface due to being pressed against the ribs and vertebrae. Such displacement deforms the vessels and produces increased stress at the points of fixation. This characteristic pattern of displacement was reinforced by the typical pattern of injury observed in the vessel walls. The tears were found characteristically on the posterior wall of the aorta, never on the anterior wall.

The theory that displacement of the heart and great vessels by the shoveling effect contributes to aortic rupture was also verified by Voigt and Wilfert [36]. Postmortem investigations were carried out on 82 drivers fatally injured in head-on collisions. The findings were compared with the damage to the interior components of the car, and the final positions of the victims were reconstructed by means of a simple dummy. These studies demonstrated that the lower part of the rim of the steering wheel was deflected in a forward direction and that the impact force transmitted from the steering assembly may act on the body and heart in different ways (Fig 1-2).

Variations in force application are obvious. We may have (1) blast waves acting on large parts of the body; or (2) force applications to local areas,

as in the case of impacting missiles; or (3) inertial forces resulting from motion of the body as a whole acting on all tissues, including the deep-seated organs. When large blasts are involved, all three types of force may be combined. Crash or impact injury usually involves forces of the second and third types. Acceleration forces encountered in aerospace flight are predominantly of the third type. In the mode of force transmission, in the time function, and in the specific biological reaction of concern, there are many findings that apply to several or all of these problem areas. In practically all cases it is not the pressure but the resulting relative displacement of adjacent tissue that leads to the stimulation of various receptors as well as to ultimate injury. Psychological reaction, physiological stimulation and reaction, and the overall clinical injury are responses secondary to the primary body deformation. Von Giérke believes that it is through this area of the body's mechanical response to the various force environments that the several technical fields concerned hang together and can benefit from one another.

REFERENCES

1. Amato JJ, Billy LJ, Gruber RP, et al: Temporary cavitation in high velocity pulmonary missile injury. Ann Thorac Surg 18:565, 1974
2. Amato JJ, Billy LJ, Lawson NS, et al: High velocity missile injury. Am J Surg 127:454, 1974
3. Anderson AE, Doty DB: Cardiac trauma: an experimental model of isolated myocardial contusion. J Trauma 15:237, 1975
4. Beckman DL, Palmer MF: Response of the primate thorax to experimental impact, in Proceedings of the 13th Stapp Car Crash Conference

New York, Society of Automotive Engineers, 1969

5. Cammack K, Raport RL, Paul J, et al: Deceleration injuries of the thoracic aorta. Arch Surg 79: 244, 1959

6. Clemedson CJ: Blast injury. Physiol Rev 36:336, 1956

7. Clemedson CJ, Hillstrom G, Lindgren A: The relative tolerance of the head, thorax, and abdomen to blunt trauma. Ann NY Acad Sci 152: 187, 1968

8. Daughtry DC: Unpublished correspondence, 1979

9. DeCandole CA: Blast injury. Can Med Assoc J 96:207, 1967

10. Desforges G, Strieder JW, Lynch JP, et al: Traumatic rupture of the diaphragm: clinical manifestations and surgical treatment. J Thorac Surg 34:779, 1957

11. Evans FG: Discussion in Impact Injury and Crash Protection. Springfield, ILL, Thomas, 1970

12. Goldsmith W: Biomechanics of head injury, in YC Fung et al. (eds.), Biomechanics, Foundations and Objections. Englewood Cliffs, N.J.: Prentice-Hall, 1970

13. Greendyke RM: Traumatic rupture of aorta. JAMA 195:527, 1966

14. Hanson PG: Radiographic studies of cardiac displacement during abrupt deceleration, in Proceedings of the 10th Stapp Car Crash Conference. New York, Society of Automotive Engineers, 1966

15. Jones JW, Hewitt RL, Drapañas T: Cardiac contusion: a capricious syndrome. Ann Surg 181:567, 1975

16. Kemmerer WT, Eckert WG, Gathright JB, et al: Patterns of thoracic injuries in fatal traffic accidents. Trauma 1:595, 1961

17. Klotz O, Simpson W: Spontaneous rupture of the aorta. Am J Med Sci 184:455, 1932

18. Kroell CK, Gadd CW, Schneider DC: Biomechanics in crash injury research. ISA Trans 13:183, 1974

19. Liedtke AJ, DeMuth WE, Jr.: Nonpenetrating cardiac injuries: a collective review. Am Heart J 86:687, 1973

20. Life JS, Prince BW: Response of the canine heart to thoracic impact during ventricular diastole and systole. J Biomech 1:169, 1968

21. Lloyd JR, Heydinger DK, Klassen KP, et al.: Rupture of the main bronchi in closed chest injury. Arch Surg 77:597, 1958

22. Lundevall J: The mechanism of traumatic rupture of the aorta. Acta Pathol Microbiol Scand 62:34, 1964

23. Marchand PA: Study of the forces productive of gastroesophageal regurgitation and herniation through the diaphragmatic hiatus. Thorax 12:189, 1957

24. McKnight JT, Meyer JA, Neville JF: Nonpenetrating traumatic rupture of the thoracic aorta. Ann Surg 160:1069, 1964

25. Moritz AR: Medionecrosis aortae idiopathica cystica. Am J Pathol. 8:717, 1932

26. Mosley RV, Vernick JJ, Doty DB: Response to blunt chest injury: a new experimental model. J Trauma 10:673, 1970

27. Nahum AM, Kroell CK, Schneider DC: The biochemical basis of chest impact protection. II. Effects of cardiovascular pressurization. J Trauma 13:443, 1973

28. Oppenheim F: Gibt es eine spontanruptur der gesundern aorta und wie kommt sie zustande? Munch Med Wochenschr 65:1234, 1918

29. Parmley LF, Manion WC, Mattingly TW: Nonpenetrating traumatic injuries of the heart. Circulation 18:371, 1958.

30. Patrick LM, Mertz HJ, Jr., Kroell CK: Cadaver knee, chest, and head impact loads, in Proceedings of the 11th Stapp Car Crash Conference. New York, Society of Automotive Engineers, 1967

31. Roberts VL, Beckman DL: The mechanisms of chest injuries, Impact Injury and Crash Protection. Springfield, ILL, Thomas, 1970

32. Roberts VL, Jackson FR, Berkas EM: Heart motion due to blunt trauma to the thorax, in Proceedings of the 10th Stapp Car Crash Conference. New York, Society of Automotive Engineers, 1966

33. Rutherford RB: Thoracic Injuries in the Management of Trauma. Philadelphia, Saunders, 1973

34. Stapp JP: Voluntary human tolerance level, Impact Injury and Crash Protection. Springfield, Ill, Thomas, 1970

35. Trinkle JK, Furman RW, Hinshaw MA: Pulmonary contusion. Ann Thorac Surg 16:568, 1973

35a. Turnery, SZ, Attar, S, Ayella, R, Crowley RA. Traumatic rupture of the Aorta. J Thorac Cardiovasc Surg 72:661, 1976

36. Voigt GE, Wilfert K: Mechanisms of injuries to unrestrained drivers in head-on collisions, in Proceedings of the 13th Stapp Car Crash Conference. New York, Society of Automotive Engineers, 1969

37. Wise L, Connors J, Hwang YJ, et al: Traumatic injuries to the diaphragm. J Trauma 13:946, 1973

38. Zehnder MA: Delayed post-traumatic rupture of the aorta in a young healthy individual after closed injury. Angiology 7:252, 1956

2. THE INITIAL MANAGEMENT OF THORACIC TRAUMA

DeWitt C. Daughtry
James DeWitt Daughtry

Approximately 50,000 people die each year from automobile accidents [37]. Some 3 to 4 million people are injured each year, and a high percentage of these sustain multiple trauma [22, 31]. As we review statistics it becomes obvious that trauma is a big killer and is surpassed only by cardiovascular disease and cancer in the United States [35, 37]. Fifty percent of all deaths in the age group of 15 to 24 are due to highway accidents [27]. Approximately 50 percent of fatalities from vehicular accidents have sustained injury to the thorax, and the chest injury is the primary cause of death in 25 percent of these fatalities [26]. It is quite difficult to determine or even to estimate the amount of morbidity and mortality attributable to chest injury itself when multiple organ trauma is present. It is known that the chest trauma alone contributes much morbidity and is a decided factor in mortality in multiple system injuries. Additional insight was gained when Kemmerer and co-workers [26] stated that of 585 traffic fatalities in a metropolitan area during a five-year period there was significant thoracic trauma in 294, and 133 of these died primarily of their thoracic injury. It is significant that less than half the fatalities due to thoracic injury survived long enough to reach a hospital and that blunt trauma produces a higher mortality than penetrating trauma [23]. Most thoracic injuries found in patients taken to rural hospitals are from vehicular accidents, whereas in many metropolitan hospitals patients with penetrating injuries compose a larger percentage.

According to Davis (Chapter 21) 72 percent of the people who died in vehicular accidents in Dade County, Florida, had sustained major thoracic injury. Present trends indicate that less severe injuries and a lower mortality rate are occurring since the legal speed limit was lowered [37].

A well-organized transport system, both surface and air, and well-trained auxiliary personnel contribute greatly to the arrival of the critically injured at the emergency treatment center in optimum condition. An adequate transport system includes two-way radio communication and the accident victim being taken to a hospital well enough equipped to manage the particular injury, thus assuring prompt quality treatment. Decreased morbidity and mortality result from an improved understanding of the deranged physiology involved and a multidisciplinary team approach for early optimum management. The American College of Surgeons has been very active for many years in establishing guidelines relative to transportation and treatment at the scene of the accident and in establishing standards in emergency treatment centers.

Successful resuscitation and coordinated team work, including qualified first aid personnel at the scene of the accident and of quality medical and other personnel at the emergency treatment center, are obvious necessities for the best care of critically injured patients [34]. It is important to obtain proper consultation. We strongly agree with Shires [44] in his plea for more training of personnel and research in the emergency-room care of the injured.

Since metropolitan hospitals receive a large volume of trauma patients, they usually have special observation and treatment units to which the critically injured are admitted. It is important to remember that proper management of the injured is a continuous process, starting at the scene of the accident and continuing until the patient is rehabilitated back to his usual status.

PERTINENT HISTORY

The immediate total appraisal of the patient and his injuries should include as much history as is obtainable. Top priority problems will obviously need immediate attention, and thus a detailed history may have to be delayed in the face of difficulties such as airway obstruction, acute hemorrhage, tension pneumothorax, a sucking wound (open pneumothorax), or the need for cardiorespiratory resuscitation. The past medical history is important, especially as it relates to chronic preexisting or coexisting disease processes, particularly of the cardiorespiratory system. Fragile or elderly

11

people or the patient who has been a heavy smoker or one who has chronic bronchitis or asthma, tolerate thoracic trauma poorly. They may thus need to be treated more actively than a previously normal person. Information should also be obtained regarding such chronic diseases as diabetes, hypertension, renal disease, Addison's disease, malignant disease, alcoholism, liver disease, Marfan's syndrome, and neurological and psychiatric problems. Also, a history relative to allergies and drugs being used should be obtained.

The chain of events that occurred prior to the patient's arrival in the emergency room also comprise relevant data. The ambulance attendants are usually available to describe the scene of the accident and report on whether the victim was the driver of a car and whether he was ejected from the vehicle. It is important to know if the victim was a pedestrian, had a fall, or sustained his injury in some other manner. The type of weapon used in shootings or stabbings also helps guide the physician's management. Entrance and exit sites and direction of penetrating forces are significant. Whether or not alcohol has been ingested and the time of the patient's last meal should be established. Any vomiting, dislodged teeth, and bleeding from the nose, mouth, or pharynx are important data. A blast injury, even though there is little evidence of trauma, alerts the physician to the possibility of pulmonary parenchymal hemorrhage and edema, which may rapidly progress to pulmonary insufficiency.

Conscious patients are usually accurate in relating pertinent data. Complaints of being cold or of having an intense thirst may alert the physician to blood loss and impending shock. Severe interscapular pain suggests aortic injury. Severe apprehension and extreme restlessness often suggest significant injury even though it may not be obvious. Stabbing pain in the thorax when the patient swallows suggests perforation or rupture of the esophagus. Coughing concurrent with swallowing suggests a tracheoesophageal fistula. Careful recording of the initial physical findings and what drugs were administered during early emergency care are of great value in later care of the patient.

FURTHER EVALUATION AND GENERAL MANAGEMENT

An organized method of evaluating a thoracic injury should include in addition to the detailed history, performing a thorough and complete physical examination, and obtaining a portable upright or semi-erect roentgenogram of the chest, an electrocardiogram, an arterial blood gases series, blood typing, and any other laboratory data that specific circumstances may require. A gastric suction tube should be inserted early in treatment to prevent gastric dilatation and subsequent vomiting that may cause aspiration pneumonia, sometimes a lethal complication. Of course top priority actions such as cardiopulmonary resuscitation, relief of obstructed airways, and correction of hypovolemic shock take precedence and must interrupt the routine evaluation and management whenever necessary [34].

The examining physician must not become preoccupied with any single injury but should evaluate the whole patient to determine the presence of multiple-system trauma. Cyanotic or reddish discoloration of the upper half of the body, distention of neck veins, a tender, resistant abdomen, painful and deformed extremities, unequal pupils, and restlessness with abnormal neurological findings may require attention by someone from another specialty. In 1955 Daughtry [10] emphasized the need to utilize a multidisciplinary approach to provide the best care for the severely injured. This is again stressed. It is in the best interest of the patient for the primary physician to be in charge of treating the most major life-threatening injury, with the other required physicians acting as consultants. Major changes or additions to therapy should be cleared through him. In 1952 Daughtry and Chesney [12] stated that few other conditions require as much of the surgeon's undivided attention as major thoracic injuries. Casual observation and management invite catastrophe. In a survey of 950 trauma deaths in the United States, it appeared to Fitts [19] that 51 percent might have been prevented by ideal medical care.

The thoroughness of the initial evaluation and early management often determines whether patients will survive, and whether they will have a relatively smooth convalescence or a complicated and prolonged recovery. Considerable skill is necessary for adequate management of individuals with limited cardiorespiratory reserve. Even a minor chest injury in such a person may be quite serious. Patients with apparently uncomplicated rib fractures should be admitted and observed for at least a few hours, since intrathoracic injuries and complications may not become manifest for many hours.

During transportation the patient's head should be turned to one side to minimize flooding of the respiratory system with vomitus or blood from an injured nose, mouth, or pharynx. This plus the removal of particulate material from the patient's mouth is of considerable value when suction equipment is not available. Elevation of the chin and insertion of a pharyngeal airway may promptly improve breathing. Bleeding from the posterior nasal and upper pharyngeal areas may be controlled by placing traction upon a Foley catheter that has been inserted through a nostril and the balloon inflated. Bronchoscopy is often used when food particles, blood, or other material have been aspirated into the tracheobronchial system, and when large amounts of blood or other material are otherwise present in the bronchial tree. This helps assure an adequate airway and helps prevent atelectasis and subsequent pulmonary suppuration. As an extra precaution we also feel that administering corticosteroids lessens the deleterious effects of exposure to aspirated gastric contents upon the lungs. If it appears that the airway obstructed by secretions will require repeated or frequent suctioning, tracheal intubation should be performed, using a low-pressure, high-volume cuff that reduces injury to the tracheal mucosa. This permits the use of a mechanical respirator, if its use becomes necessary, and also gives easy access for repeated aspiration of secretions from the tracheobronchial tree. Tracheostomy need not be done early in treatment but can be delayed for a few days.

HIGHEST PRIORITIES

Since the seriousness of chest injury depends primarily upon the degree of derangement of pulmonary and cardiovascular function, initial care should be directed toward rapidly restoring these functions to normal. This goal is accomplished by establishing a clear airway; stabilizing and reestablishing the integrity of the chest cage; correcting a sucking chest wall defect or open pneumothorax; decompressing a pneumothorax, hemothorax, or combined hemopneumothorax; restoring adequate blood volume; and eliminating pericardial tamponade. Body functions are dependent on optimum tissue perfusion and perfusion cannot be restored unless shock is prevented or controlled by ade-

quate blood volume replacement and the elimination of the causes of shock. Relief of airway obstruction, cardiopulmonary resuscitation, and control of massive hemorrhage and correction of hypovolemic shock assume high priorities in emergency care. A sucking chest wound requires immediate control by pressure with a dressing and the introduction of a closed thoracotomy decompression tube to correct and prevent recurrence of pneumothorax. Tension pneumothorax may occur rapidly if the surface of the lung has been torn or penetrated and a thoracostomy decompression tube has not been inserted.

Shock

Apprehension, combativeness, profuse perspiration, cool skin, hypotension, tachycardia, tachypnea, cyanosis or pallor, and, later, restlessness are signs of shock that may be due to extensive trauma, major hemorrhage, airway obstruction, tension pneumothorax, pericardial tamponade, cardiac contusion, or progressive respiratory insufficiency. Often the welfare of the patient depends on several problems being controlled simultaneously since many of them may be interrelated in extensive trauma. Since subtle changes and sometimes even major deterioration may occur rapidly and even go undetected, during the process of management of major thoracic injury, continuous monitoring and reevaluation of all variables are very important. Serial chest roentgenograms, continuous electrocardiogram monitoring, blood gas measurements, and continuous close observation by the attending surgeon and other consultants are all vital for adequate care of severe trauma. Early intravenous, pulmonary, arterial wedge pressure, and systemic arterial pressure monitoring are necessary in selected cases. These invasive techniques provide data that help differentiate between shock from blood loss and other types of shock and provide information relative to cardiorespiratory function. They also provide a route for administering blood, fluids, and medications. By preventing or combating shock, or both, early, the need for later resuscitation is usually prevented.

BLOOD VOLUME. Hypovolemia is treated with a balanced salt solution to help maintain an adequate arterial pressure and tissue perfusion while blood is being made available. It has been emphasized by Trinkle, Furman, and Hinshaw [49] that a contused lung is very sensitive to the administration of noncolloid fluids. Hypovolemia or persistent bleeding, as indicated by the thoracotomy tube drainage, not responsive to blood and other volume expanders often requires surgery for resuscitation and definitive control of hemorrhage. A catheter in the urinary bladder is another guide in monitoring the adequacy of tissue perfusion; a 30- to 40-ml urine output usually indicates adequate perfusion. It should be remembered that not all cases of shock are due to hypovolemia and that the injudicious administration of excessive amounts of intravenous fluids and blood in the presence of lung contusion, the wet lung syndrome, or progressive respiratory insufficiency may be harmful [49]. This situation is common following blunt or crushing injuries to the thorax. A broad-spectrum antibiotic is often indicated on a prophylactic basis, particularly for those who have received a gunshot blast at close range or injuries to the airways or other viscera, and those who have extensive soft tissue injury or are in shock [20, 33]. The penicillins are widely used prophylactically because of their wide spectrum of activity and bacteriocidal action, their excellent distribution throughout the body spaces, and the fact that they are relatively cheap. They are also relatively free of untoward reactions. Bacteriological cultures from the injured tissues and body secretions should be obtained early in treatment to serve as a guide to specific antibiotic therapy. Tetanus toxoid may be indicated, depending on the type of wounding force or object. Steroids may be helpful in the management of shock, aspiration (of gastric contents), pneumonitis, fat embolism, and pulmonary insufficiency.

Roentgenograms

Frequent auscultation of the thorax offers information relative to the adequacy of lung expansion, the extent of congestion, and the aeration or movement of air in the lungs during both spontaneous breathing and when a respirator is being used. The initial upright portable roentgenogram of the chest is sufficient to make the diagnosis of pneumothorax, hemothorax, pneumomediastinum, or widening of the mediastinum. This type of study often demonstrates free air in the soft tissues of the neck, the mediastinum, and beneath the diaphragm, suggesting other major injuries.

The chief concern at this time is with visceral injury rather than the number of ribs that may have been fractured. Fractured ribs can be documented by additional roentgenograms later, be-

fore the patient's discharge from the hospital. Other special roentgenograms such as esophagograms and aortograms may be requested by the attending thoracic surgeon, however. It is fortunate that he is usually trained and experienced in roentgenogram interpretation because most of these patients arrive in the emergency room at times when the staff radiologist is not in the x-ray department. The attending thoracic surgeon thus correlates the history, physical findings, roentgenograms, electrocardiograms, laboratory reports, and other pertinent findings in assessing and treating the injuries and their complications.

Flail Chest

Tracheal intubation and the use of a volume respirator are usually the treatment of choice for a "flail chest cage" complicated by respiratory distress. The physiological significance of flail chest depends upon the size of the flail segment, the extent of other tissue injuries, and the prior stamina of the patient. If intubation equipment and a respirator are not immediately available, or when the patient has to be transferred some distance to a properly equipped facility, either localized pressure over the mobile segment of the chest cage or the application of traction to a towel-clip that grasps the central area of the unstable defect, be it ribs or sternum, is useful as a temporary measure. If an anesthesia-type endotracheal tube is not available, emergency tracheostomy may be necessary but it is much more hazardous than when performed electively and under much better operative conditions.

The pain accompanying fractured ribs may be controlled by intercostal nerve block or small titrated doses of narcotics, or both. This improves pulmonary function and facilitates coughing up secretions. Early tracheal intubation and the use of positive end-expiratory pressure has been very helpful in the immediate treatment and in the prevention of postoperative complications. Schackford, Smith, and Zarin [42] concluded from a study of 42 patients with flail chest that mechanical ventilation is not necessary unless the patient has significant pulmonary dysfunction. Their criteria for the use of mechanical ventilation are: tachypnea, dyspnea, air hunger, agitation, arterial Po_2 of less than 60 mm Hg, or Pco_2 of more than 60 while breathing room air. The patient of course has received chest physiotherapy and intercostal nerve blocks before the decision is made to use the mechanical respirator. They also use the return of blood gases to normal to determine when to discontinue the use of a respirator. Trinkle and associates [50] have shown by comparative studies that the flail area of the chest wall is not as harmful to respiratory mechanics as has been claimed for the past 20 years. They have shown that the amount of lung contusion is a major factor in thoracic injury and should be treated as a separate injury by limiting noncolloid fluids and by administering furosemide, methylprednisolone, and intravenous albumin, all of which lessen the pulmonary lesion anatomically and physiologically. Their studies [49] show better results and fewer complications when mechanical ventilation is not used (see Chapters 4 and 8 for additional details).

Pneumothorax and Hemothorax

Tension pneumothorax can be managed temporarily by aspirating air through a large-bore needle. One should not await the completion of a roentgenogram if the tension pneumothorax is life-threatening. The ideal treatment is tube thoracostomy decompression, using at least a No. 28 French tube inserted through an intercostal space at the upper level of the pneumothorax. A small pneumothorax may need only close observation unless the patient is to have surgery under general anesthesia or a respirator is to be used. The closed thoracostomy tube decompression should be performed to prevent possible tension pneumothorax during anesthesia or from the use of other means of mechanical respiratory support.

The closed thoracostomy tube for the decompression of hemothorax is placed in the most dependent position of the hemothorax space. The size should be as large as is practical (we prefer a No. 32 to 36 French). If hemopneumothorax is present, it is preferable to insert two large tubes to assure optimum decompression of both processes and lessen the risk of blockage of the tubes by blood clots. One must be sure that both tubes are functioning well, otherwise an additional tube or tubes may need to be inserted. Decompression thoracostomy tubes are not only useful for reexpansion of the lung but are also valuable monitoring devices to help determine the amount of continued air leakage or the amount of continued bleeding. The amount of escaping blood should be measured hourly. This type of monitoring helps one to determine whether additional studies may be necessary and whether immediate thoracotomy is

indicated for control of hemorrhage or repair of fracture or laceration of a bronchus or of the trachea (Fig. 2-1A). Some of those with continued air leakage from airway trauma, however, may require only tracheostomy or tracheal intubation with an anesthesia-type tube as the only necessary treatment; such procedures may be adequate for a small tear or small penetrating wound of the trachea. The use of a Heimlich valve* attached to the thoracotomy tube allows uninterrupted functioning of the tubes when a patient needs to be transferred to another area for study or to another facility for more adequate management (for further details see Chapters 5 and 6).

Injury to Lung and Tracheobronchial Tree

Although major injury to the lungs and tracheobronchial tree are rather rare because the structures are pliable, somewhat mobile, and have reasonable protection because of their location, such injury, either blunt or penetrating, is possible. It is less often suspected following blunt trauma or acute extension of the neck.

Our experience with the emergency management of fracture or laceration of the trachea (Fig 2-1 A,B), larynx, and bronchi dates back to 1950 [9]. These injuries usually require emergency surgical repair, though there may be enough time to perform a diagnostic bronchoscopy. We have, however, treated a few small injuries to the trachea without resorting to direct tracheal repair. Most of these have been in children who have fallen on a sharp object such as a stick or the edge of a brick and showed marked subcutaneous emphysema of the tissues of the neck when seen. Several of these have been treated with tracheostomy as the only treatment but only after the extent of injury had been determined by bronchoscopy.

In rare instances continued air leakage may be due to the rupture of a preexisting pulmonary bleb or cyst. This is usually not of serious significance because the lung can be reasonably well reexpanded by use of a thoracostomy tube. Occasionally one of these reexpanded lungs will require open thoracotomy some days later to suture the leaking surface of the lung. It should be repeated that thoracostomy decompression tubes must not be clamped in the presence of air leakage, otherwise a life-threatening tension pneumothorax may occur. The connection of a Heimlich valve to

* Manufactured by the Bard Parker Division of Dickinson and Co., Rutherford, N.J.

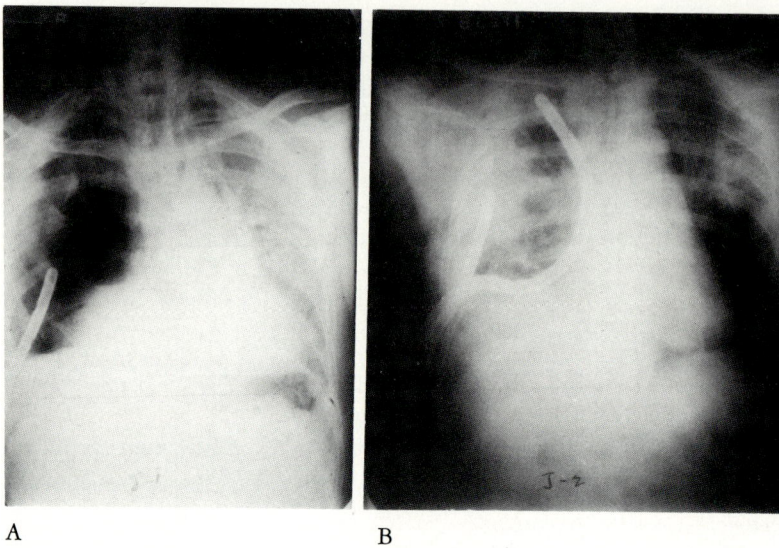

A   B

the thoracotomy or thoracostomy decompression tube permits the safe and convenient moving of the patient (detailed management of tracheo-bronchial injury is found in Chapter 7).

Fig 2-1. (A) Blunt force transection of the lower thoracic trachea, producing right tension pneumo-thorax and airway obstruction. (B) Roentgenogram taken immediately after postoperative tracheal repair.

Bleeding

Early massive or continued brisk bleeding of 500 cc per hour for three hours or longer would suggest damage to the heart or a major intrathoracic vascular structure. The initial large amount of blood that escapes through the intrapleurally placed decompression tubes may be less significant than the continued bleeding of several hundred cc of blood per hour. Massive bleeding requires immediate thoracotomy whereas continued bleeding at a slow rate may allow enough time for a diagnostic angiogram if it appears that the source of bleeding is from one of the major intrathoracic vascular structures. If time permits, an angiogram will often give valuable information toward a more definitive approach to the particular lesion. Laceration of the internal mammary artery and/or deep laceration of the surface of the lung, usually in penetrating type injuries, may be the sources of major bleeding. About approximately 25 percent of people who die from automobile accidents have a major vascular injury. Most who sustain rupture of the aorta do not survive long enough to reach a hospital. Some 20 percent who receive a major vascular injury reach the hospital alive, thus presenting an opportunity for salvage of the patient. Reul, Mattex, and Beall [41] are advocates of aggressive operative management for extensive in-

trathoracic trauma and their salvage rate has been impressive.

The entire surgical team should be alerted when a patient is taken to the special procedure unit for the performance of an angiogram. If the source of bleeding is an injury to the heart, the only findings may be those of hemorrhage and hypovolemia. However, injury to a heart with a relatively intact pericardium may produce a life-threatening pericardial tamponade because of the accumulation of blood in the pericardial cavity. This usually produces arterial hypotension, increasing central venous pressure and decreased pulse pressure. Pericardiocentesis may produce temporary relief while the patient is prepared for surgery. The most common cardiac injury is myocardial contusion, which often produces multiple arrhythmias and congestive failure; the clinical picture and management is that of a myocardial infarction.

A rare cardiac emergency may arise when the heart herniates through a tear or long laceration of the pericardium, usually occurring from blunt trauma. It causes a wide cardiac shadow on a roentgenogram, while an electrocardiogram shows rotation of the left ventricle. Angina often occurs, venous pressure increases, and the arterial pressure drops. Cardiac failure usually ensues and death usually occurs unless surgery is performed promptly to reduce the herniation of the heart and to repair the pericardium. Having the patient lie on the contralateral side while emergency surgery is being arranged may afford him some temporary relief. Surgery can best be performed in the emergency room area in acute, life-threatening conditions (see Chapters 9, 10, and 11 for detailed management of cardiovascular injuries).

Bronchial Hemorrhage

On a few occasions we have seen serious, otherwise uncontrollable hemorrhage into the tracheobronchial tree. Bronchoscopy was performed using a Fogarty embolectomy catheter, and the hemorrhage was confined to one lung, a lobe, or even a segment by placing the catheter through the bronchoscope and inflating the balloon while the patient was being prepared for an emergency operation.

Perforation or Rupture of the Esophagus

Perforation or rupture of the esophagus should usually be repaired promptly and the ipsilateral pleural space drained with a large thoracostomy tube. Spontaneous rupture of the esophagus is even more devastating than iatrogenic rupture because it occurs at the esophagogastric juncture (Fig 2-2). Because the tear also involves the upper portion of the stomach, the mediastinum is bathed with gastric juice; this produces a fulminant chemical mediastinitis that is usually rapidly fatal if not properly treated. The pleural cavity and the mediastinum should be thoroughly irrigated with saline during operative repair of the area of rupture. The catastrophe is caused by violent retching or vomiting by the patient usually while the stomach is full. It usually leads to severe pain, shock, and acute prostration, the vomitus frequently contains blood. Other diagnoses often given are myocardial infarction, dissection of the aorta, or perforation of a peptic ulcer. The diagnosis is confirmed when radiopaque medium is seen to escape through the perforation during an esophagogram.

Subcutaneous emphysema, often seen in the mediastinum and in the neck, is associated with tenderness and painful manipulation of the larynx, particularly if the lesion is in the upper esophagus. If the abdomen is explored due to a mistaken diagnosis, the observation of retroperitoneal bubbles of

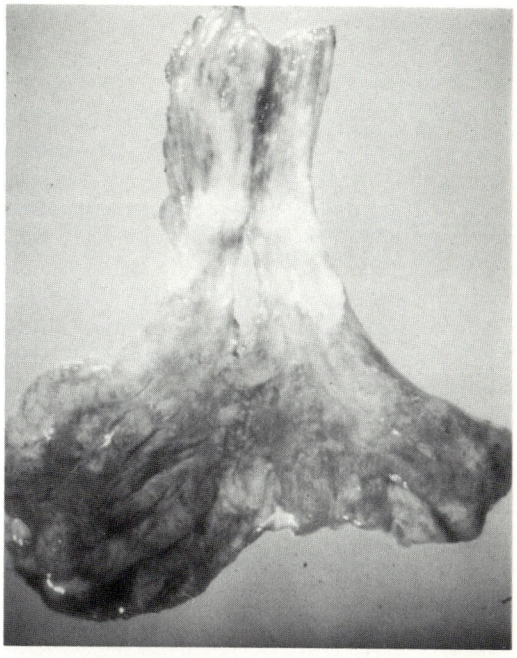

Fig 2-2. Typical spontaneous rupture of the esophagogastric juncture. Mucosal delineation between esophagus and stomach is clearly seen.

air overlying the area of the pancreas is usually diagnostic of perforation of the lower esophagus (for further discussion see Chapter 12).

INDICATIONS FOR EMERGENCY THORACOTOMY

The following conditions or events usually require emergency or early thoracotomy [18, 28]:

1. Cardiac hemorrhage
2. Pericardial tamponade
3. Major trauma of the great vessels
4. Rapid and continued hemorrhage
5. Major rupture of a diaphragm
6. Tracheobronchial or esophageal rupture
7. Torsion of the lung
8. Removal of objects on which victim is impaled
9. Removal of knife blades embedded into the area of the heart or major vascular structures
10. Persisting arrhythmia produced by foreign bodies embedded in the myocardium
11. Large, deep laceration of the lung

12. A large, destructive injury to the lung by high-velocity missiles
13. Close range shotgun wounds
14. Considerable loss of chest wall, either soft tissue and/or bony cage

Penetrating wounds are four or five times as likely to require an immediate thoracotomy than blunt-type injuries. Resuscitation for intrathoracic injury, especially if it is due to blood loss, should usually be performed by the open technique, ideally in an emergency operating room setting. It is obvious that greater patient salvage is possible if the patient does not have to be moved some distance to an operating room in another area of the hospital for emergency procedures. In addition to the resuscitation, definitive corrective surgery may be performed at the same time, thus increasing the percentage of salvage of patients, especially those with massive hemorrhage.

AUTOTRANSFUSION

In 1818 Blumdel [3] reported having treated 10 women with severe postpartum hemorrhage with autotransfusion of blood collected from vaginal bleeding. In 1860 Brainard [4] collected blood during a leg amputation, defibrinated it, and reinfused it into a patient. Over the next 25 years Miller [36] in 1885 and others [32, 48] used autotransfusion. In 1917 Elmendorf [17] reported the first autotransfusing of blood taken from the thoracic cavity.

We have used autotransfusion for over 30 years and agree with some of the more recent advocates—Symbas and colleagues [47], Duncan, Klebanoff, and Rogers [15, 16], and Couch, Laks, and Pilon [8]—that it has considerable value in the management of massive hemorrhage following trauma, in addition to its use in elective and other emergency surgery. Our early experience with autotransfusion was due primarily to the unavailability of large amounts of banked blood rather than its other advantages.

A large volume of trauma cases places a big burden on blood banks, depleting them to the extent that it may be disruptive to electively scheduled surgery. It has been obvious for many years that transfusion of banked homologous blood is not infrequently followed by a significant incidence of hepatitis and other serious and relatively minor transfusion reactions [8, 14, 45, 46]. These

transfusion and posttransfusion reactions cause much morbidity and a significant number of deaths each year. In addition to the untoward reactions related to transfusions, one should be acutely aware of the considerable inconvenience and vast cost of procuring and processing banked homologous blood. The availability and compatibility of blood are assured with the use of autotransfusion. It also helps in replacing and maintaining blood volume earlier and prevents unnecessary delay in emergency surgery. Following are some indications for autotransfusion [1, 6, 13, 14, 16, 38, 39, 45, 46]:

1. Actual or expected blood loss exceeding 1500 cc.
2. Extensive surgery
3. Inability to obtain adequate banked blood
4. Rare blood types
5. Previous transfusion reaction
6. Religious prohibition against regular blood transfusions
7. Bleeding diathesis

There are no absolute contraindications, although one should not use blood that is contaminated by intestinal tract contents except under extreme emergency conditions. It is also hazardous to use systemic heparinization as the anticoagulant technique in the presence of obvious or suspected brain injury.

If the type of injury does not require the use of extracorporeal circulation, it may not be advisable to use heparin systemically because of the possible or probable complication of hemorrhage into areas not being treated surgically. Trauma is often extensive or involves many systems, some of which may not be obvious at the outset of treatment. Patients with suspected brain injury should not have systemic heparinization as an elective technique, though in some instances there may not be any choice.

Alternate techniques, particularly applicable to patients with trauma, are available. Acid citrate dextrose solution, acid phosphate dextrose solution, or heparin may be used as additions to the blood or to prime the equipment being used for autotransfusion. These alternate techniques have been used in collecting blood from the pleural cavity and administering it to the patient preoperatively or intraoperatively. Symbas and associates [47] in emergency situations have collected blood from the thoracic cavity and reinfused it into patients without the use of an anticoagulant. The defibrinated blood from the thoracic cavity does not clot and can be given in this manner through a filter. Similarly, Reul [40] described a simple technique of collecting blood from the pleural cavity through a thoracostomy tube into standard blood transfusion bags containing citrate phosphate dextrose solution and then reinfusing it through a fine filter. Intraoperatively he uses a standard Bentley autotransfusion system with an acid phosphate dextrose solution as the anticoagulant. He believes that this is a safer procedure in trauma patients. Raines and co-workers [38] and Reul [40] recommend the administration of calcium when using those anticoagulants in over 5 units. Many others avoid the use of systemic heparin in autotransfusions, particularly in trauma patients, and some also believe that the coagulopathies are not only volume-related but also may be heparin-related [6, 7, 13, 15, 38, 40].

Complications of Autotransfusion

Adverse effects upon the blood (which will be discussed later) are due to a combination of factors. The most important single factor is the reaction of the blood to the exposed tissues [13]. Another factor is trauma to the blood during its salvage by suction and contact with the autotransfusion system [6–8, 15, 16, 39]. The salvage of blood should be by gentle suction from a blood pool, and skimming the wound or other tissues with the aspirator tip should be avoided.

Rakower and Worth [39] reported that in 93 percent of their patients there was continued, troublesome oozing due to defibrination and systemic heparinization, particularly in patients who had received massive autotransfusion. This oozing caused considerable additional blood loss and delayed completion of surgery. Their patients required transfusion of large quantities of banked blood. Because of these problems Rakower suggested that an alternate technique of administering anticoagulant might be preferable. Some of the decrease in blood elements is due to failure to salvage all of the blood lost and also because of the hemodilution factor due to the use of anticoagulant solutions and other fluids that may be given while autotransfusion is being performed [8, 40].

The major complications of autotransfusion are primarily the effects upon the formed blood elements and the coagulation process [1, 2, 7, 13, 16, 38, 39]. Most all autotransfusion patients have a reduction in the red blood cell mass, in hematocrit,

in hemoglobin, and in the platelet count, and have decreased fibrinogen. Conversely, most have an increase in serum bilirubin and free hemoglobin. The majority of those who have more than 2000 cc of blood in autotransfusions develop hemoglobinuria, which, however, does not seem to adversely affect renal function [6]. The red blood cell survival time remains near normal [4]. Experimental studies by Bennett and Geelhoed [1] indicate that microaggregates that form in 3-week-old banked blood are more damaging to the morphology of perfused lungs than autotransfused blood. Microfilters of the 150-micron size remove clots and particles of matter of a size that could harm the lungs but allow normal blood elements to pass through [6]. Aggregation of platelets is common but they soon deaggregate after being reinfused into the patient. Most of the adverse effects upon the blood elements are self-correcting or reverse themselves in 2 to 5 hours and the others within 2 or 3 days [2, 6–8, 14, 16, 39].

Hemorrhagic coagulopathies are closely related to the autotransfusion of a massive quantity of blood. It seldom occurs unless the amount of blood autotransfused exceeds 5000 cc. They usually respond to the vigorous infusion of fresh frozen plasma, fresh whole blood, and epsilon aminoproprionic acid. Air embolism, which rarely occurs, can be prevented by clearing the lines and other equipment of air bubbles and by maintaining 200 cc of solution in the reservoir at all times during autotransfusion. Infection has not been a problem even when it has appeared that the blood pool might have been contaminated.

One might conclude by stating that autotransfusion seems to be a safe, relatively cheap, and valuable adjunct to the management of trauma and other types of surgery in which massive hemorrhage may occur [29]. Autotransfusion not only conserves resources but saves lives, and it does not seem to be damaging to the body's major organs. Major complications are rare and are usually volume-related [15, 39]. It is suggested that a Bentley autotransfusion system or similar equipment be available whenever one suspects hemorrhage of more than 1500 cc. The equipment is easy to use and does not require highly technical personnel.

TORSION OF THE LUNG

Torsion of the lung or a portion of a lung, a rare condition, may be caused by a marked degree of

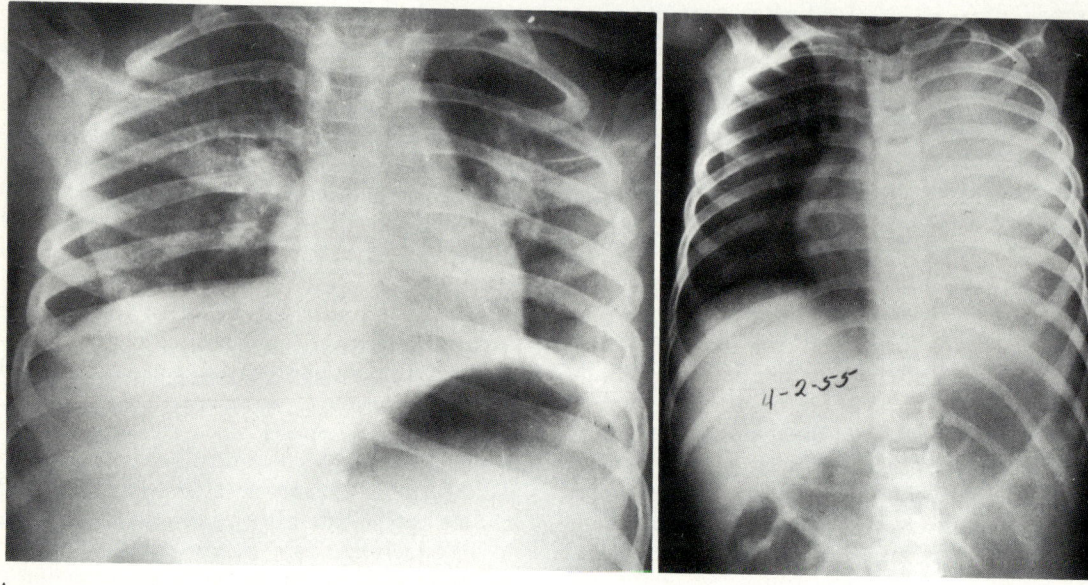

A

B

Fig 2-3. (A) Torsion of left lung, bronchovascular pattern is directed superiorly and laterally. (B) Atelectasis of lung that underwent 180 degree clockwise torsion. Gangrene is now present. Note the obvious shift of the mediastinum toward the right.

compression of the lower thorax. The lung rotates 180° clockwise after disruption of the inferior pulmonary ligament and then suddenly becomes engorged with blood. Lung infarction and gangrene occur in rapid succession. The diagnostic x-ray finding is a reversal of the bronchovascular pattern or shadow on chest roentgenogram. The bronchovascular pattern assumes a superolateral direction (Fig 2-3) rather than the usual inferolateral distribution. Subsequent roentgenograms show a rapidly developing "ground glass" appearance, which progresses to solid opacification (Fig 2-3 B) as well as a shift of the mediastinum toward the contralateral side. As necrosis of the lung occurs, small air pockets without fluid levels may develop in the involved portion or all of the lung that may have undergone torsion. The diagnosis can be confirmed by the visualization of bronchial torsion and obstruction through a bronchoscope. Immediate surgery is necessary to salvage the lung and the life of the patient. Most of these have been fatal due to delayed diagnosis or nondiagnosis during life. In 1957 Daughtry [11] reported the successful treatment of torsion of the lung in a six-year-old child. In 1967 Selmonsky and co-workers [43] reported the successful management of torsion of the right middle lobe due to blunt thoracic trauma. Torsion of a lobe, most often the middle lobe, can occur in nontrauma patients after a lobectomy is performed.

FOREIGN BODY OBSTRUCTION

On occasion an emergency arises when a foreign body of sufficient size to obstruct the airways is inhaled or aspirated into the larynx or the trachea. Immediate removal or dislodgement of that body is a life-saving measure. Aspiration of a solid object that fits into the lung or trachea in such a manner as not to permit the exchange of air is more likely to occur in small children. Placing the child in the upside-down position plus exploring the pharynx with a finger is often effective in relieving the obstruction. Also the Heimlich maneuver [24, 25] that has been proposed for the management of the café coronary syndrome should also be tried. If the obstruction cannot be completely relieved immediately, place the child in any position that allows the best possible respiratory exchange. An endoscopist should be alerted of the emergency and be available in the emergency room when the patient arrives in the hospital. (Details of management of foreign bodies in the air and food passages are to be found in Chapter 13.)

Café Coronary

Café coronary is obstruction of the airway due to the aspiration of a large bolus of poorly chewed meat into the pharynx, larynx, or trachea. It is the most common fatal type of acute airway obstruction. Statistically it is the sixth leading cause of accidental death, according to Heimlich [24, 25]. Some 3900 deaths per year are attributed to this cause, but it is likely that it causes far more because many of these deaths are attributed to cardiac origin until or unless a complete postmortem examination is performed.

It most often occurs in middle-aged or older individuals who are attending a party and who have been drinking cocktails or eating a meal while laughing or talking. Many of the victims are on sedatives and/or have dentures. They fail to masticate meats properly, and a large, poorly chewed piece of meat finds its way into the upper major air passages. The victim suddenly becomes cyanotic, clutches at the throat, becomes motionless, and cannot utter a sound. Unless someone suspects the cause of the problem and proceeds to correct it, the patient dies immediately. Initially a blow on the back may be adequate. Finger removal of the bolus of meat, too, can usually be accomplished, thus clearing the airway. The Heimlich maneuver which dislodges the bolus [24, 25] has been widely publicized and is highly successful in resuscitation or salvage of these people. The procedure consists of approaching the patient from behind and placing both arms around him or her; one fist is clenched and with the other open hand placed over the fist a quick upward thrust is made over the epigastrium. It may be repeated several times or until air exchange is normal. If the patient has been anoxic for several minutes prior to proper management, cardiopulmonary resuscitation should be performed and may be successful if it is performed within the first 4 to 5 minutes. This can restore pulmonary and cardiac function that has ceased but is only effective after the airway obstruction has been removed.

REFERENCES

1. Bennett SH, Geelhoed GW: Pulmonary effects with and without filtration. Presented at the Second Annual Bentley Autotransfusion Seminar, Chicago, October 13, 1973

2. Bennett SH, Geelhoed GW, Gralnick H, et al: Effects of autotransfusion on blood elements. Am J Surg 125:273, 1973

3. Blumdel J: Experiments on transfusion of blood. Med Chir Trans 9:56, 1818

4. Brainard DM: Amputation of the thigh for disease of the knee joint: transfusion of blood. Chicago Med Soc 18:1016, 1860

5. Bregman D, Pavodi EN, Hutchinson JE, et al: Intraoperative autotransfusion during emergency thoracic and elective open-heart surgery. Ann Thorac Surg 18:590, 1974

6. Brener BJ, Raines JK: Intraoperative autotransfusion and clinical surgery. Presented at the Second Annual Bentley Autotransfusion Seminar, Chicago, October 13, 1973

7. Buth J, Raines JK, Kolodny GM, et al: The effect of intraoperative red cell mass and red cell survival. Surg Forum 26:276, 1975

8. Couch NP, Laks H, Pilon R: Autotransfusion. Arch Surg 108:121, 1974

9. Daughtry DC: Bronchial anastomosis and broncho-plastic procedures in the interest of preservation of lung tissue. Discussion of a paper presented by D. Paulson, et al. J Thorac Cardiovasc Surg 29:238, 1955

10. Daughtry DC: Management of non-penetrating injuries. Am Surg 23:462, 1957

11. Daughtry DC: Traumatic torsion of the lung. N Engl J Med 256:385, 1957

12. Daughtry DC, Chesney JG: Advancing field of thoracic surgery. J Fla Med Assoc 38:541, 1952

13. DiOrio DA, Symbas PN: The effects of tissue surfaces and anticoagulants upon blood components recovery during autotransfusion. Presented at the Second Annual Bentley Autotransfusion Seminar, Chicago, October 13, 1973

14. Dowling J: Autotransfusion: its use in the severely injured patients. Presented at the First Bentley Autotransfusion Seminar, San Francisco, October 12, 1972

15. Duncan SE, Klebanoff G, Rogers W: Clinical experience with intraoperative autotransfusion. Presented at the Second Annual Bentley Autotransfusion Seminar, Chicago, October 13, 1973

16. Duncan SE, Klebanoff R, Rogers W: Clinical experience with intraoperative autotransfusion. Ann Surg 180:296, 1974

17. Elmendorf N: Ueber wieder infusion nash punktion eines frischen Hamaothorax. Munch Med Wochenschr 64:36, 1917

18. Ferguson TB: Emergency treatment of chest injuries. J Fla Med Assoc 54:120, 1967

19. Fitts WT: The annual Scudder oration on

trauma. Medical Tribune World Wide Report, June 7, 1970

20. Freeark RJ: Antibiotic prophylaxis in trauma patients. Contemp Surg 10:59, 1977

21. Geelhoed G, Wright CB, Mason KG, et al: The physiology of autotransfusion in the heparinized baboon. Presented at the Second Annual Bentley Autotransfusion Seminar, Chicago, October 13, 1973

22. Gurdjian ES: Impact Injury and Crash Protection. Springfield, ILL, Thomas, 1970

23. Harrison WH, Gray AR, Couves CM, et al: Severe non-penetrating injuries to the chest, clinical results and the management of 212 patients. Am J Surg 100:715, 1960

24. Heimlich HJ: A life-saving maneuver to prevent "food choking." JAMA 234:398, 1975

25. Heimlich HJ, Hoffman KA, Canestri FR: Food choking and drowning deaths prevented by external subdiaphragmatic compression, physiological basis. Ann Thorac Surg 20:188, 1975

26. Kemmerer WT, Eckert WG, Gathright JB, et al: Patterns of thoracic injuries and fatal traffic accidents. J Trauma 1:595, 1961

27. Kilman JW, Charnock E: Thoracic trauma in infancy and childhood. J Trauma 9:863, 1969

28. Kish G, Kozloff L, Joseph WL, et al: Early thoracotomy in the management of chest trauma. Ann Thorac Surg 22:23, 1976

29. Klebanoff G: Summary and review. Presented at the Second Annual Bentley Autotransfusion Seminar, Chicago, October 13, 1973

30. Klebanoff G, Phillips G, Evans W: Use of a disposable autotransfusion unit under varying conditions of contamination. Am J Surg 120:351, 1970

31. Kulowski G: Crash Injuries: The Integral Medical Aspects of Automobile Injuries and Death. Springfield, Ill, Thomas, 1960

32. Lockwood CD: Surgical treatment of Banti's disease, report of three cases. Surg Gynecol Obstet 25:188, 1917

33. Love JW: Chest injuries. JAMA 232:285, 1975

34. Lucas CE: Early care of the critically injured patients. Hosp Med 13:31, 1977

35. Meade RH: A History of Thoracic Surgery. Springfield, Ill, Thomas, 1961

36. Miller AG: Case of amputation of the hip joint

in which reinjection of blood was performed and rapid recovery took place. Edinb. Med J 31:721, 1885

37. National Safety Council: Accident Facts. 1976 Edition. Chicago, National Safety Council, 1976

38. Raines J, Buth J, Brewster DC, et al: Intraoperative autotransfusion: the equipment, protocols and guidelines. J Trauma 16:616, 1976

39. Rakower SR, Worth MH, Jr.: Massive intraoperative autotransfusion. Presented at the Second Annual Bentley Autotransfusion Seminar, Chicago, October 13, 1973

40. Reul GJ, Jr.: A safe technique for autotransfusion in trauma. Presented at the Second Annual Bentley Autotransfusion Seminar, Chicago, October 13, 1973

41. Reul GJ, Jr., Mattex KL, Beall AC: Recent advances in operative management of massive chest trauma. Ann Thorac Surg 16:52, 1973

42. Schackford S, Smith DE, Zarin SC, et al: Ventilatory and nonventilatory treatment in patients with flail chest. Am J Surg 132:759, 1976

43. Selmonsky CA, Fledge JB, Jr., Ehrenhaft JL: Torsion of a lobe of the lung due to blunt thoracic trauma. Ann Thorac Surg 4:166, 1967

44. Shires T: Trauma symposium. Bull Am Coll Surg 58:7, 1973

45. Symbas PN: Autotransfusion from hemothorax: experimental and clinical studies. J Trauma 12:689, 1972

46. Symbas PN: Experimental and clinical experience with autotransfusion. Presented at the First Annual Bentley Autotransfusion Seminar, San Francisco, October 12, 1972

47. Symbas PN, Levin JM, Ferrier FL, et al: A study on autotransfusion from hemothorax. Southern Med J 62:671, 1969

48. Thies J: Zur Bheantlung der Extravteringravieitat. Zentralb Gynaeckol 38:11, 1914

49. Trinkle JK, Furman RW, Hinshaw MA: Pulmonary contusion. Ann Thorac Surg 16:568, 1973

50. Trinkle JK, Richardson JD, Franz JL, et al: Management of flail chest without mechanical ventilation. Ann Thorac Surg 19:355, 1975

51. Wright CB, Geelhoed GW, Mason KG: Autotransfusion in subhuman primate. Am J Surg 128:49, 1974

3. TRACHEOSTOMY

Paul C. Samson

Tracheostomy derives from ancient medical practice and may well be one of the oldest of surgical procedures for maintaining life under emergency conditions. Some Egyptian scholars believe that hieroglyphics on the wall of a tomb at Sakkara (ca. 3000 B.C.) depict a tracheostomy [10]. It was described and probably attempted in 124 B.C. by Asclepiades of Bithynia and later discussed, if not actually performed, by Antyllus in A.D. 198, Paul of Aegina in A.D. 690, and Rhazes in the ninth century. Apparently no instrument of any kind was passed into the trachea during these early operative attempts. A straight tube was first used by Placentibus in the sixteenth century, and his procedure was described repeatedly during the succeeding two hundred years, although Casserius suggested a curved tube in the 1600's. In 1620, Habicot of Paris reported on four successful operations and published the first monograph on the subject. Each of his cases represented an aspect of upper airway obstruction due to injury [26, 35].

The ancients used the term *bronchotomy;* in 1718 Heister introduced *tracheotomy,* and this was later popularized by Trousseau. In 1938 Negus suggested *tracheostomy* to describe the maintained opening in the trachea, a term now universally accepted as correct [22, 44].

It is important to remember that initially tracheostomy was employed almost entirely for airway obstruction at or above the level of the larynx. In the early part of this century, Jackson performed a few *tracheostomies* for the removal of excessive secretions; later, however, in 1911 [29], he introduced bronchoscopy as a new and important method for achieving the same purpose. (It is remarkable that so astute an observer should have regarded tracheostomy primarily as a means of correcting upper airway mechanical obstruction while ignoring the indications for which it is frequently used today.) Also in 1911, St. Claire Thompson [43] considered *tracheotomy* to be indicated in cases of injury or major surgery on the head and neck, primarily to prevent blood and excretions from entering the airway. In 1943, Galloway [21] recommended tracheostomy in patients with bulbar poliomyelitis to facilitate the aspiration of tracheobronchial secretions.

In World War II, references to tracheostomy in trauma were few [32]. It was mentioned as possibly being indicated in some cases of traumatic wet lung, flail chest, mediastinal emphysema, tension pneumothorax, and tracheoesophageal wounds. In the history of the Second Auxiliary Surgical Group [34], it was described only in connection with maxillofacial wounds and trauma to the larynx. The excessive secretion problem (traumatic wet lung), now such a common indication for tracheostomy, was handled exclusively by bronchoscopy, repeated tracheobronchial catheter aspirations, and, from time to time, by positive-pressure oxygen [9].

Shortly after World War II, the indications for tracheostomy in trauma broadened rapidly. In 1950 Baronofsky and associates [3] stressed the importance of tracheostomy in handling excessive bronchial secretions, particularly if the patient was comatose. Carter and Giuseffi [11] the following year demonstrated clearly the value of tracheostomy in severe crushed-chest injuries. In a later publication [12] the same authors also showed that a number of thoracic surgeons had commenced independently and roughly simultaneously to employ tracheostomy in trauma treatment shortly after their return to civilian life.

Two classic papers then set the stage for tracheostomy to be combined with mechanical ventilation in cases of crushed chest with flailing. In 1956 Avery and co-workers [2] described their combination of an "uncuffed" tube with a Mörch respirator to produce alkalotic apnea and "internal pneumatic stabilization." In 1957 Björk described the use of a cuffed tube with an Engström volume-cycled ventilator [6].

In more recent years, tracheostomy for trauma has formed an appreciable segment of any tracheostomy series. The percentage depends, of course, on the type of hospital from which the reports have emanated—relatively low in Veterans Administration hospitals, much greater in city and county hospitals. Our own survey [17] of sixteen years ago showed 18 percent while a later report [5] revealed that 26 percent of 1000 tracheostomies were carried out because of trauma.

SYMPTOMS AND SIGNS PORTENDING RESPIRATORY INSUFFICIENCY

Any of the symptoms and signs of respiratory insufficiency presented below may develop during examination or treatment of the patient, and the examiner should be aware that some type of respiratory assistance may become necessary at any time. Such assistance usually consists of giving oxygen by nasal catheter or mask, relief of chest-wall pain (commonly by regional intercostal nerve block), tracheobronchial catheter aspiration, bronchoscopy, insertion of an endotracheal tube, tracheostomy with an uncuffed tube, or tracheostomy with a cuffed tube and a mechanical respirator. The symptoms and signs are:

1. Dyspnea.
2. Hyperpnea, particularly if the secondary muscles of respiration are being used. True air hunger should be regarded as a danger sign.
3. Croupy respirations with a marked inspiratory crow localized over the larynx are characteristic of worsening upper airway obstruction.
4. A continuous hacking, poorly productive cough indicates excessive secretions in the tracheobronchial tree. The patient succeeds in raising only small amounts of sputum, and when the patient is examined there are continually shifting rhonchi.
5. Pallor, tachycardia, and an early increase in blood pressure are signs of beginning hypoxia and hypercapnia.
6. Manic excitement followed by coma usually means severe hypoxia. In the past this was frequently attributed to pain; large doses of morphine were often given for its relief with the occasional development of cardiac arrest. Other symptoms of hypoxia are fatigue, headaches, loss of judgment, and personality changes.
7. Cyanosis is a late sign of hypoxia. It should never be allowed to supervene in a patient under observation and treatment.
8. Delayed shock in the absence of obvious hemorrhage, a mangled limb(s), or peritoneal contamination often signifies severe respiratory insufficiency (adult respiratory distress syndrome) with total vascular collapse and impending cardiac or respiratory arrest, or both.

Symptoms and signs should be correctly interpreted, but arterial blood gases must be frequently monitored to provide warning of a subtle worsening in ventilatory capacity. In most instances, such changes indicate ventilation-perfusion abnormalities or right-to-left shunts (either gross or microatelectasis). If only the PaO_2 is decreased and other values are normal, oxygen administration may suffice although a decrease in the dead space may be warranted. The development of acute respiratory failure is indicated by a PaO_2 value below 60 mm Hg and a $PaCO_2$ above 49 mm Hg (hypercapnea) [5]. More often than not, respiratory acidosis will also be present, as shown by a pH below 7.3. Critical levels of these three measurements are commonly listed as: PaO_2, 45 mm Hg; $PaCO_2$, 76 mm Hg; pH, 7.25. The situation becomes more dangerous if the levels shown are reached rapidly; assisted respiration is in order *at once* if they are reported.

Ventilatory failure may also occur when the lungs are morphologically normal. Injury to the chest wall and abdomen or laryngotracheal obstruction may all interfere with adequate ventilation. These disorders may not at first result in marked blood gas changes; if dyspnea is an early feature, however, it may be so prominent a symptom that immediate remedial treatment will have to be undertaken.

INDICATIONS FOR TRACHEOSTOMY

The indications for tracheostomy in the injured patient are basically the same as those in patients with disease, i.e., laryngeal obstruction, the desirability of decreasing anatomical dead space, excessive secretions in the tracheobronchial tree, and problems associated with poor gas transport across the alveolar-capillary membranes. It is in this last situation particularly that the combination of cuffed tubes and mechanical respirators continue to prove their worth. The injury necessitating tracheostomy may be thoracic or nonthoracic. Likewise, the condition of the patient prior to injury has considerable bearing on the decision to perform the operation. Thus, a young, healthy adult may be able to cough and raise excessive secretions while an older individual with emphysema and bronchitis whose gas exchange is significantly impaired may be thrown into sudden respiratory failure with what might appear at first to be rather minimal chest injury. The attending physician can easily avoid embarrassment by keeping these possibilities in mind.

What follows are particular situations in three types of trauma—nonthoracic, combined thoracic/nonthoracic, and thoracic—for which tracheostomy may be indicated. Also included is a discussion on the role of the endotracheal tube and its use in relation to tracheostomy.

Nonthoracic Trauma

Indications for tracheostomy in nonthoracic trauma would be as follows:

1. Laryngeal edema with obstruction due to a crushing or penetrating injury or to a foreign body.
2. Penetrating or crushing wounds of the cervical trachea.
3. Head injury with unconsciousness.
4. Severe maxillofacial injuries.
5. Cervical cord injury with poor ventilatory capacity.
6. Stretch injury of the neck with phrenic paralysis.
7. Secondary lung damage associated with trauma elsewhere. In this instance, some of the pertinent factors are: shock with slowing of circulation and sludging; pulmonary edema from excessive administration (in time and amount) of electrolytes or blood; and fat embolism.

Combined Thoracic/Nonthoracic Trauma

Patients with minor thoracic trauma but a tremendous secretion problem made worse by preexisting emphysema and "bronchitis" fall into this combined category. The need for tracheostomy may become paramount if general anesthesia is necessary for abdominal exploration, for control of hemorrhage, or for major limb repair.

Thoracic Trauma

There are many indications for tracheostomy in thoracic trauma. These are gone into in detail below:

1. Tears or complete ruptures of the tracheobronchial tree always necessitate tracheostomy plus early thoracotomy and repair.
2. Burns of the airway may require tracheostomy under certain circumstances [37, 42]. Before the procedure is undertaken, it is advised that the following measures be employed: early endotracheal intubation; oxygen administration under high humidification; ventilatory assistance as indicated; and for early unrelenting bronchospasm, a single, large intravenous dose of steroids, perhaps repeated two or three times [4].

Recent published reports have stressed that it is highly undesirable to perform early tracheostomies "on suspicion," except when specific criteria are met. These comprise: undoubted evidence of pulmonary burn, especially if the burn is sustained in a closed space (severe smoke inhalation); evidence of a tracheobronchial pseudomembrane that cannot be completely cleared by suction-bronchoscopy; and progressive uncontrolled respiratory insufficiency.

3. Accidental gassing is an indication since mustard gases and lewisite, which are vesicants, can cause severe inflammation and even sloughing of the respiratory mucosa, while lung irritants such as chlorine and phosgene exert their main action deeper and may cause severe pulmonary edema. Tracheostomy may become indicated for continuing tracheobronchial toilet following bronchoscopy if there is upper airway obstruction. Ventilatory assistance with a respirator may also be indicated.

4. Indications for tracheostomy in chest wall trauma are "crushed chest syndrome" with flail segments and traumatic asphyxia. Perhaps one of the greatest advances of treatment of crushed chest syndrome with flail segments is the use of a cuffed tube with mechanical ventilation. This has been called internal fixation. It may not be redundant to stress the emergency insertion of an endotracheal tube and the emergency external application of towel clips, Levin forceps, or available hooks to stabilize a severely flailing chest. Even without flailing, a fractured sternum and ribs may cause poor air exchange because of impaired ventilatory motion.

Traumatic asphyxia may dictate tracheostomy for ventilatory support, but more often it becomes necessary because of associated injuries rather than the asphyxia or "masque ecchymotique" itself.

5. In the mediastinum, a traumatic tracheoesophageal fistula probably will require tracheostomy. Severe progressive mediastinal emphysema from whatever cause may lead to respiratory embarrassment, requiring subsequent tracheostomy.

6. The spectrum of posttraumatic pulmonary insufficiency (traumatic wet lung) or posttraumatic respiratory distress syndrome may be indications

for tracheostomy, as are severe contusion [16], "blast lungs," and aspiration pneumonitis, particularly in the unconscious patient.

Role of Endotracheal Tubes

At this time, it seems appropriate to discuss the role of endotracheal tubes as, first, emergency substitutes for tracheostomies in patients in acute respiratory failure whose intensive ventilatory supervision will presumably last longer than from 10 to 12 days, and, second, their use for an unspecified period pending a decision as to the need for tracheostomy. In the first situation, the immediate insertion of an endotracheal tube should replace the emergency tracheostomy. Any modern emergency department will have the tools and the expertise necessary to establish good control of ventilation in a few seconds. Tracheostomy can then become an urgent but not an emergency procedure. There is also no question that the endotracheal tube can be used for temporary respiratory assistance and is frequently employed under these circumstances as a definitive measure. For instance, in the "pure" adult respiratory distress syndrome with minimal secretions, endotracheal intubation is almost always employed when ventilatory assistance is needed [41].

The disadvantages of an endotracheal tube are pain and discomfort for the patient and possible contamination of the lower airway. An endotracheal tube precludes oral alimentation, and, most important, since it is difficult to suction and clean, it is more likely to be occluded with mucus plugs.

Moore and colleagues [33] advise that all patients for whom tracheostomy is being considered should first be tested by trial endotracheal intubation. I do not agree completely. When the patient is overwhelmed by excessive tracheobronchial secretions as a prominent part of his problem, tracheostomy should be done expeditiously. An indwelling endotracheal tube is not an efficient nor certain conduit for successful suctioning. If there is lobar atelectasis or if there has been aspiration of stomach contents or similar circumstances, bronchoscopy followed immediately by intubation and tracheostomy is the first choice rather than a trial of endotracheal intubation.

TRACHEAL CANNULAS

A wide assortment of tracheostomy tubes is available. They differ in material, neck plate, size,

length, and angle between neck plate and tube. Metal tubes should be of stainless steel. It is important that the metal tracheal cannulas throughout a given institution be of the same make so that tubes of the same size are interchangeable. Two complete sets (sizes 0 to 6) should be available in the operating room, the intensive care unit (ICU), and in the emergency department. The neck plate is a matter of choice, although I prefer a relatively unobstructed surface such as that found in the C. L. Jackson model. The adult-sized tubes are almost always 90° between neck plate and cannula.

The angle and length of tube are especially important factors when used for the younger age group. At Children's Hospital Medical Center of Northern California there is a preference for the Holinger metal tube, which has a 65° angle and is available in two lengths.

As a rule, I do not insert the largest uncuffed tube possible. Continued ability to speak is important, and even in children the feeling that air is passing through the larynx is reassuring. Also with larger tubes, there is a greater risk of tracheal wall pressure and erosion. An exception to this is in children with burns of the airway in whom a larger than usual tube will diminish the chances of obstruction by tenacious secretions [37, 42].

When the respirator is necessary, a relatively large cuffed tube is inserted. Only in the Mörch type of respirator is a cuffed tube unnecessary. By present-day standards, however, accurate measurements of inspiratory pressure, delivered volume, and oxygen percentage are not possible unless a cuffed tube is employed. The use of the slip-on cuff with a metal tracheostomy tube is presently obsolete. When a mechanical respirator is used, an adaptor must be available to fit the type of tracheal tube employed. Most if not all of the modern cannulas now have universal adaptors.

Several types of nonmetallic cuffed tubes are now commercially available. The relatively new Portex Blue Line disposable tracheostomy tube featuring the cylindric, low-pressure Soft Seal cuff is now widely used. All of the newer tracheostomy tubes emphasize the principle of the sausage-shaped, low-pressure cuff: the Lanz tube; the Kamen Wilkinson Fomecuf tube; and the self-inflating cuff, Sin Cuf [1]. In an attempt to correct some of the deficiencies inherent in many of the cuffed tubes, a new tracheostomy cannula was

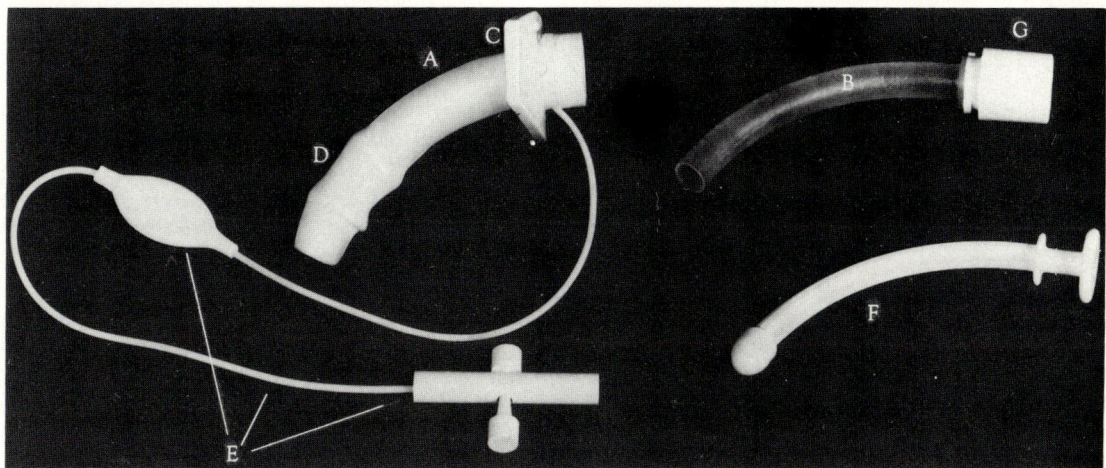

Fig 3-1. The component parts of the new tube: (A) *outer cannula,* (B) *inner cannula,* (C) *"hinge-joint" neckplate,* (D) *sausage-shape cuff (deflated),* (E) *inflation system (the line, test balloon, pressure retention device),* (F) *obturator, and* (G) *"twist-lock" adaptor. (From P. C. Samson,* Ann Thorac Surg *10:58, 1970. By permission.)*

evolved, described and used extensively by Hardy, Fettel, and Shiley [27, 28] (Fig 3-1).

THE OPERATION

However ancient in concept, the operation of tracheostomy is still fraught with difficulties, usually because it is performed too late, because of technical misadventures, or because of poorly managed aftercare. Eiseman and Spencer [18] rightly emphasize that tracheostomy is often underrated as a surgical procedure and that the details of the operation are often dismissed as too simple to warrant serious study. It is to be hoped that as the number of tracheostomies increase, so will the sense of timing become more accurate and lead to a larger number of elective procedures. We strongly prefer to perform tracheostomies in the operating room, although obviously facilities should also be available in an ICU or in a busy emergency department.

There are, in essence, three kinds of tracheostomy: (1) orderly or elective (some authors term this *prophylactic*), (2) hurried or urgent (also known as *therapeutic*), and (3) a true emergency operation. Whether the operation is elective or urgent, it can nearly always be performed in the operating room; and we believe there is little justification these days for an emergency tracheostomy at the bedside. If one is faced with the necessity of securing an adequate airway, the insertion of an endotracheal tube will almost always stave off the acute emergency until facilities for an orderly operation can be arranged. The "midnight tracheostomy" performed with poor lighting and inadequate help on a writhing and anoxic patient constitutes a harrowing experience for the physician and may well be fatal for the patient.

Techniques

The recent report of 655 "cricothyroidotomies" (more properly called *cricothyroidostomy*) has now been published [8]. There were no postoperative subglottic stenoses in spite of dire warning by Chevalier Jackson [30]. Many of us attending the meeting at which the report on cricothyroidotomy was first made have now had increasing experience with the operation. Nevertheless, it still seems advisable to describe the far more frequent standard tracheostomy.

The patient is placed supine on the operating table with a flat roll under the shoulders so that the neck is moderately extended (Fig 3-2). The chin is pointed toward the ceiling and kept in the midline at all times. I usually prefer light general anesthesia, although local infiltration can be used; in either case high oxygen concentrations must be maintained. Since so many of our trauma patients' problems have to do with excess secretions, bron-

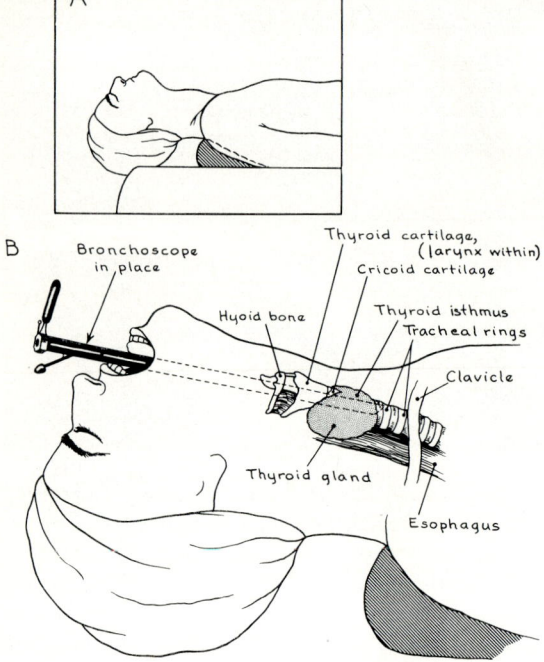

Fig 3-2. Preparing the patient. (A) The patient is in the proper position with a roll placed under the shoulders to hyperextend the neck. (B) Bronchoscope is in place for aspiration of excessive secretions just before tracheostomy procedure. (From P. C. Samson. In G. F. Madding and P. A. Kennedy (eds.), Atlas for Attorneys—Surgical Techniques. San Francisco: Bancroft-Whitney, 1968.)

choscopy is frequently performed just prior to the tracheostomy so that a clear airway will be assured. The bronchoscope may then be left in place as a stent and for the delivery of oxygen, or it may be replaced with an endotracheal tube. By this time no emergency exists.

A 3 to 4 cm horizontal incision is made between the anterior borders of the sternocleidomastoid muscles, 2 cm above the sternal notch (Fig 3-3). The investing layer of the deep cervical fascia and the strap muscles are dissected longitudinally in the midline. Large branches of the anterior jugular veins may need ligation. Meticulous hemostasis is essential, and in this connection the high-frequency cautery saves considerable time.

The pretracheal fascia is then split longitudinally, exposing the thyroid isthmus (Fig 3-4). When the isthmus is enlarged and is truly in

midincision, it should be divided between suture ligatures. Much more often, it can be retracted superiorly and thus moved out of the way. The tissues are separated at each side of the now-exposed trachea just enough to allow the shallow insertion of two small retractors; this gives further immobilization. The cricoid cartilage and the first tracheal ring are identified so that they will not be injured. A longitudinal incision is made through the second, third, and perhaps fourth tracheal rings. Care must be taken not to incise too deeply because the scalpel could injure the esophagus. I can see no useful purpose in taking a button out of the trachea or in making T, U, inverted U, or cruciate incisions as these take a little extra time and not infrequently cause the tube to be inserted off center. From time to time, one can insert 00 silk mattress sutures through each edge of the incised trachea to simplify exposure during the immediate postoperative period either for changing the tube or for bronchoscopy. These traction sutures are brought out loose through the incision and fastened to the neck. The tracheal incision is spread by curved forceps or a dilator.

The end of the tracheal cannula is pointed into the trachea at the start of insertion and not parallel with it. The neck plate is next rotated upward 90° as the tube is advanced. The endotracheal catheter should not be completely withdrawn until it is certain that the tracheal cannula is in place (Fig 3-5). The same techniques would be used to insert a cuffed tube except that a lengthier incision in the trachea might be necessary.

Careful check of the tube's position must now be made. If the tube is fitting correctly, the neck plate will remain flush on the neck without pressure, the aspirating catheter can easily be passed without obstruction, and the patient will breathe freely without stridor or cough. If these criteria are not met, it means that the tube is either not fitting properly or that a false passage has been made into the mediastinum.

No deep sutures are used to close the dead space. One or two fine sutures through the skin and subcutaneous tissue are sufficient, with the space immediately surrounding the cannula left open. A square gauze moistened with saline is cut and slipped under the neckplate before the tapes are tied. The tube may be made more secure by actually suturing it to the skin rather than depending upon the tape.

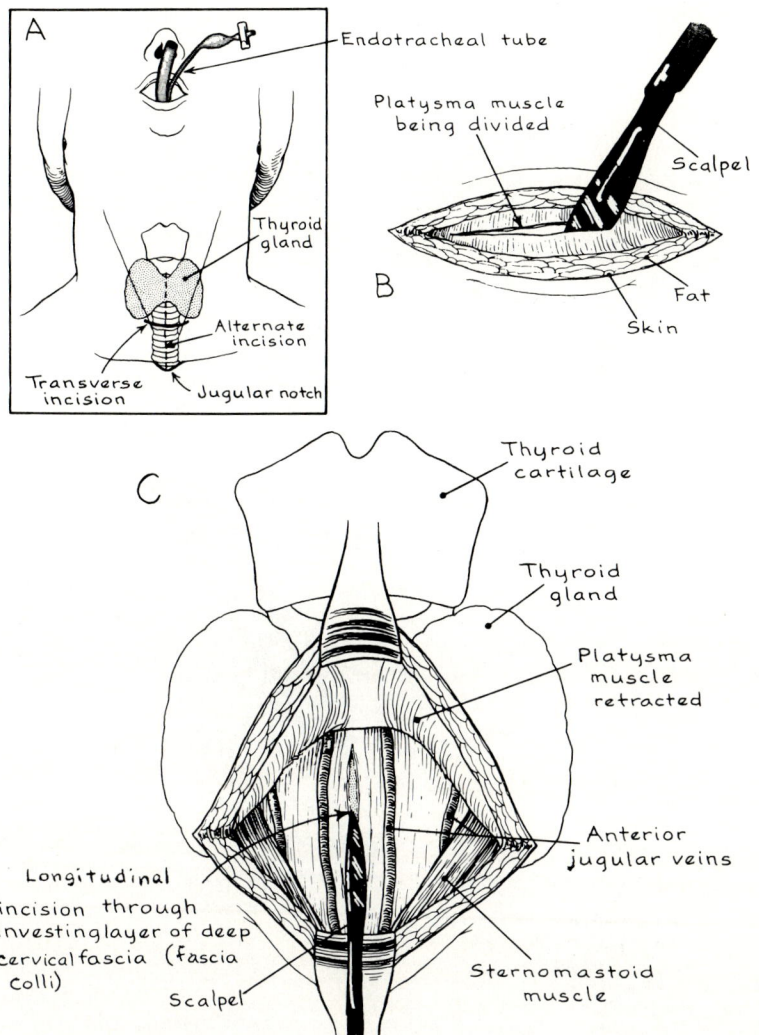

Fig 3-3. The initial incision. (A) An endotracheal tube has now replaced the bronchoscope. The site of the preferred transverse incision is shown. The vertical incision site often used in emergencies is indicated by the dashed line. (B) The transverse incision extends through the platysma muscle. (C) With the platysma muscle retracted, a vertical incision is made through the investing layer of the fascia colli. (From P. C. Samson. In G. F. Madding and P. A. Kennedy (eds.), Atlas for Attorneys—Surgical Techniques. San Francisco: Bancroft-Whitney, 1968.)

True Emergency Tracheostomy

A true emergency tracheostomy is undertaken only when there is severe laryngeal obstruction with im-

pending or actual cessation of respirations. The operation has been described by Jackson and Jackson [30]. The neck is quickly extended, and the fingers of the left hand immobilize the laryngeal cartilage and upper trachea. A vertical midline incision is made from just below the cricoid cartilage to the suprasternal notch. Hemostasis is ignored. The left index finger then describes the trachea, and the midline cut is deepened with the trachea well outlined. The left index finger is shifted just to the left and with this guide, a vertical midline incision is made through the tracheal rings, usually the second and third. The tracheal incision is spread, a cannula is rapidly inserted, and appropriate ventilation is commenced. Local external pres-

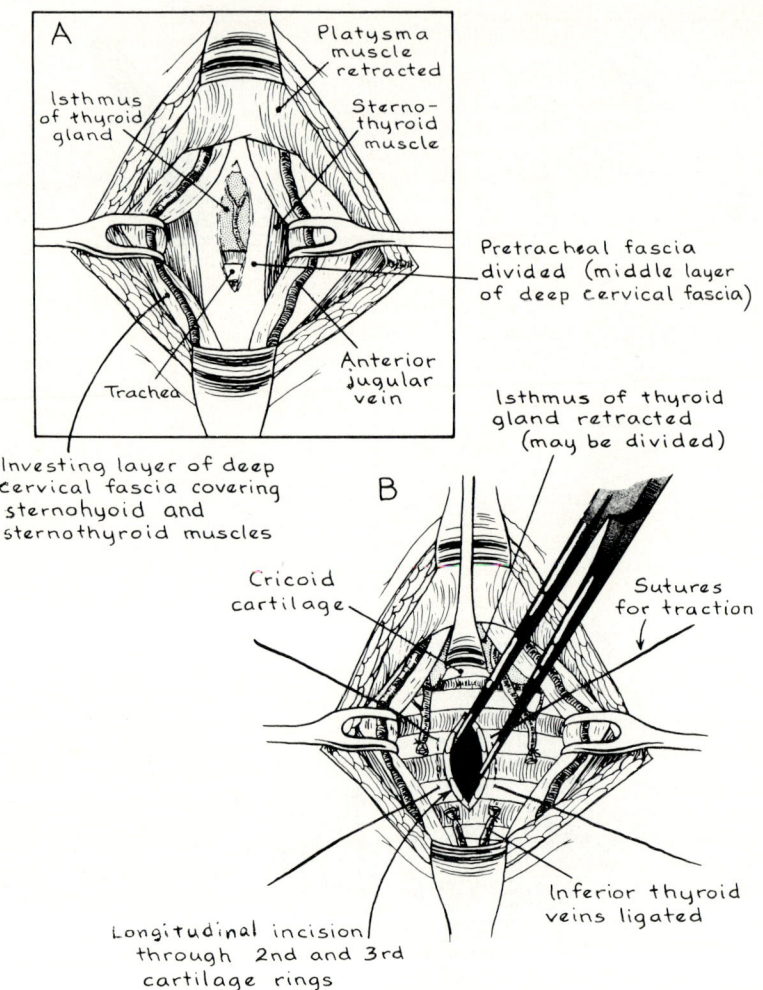

Fig 3-4. Exposing and incising the trachea. (A) The pretracheal fascia is exposed and incised longitudinally after the sternohyoid and sternothyroid muscles have been retracted. (B) The thyroid isthmus is freed and retracted superiorly. A longitudinal midline incision is made through the second and third cartilage rings of the trachea. Optional traction sutures are inserted. (From P. C. Samson. In G. F. Madding and P. A. Kennedy (eds.), Atlas for Attorneys—Surgical Techniques. San Francisco: Bancroft-Whitney, 1968.)

sure on either side of the main incision will control bleeding until a later time when deliberate hemostasis can be undertaken.

One must emphasize again that an emergency operation is rarely indicated under present-day conditions. The ready availability of a direct laryngoscope and endotracheal tubes in strategic locations will obviate all but the rarest of emergency tracheostomies.

SURGICAL RISKS, ACCIDENTS, AND ERRORS

Operative and postoperative complications of tracheostomy as high as 33 percent have been reported. Some have been lethal. There are more complications when the operation is performed on infants and small children. Probably the main surgical error is in not operating promptly when obvious indications exist. There is ample evidence that both complications and death rates are signifi-

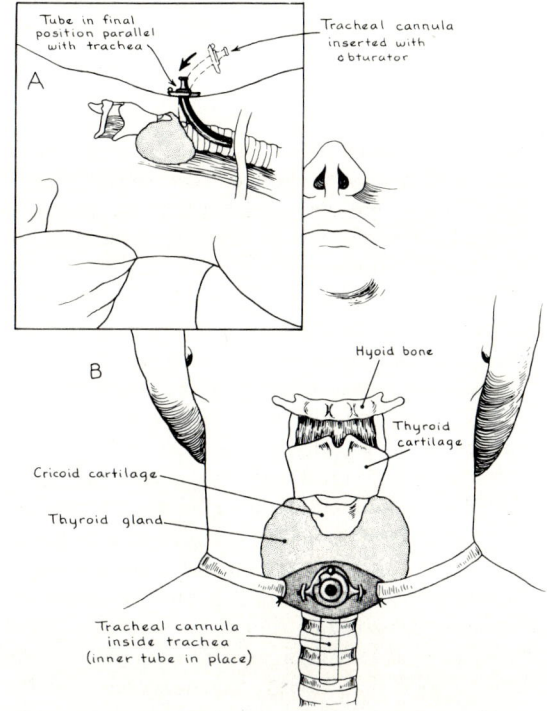

Fig 3-5. Technique of cannula insertion. (A) The outer tube with obturator is pointed into the trachea. The neckplate is rotated upward 90 degrees, and the tube advanced and slipped down the trachea. (B) The tracheal cannula with inner tube inserted is held tightly in place by a tape tied around the neck. (From P. C. Samson. In G. F. Madding and P. A. Kennedy (eds.), Atlas for Attorneys—Surgical Techniques. San Francisco: Bancroft-Whitney, 1968.)

cantly increased when tracheostomy becomes an emergency procedure performed under less than ideal circumstances [6, 17, 30, 44].

The following are the most common operative accidents during emergency tracheostomies, and review of them makes it obvious that complications are reduced when the procedure is unhurried.

1. *Hemorrhage.* This may only be troublesome oozing and can be minimized when the dissection is kept to the midline and the main vessels are ligated before division. Hemorrhage may be lethal, however less frequently from exsanguination than from tracheobronchial aspiration by blood and obstruction. It is more likely to occur under emergency conditions when airway obstruction is already present and the neck veins are dilated.

2. *Subcutaneous and mediastinal emphysema.* When airway obstruction leads to violent respiratory efforts, air may be sucked into the tissues of the cervical region and mediastinum. This complication can be avoided by the establishment of an adequate airway through intubation or bronchoscopy rather than tracheostomy. When cervical emphysema occurs immediately following tracheostomy, it means that the incision was closed too tightly and the skin sutures must be removed.

3. *Pneumothorax.* Mediastinal emphysema may rupture into the pleural cavity, or the apical pleural cap may be torn during dissection, particularly during emergency tracheostomy, if the patient is restless. Death is possible if a pressure pneumothorax is not recognized and treated at once by intercostal tube insertion.

4. *Air embolism.* This may occur when there is partial division of distended neck veins during inspiration. Minor degrees of air embolism probably occur commonly. Again, death may supervene.

5. *Damage to cricoid cartilage and first tracheal ring.* This occurs when a careless incision is made without locating the cricoid cartilage exactly; occasionally scarring and eventual subglottic stenosis follow.

6. *Accidental incision of posterior tracheal wall and esophagus.* A hurried and too deep incision through the anterior tracheal wall may penetrate the posterior wall and esophagus. The soft, narrow trachea of the infant is particularly vulnerable. To a large extent, this complication can be avoided by the use of an endotracheal tube or a bronchoscope as a stent in the trachea. If esophageal perforation goes unrecognized and unrepaired, the resulting esophagotracheal fistula is often fatal. In a variation of this accident the posterolateral trachea wall only was incised on a small child during an emergency tracheostomy. The rapid development of tremendous cervical emphysema prompted immediate exploration through the tracheostomy. The 9-mm iatrogenic incision was easily closed from inside the trachea.

7. *False passage of tracheal tube into the mediastinum.* Such a complication hardly seems worth mentioning, but it has happened more than once in an emergency situation. The surgeon must be convinced that there is free exchange of air before the patient leaves the operating table.

8. *Damage to recurrent laryngeal nerves.* Careless dissection too far posteriorly on the trachea

may damage one or both recurrent laryngeal nerves.

POSTOPERATIVE CARE

Constant vigilance, intelligent application, full dedication, and asepsis are the hallmarks of successful postoperative nursing care. Only by such means can most complications be avoided [23, 35].

Roentgenographic Confirmation

It is well to confirm the position of a metal cannula in the trachea by anterior and lateral roentgenograms of the neck as soon as possible following tracheostomy. This is particularly true in children but is worthwhile in adults also. X-ray visualization is the only way to make sure that the size, angle, and the length of the tube are correct for the patient.

Humidification

Ambient air passing into the tracheostomy tube is far too dry and is mainly responsible for the development of crusts and plugs in the trachea. The bubbling of oxygen or air through a standard humidifier does not moisten it sufficiently—some type of nebulization or ultrasonic mist is mandatory. Excellent commercial models are now available to achieve this. Infants and small children are usually placed in some type of mist-forming tent. More and more I depend on distilled water as the moistening vehicle rather than the various types of wetting agents.

Oxygen must be administered under carefully supervised conditions. If the patient is still dyspneic, even though the skin is pink, it may mean that he has respiratory acidosis; the use of a positive pressure respirator with a cuffed tube may then become necessary.

The Aspiration of Secretions

This constitutes one of the most important aspects of postoperative care and I emphasize again that the presence of excessive tracheobronchial secretions is a frequent indication for tracheostomy. The equipment required comprises a whistletip catheter, a Y-tube connector, and a high-vacuum pump delivering suction of 200 to 250 cm of water (150 to 175 mm Hg). We have come to demand asepsis in the handling of the catheter. A sterile catheter should be used with each aspiration. Pharyngeal aspiration is often necessary and should be done with a separate catheter and Y-tube. When secretions are excessive, suctioning may be required every 10 to 15 minutes. If the cannula contains an inner tube, it should be removed at least once an hour, cleaned, rinse-sterilized, and immediately reinserted at the end of aspiration. It is possible that the use of *two* interchangeable inner cannulas would speed this process appreciably. When the secretions are very thick, a few cubic centimeters of distilled water may be introduced into the trachea just before suctioning.

Tracheobronchial toilet (Fig 3-6) must be meticulous. The catheter is passed through the cannula as far as it will go (approximately 15 cm) with the Y-tube open and no suction [23, 35]. The Y is intermittently closed by digital pressure and the catheter rotated as it is slowly withdrawn. Full suction should never exceed 2 to 3 seconds, and intermittent make-break suction with the finger is the maneuver of choice. The catheter should be repassed as long as significant amounts of secretion are obtained, taking care, however, that the patient does not become exhausted or cyanotic. An oxygen line should be handy so that intratracheal oxygen can be given if the patient becomes obviously hypoxic during the procedure. Each stem bronchus may be entered by turning the head of the patient sharply in the opposite direction. The catheter tends to enter the right stem bronchus if the neck plate is turned clockwise, the left stem if it is rotated counterclockwise (Fig 3-7). If the patient is comatose, he should be turned from side to side and modified postural drainage employed to prevent pooling of secretions in the dependent bronchus.

The patient may continue to be dyspneic or wheeze following aspiration. This suggests the presence of crusts or plugs and indicates bronchoscopy for inspection and removal of the offending material. It can be performed either through the larynx or through the tracheostomy stoma. If the latter is fresh, it is probably better to do the bronchoscopy in a more formal way from above.

Care of Cuffed Tubes and Respirators

A few words are in order concerning the special care of cuffed tubes and respirators. It should go without saying that the cuff must be tested for leaks and stretched before the cannula is slipped into the trachea. The inserted cuff must not be subjected to undue air pressure. Experimental evi-

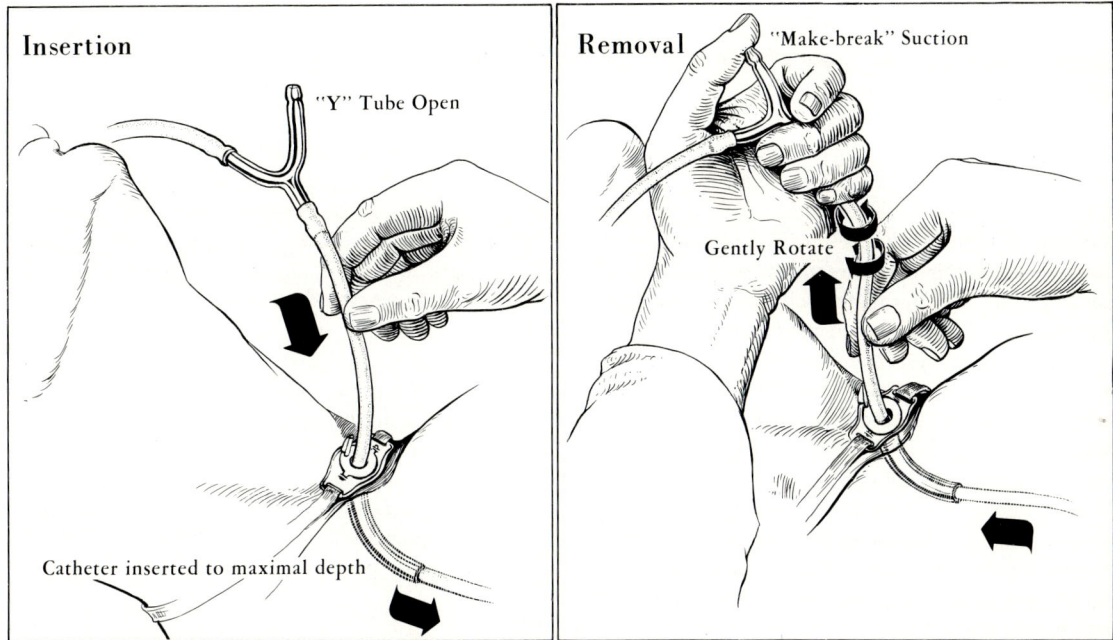

Fig 3-6. *Technique of catheter aspiration: insertion and removal of catheter. (From* Hospital Medicine *1:2, 1964, Hospital Publications, Inc. By permission.)*

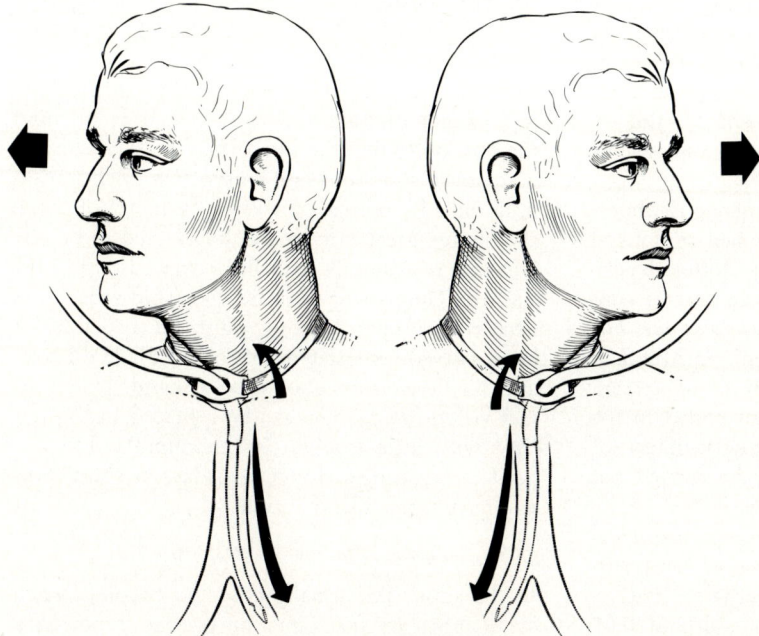

Fig 3-7. *Technique for inserting catheter into stem bronchi. The catheter tends to enter the right stem bronchus if the neckplate is turned clockwise, the left stem if it is rotated counterclockwise. (From* Hospital Medicine *1:2, 1964, Hospital Publications, Inc. By permission.)*

dence now supports the premise that overdistention is an important cause of posttracheostomy stenosis. One should determine the minimal amount of air necessary to occlude the tracheal lumen. If the patient is unconscious, the volume of air that will barely occlude the trachea during positive pressure is accurately measured by the anesthesiologist. Should the patient *remain* unconscious in the ICU, the cuff is inflated with just enough air that the ventilator is automatically cycled. If the patient is awake, he is asked to speak, and the cuff is adjusted just so phonation is barely prevented. These amounts of air are then noted for future inflations.

A cuffed tube should be deflated for at least 5 to 10 minutes every hour to prevent prolonged contact with the tracheal mucosa. The deflation should be positive, with the air actually withdrawn by syringe. This may pose great difficulty if continuous respirator treatment is needed. Nevertheless, even with the cuff uninflated, one can trigger the respirator manually and thus achieve sufficient ventilation to tide the patient over these critical few minutes. I have had no experience with the tracheostomy tube containing a double balloon. Theoretically it has the advantage that the ballons can be inflated alternately, but there is a good chance for overlapping of the sites of pressure and the tube is bulky. Furthermore, the reported stenosis following its use had one of the longer segments of stenosis [24, 39].

Care of the respirator is of tremendous importance, and this is especially true when prolonged mechanical respiration is necessary. Bitter experience has shown that the respirator can become contaminated by such organisms as *Pseudomonas*. The development of an exotic pneumonia in a patient otherwise doing reasonably well is an unpleasant occurrence and not infrequently has ended in the patient's death. Hence, continuing surveillance of the asepsis of the apparatus must be carried out [13].

In our own ICU, all tubing and equipment except the ventilator is changed, cleaned, and gas-sterilized every 24 hours. The ventilator itself is gas-sterilized between patients. In addition, 0.25 percent acetic acid (to counteract *Pseudomonas* organisms) is flushed through all nebulizers, humidifiers, and ultrasonic devices for 15 minutes twice every 24 hours. Finally, monthly cultures are made routinely from all parts of the respirator.

While respirators are discussed in greater detail in another chapter, it may not be remiss to mention them here. Numerous kinds of apparatus are available but all have certain common features: (1) they either assist or control ventilation, and (2) they restore arterial blood gases toward normal [13, 19]. There are two basic types of ventilators: (1) those that are pressure-cycled (pressure limiting/volume variable), represented by the Bird Mark 7 and 8 and the Bennett Pr2; and (2) the volume-cycled variety (volume constant/pressure variable), such as the Engström, Emerson, and Bennet Ma 1. A volume ventilator is one in which a constant volume of oxygen mix is delivered to the lungs, regardless of the pressure it takes. The pressure-controlled machines are usually adequate if oxygenation can be maintained by pressures generally under 35 mm Hg. If higher pressures are necessary, then a volume-controlled machine should be used.

Changing the Cannula

A well-fitting tracheal tube (with inner and outer cannulas) need not be changed for several days. The lumen, however, may become sticky, causing difficulty when reinserting the inner cannula. This occurs when the inner tube has not been replaced immediately after cleaning. Under these circumstances, the entire tube must be changed. With some of the cuffed tubes, such as the Portex, there is no inner cannula and one must bear in mind the possibility that the lumen may become clogged with sticky secretions and crusts. If a tracheal cannula must be reinserted within 24 hours of a tracheostomy, great care should be exerted to be certain that the cannula is in fact replaced within the trachea. The patient must be quiet and sedated, if necessary. Proper lighting must be available. A large, curved hemostat, or one of the blade-dilators, and small retractors should be at hand. Under *direct* vision the cannula can be replaced in the trachea with little trouble. If the cannula does not need to be changed for 5 or 6 days, a sinus track will have formed by that time.

Decannulation—The Art of Weaning

In the adult, this usually poses no problem when metal tubes are used and the patient is not on a respirator. If the patient can breathe comfortably around the tube when it is temporarily occluded with the finger, the tube is corked. If he has difficulty breathing around the tube, then a smaller size is inserted before corking.

The art of weaning a patient from long-continued mechanical ventilation is an entirely different matter. The following criteria have been proposed for successful weaning [38]:

1. Resting minute ventilation less than 10 liters per minute
2. Maximal voluntary ventilation more than twice minute ventilation
3. Tidal volume greater than 5 ml/kg
4. Vital capacity greater than 1 liter
5. Maximum inspiratory force less than 20 cm H_2O

It is our local custom to deflate the tracheostomy cuff and disconnect the respirator for 5 minutes out of 60 minutes, increasing the time off by 5-minute increments to a total of 55 out of 60 minutes off the respirator, as tolerated. During the first few nights the patient should be placed back on the ventilator for maximum rest. Frequent observations of pulse rate, respiration, blood pressure, and arterial blood gases are made and recorded. During spontaneous breathing, adequate oxygenation and ventilation should be provided through a T-tube connection. When the patient continues to be comfortable and all signs and symptoms are stable after 60 minutes of spontaneous breathing, the weaning process should continue, either by corking the cuffed tube or by inserting a corked metal tube. When the cork is easily tolerated for 48 hours, the patient is extubated.

As a rule the sinus closes spontaneously in 48 to 72 hours. A small wick of vaseline is inserted to keep the skin edges apart and a dry dressing applied. No further suturing is necessary at this time.

POSTOPERATIVE COMPLICATIONS

A variety of postoperative complications have been reported. These can all but be eliminated by strict adherence to the principles of postoperative care.

Undue pressure from an ill-fitting tube

A tube that is too large, too long, or at a wrong angle—creating undue pressure—has led to tracheal ulceration, obstruction, granuloma formation, and hemorrhage. Early postoperative x-ray checkup, including a lateral film, will prevent such difficulties.

Bleeding

Bleeding may appear in several guises and may be fatal if the bronchi become flooded. Immediate bleeding is always incisional. If only moderate, the loose skin sutures may be removed and the wound packed with gelfoam. If the bleeding is severe, a formal exploration of the tracheostomy incision should be carried out, hopefully with good light and good suction. Delayed and often fatal hemorrhage is usually due to pressure necrosis of the wall of a major artery. One example is erosion of the innominate artery from a tracheostomy tube that was inserted too low into the trachea [39]. In other cases, the tip of an ill-fitting tube eroded through both the tracheal wall and a paratracheal vessel [45]. Once can be forewarned by several small bleeding incidents that may precede the sudden final fatal gush.

The formation of crusts and plugs

Crusts and plugs lead to blockage of the tube and perhaps asphyxia or pulmonary atelectasis. These are primarily due to poor humidification and careless tracheobronchial toilet.

Dislodgement of cannula

Due to careless inattention, dislodgement of a cannula has resulted in death, particularly in infants and young children.

False passage into the mediastinum on attempted replacement

As stated earlier, the early replacement of a cannula should not be undertaken without proper help, lighting, and instruments. The lack of any one of these can result in a false passage into the mediastinum.

Infection

Infection may be a wound infection, usually seen when tissues are sutured too tightly around the tracheostomy tube, or infection in the tracheobronchial tree. The latter form may be introduced by those caring for the patient (unsterile and careless tracheobronchial suction) or it may be machine-induced. In either event, this can become a highly serious complication.

Tracheal stenosis

Tracheal stenosis has occurred (1) after operative injury to the cricoid cartilage; (2) at the site of the tracheostomy stoma, usually from surgical mangling of the tracheal cartilages, or the development of granulomas; (3) at the site of the cuff, from prolonged and/or too great pressure in the cuff; and (4) at the tip of the tracheostomy cannula following ulceration and necrosis of the tracheal wall from a poorly fitting cannula. Nearly all these are results of iatrogenic accidents and their prevention has been discussed in preceding sections.

The treatment of posttracheostomy tracheal stenosis is fraught with difficulty. It is apparent that repeated dilations are rarely definitive. Surgical excision is the treatment of choice and has been well described in the recent literature. Grillo [24] has successfully resected many midcervical stenoses through a modified collar incision, the longest successful one being 4.5 cm. Direct end-to-end anastomosis of the trachea was performed using interrupted fine Dacron sutures. We have closely followed Grillo's technique [25] and have now resected some 10 tracheal stenoses with success.

Fishman and Dedo and co-workers [20] also advocate a cervical approach where possible with sleeve resection of the stenosis and direct anastomosis. Apparently they gain extra length by "laryngeal release." In this technique, the thyroid cartilage and hyoid bone are exposed through upward dissection from the collar incision. Both superior cornuae of the thyroid cartilage are divided and the thyro-hyoid membrane is incised. These maneuvers lower the larynx an approximate 2.5 cm, thus significantly reducing tension on the anastomosis.

The management of healing defects

If the tracheostomy tube has been in place for a long period, the sinus between skin and trachea may become epithelialized and, under these circumstances, will not close. On the other hand, the stoma may obliterate, with the skin becoming firmly adherent directly to the trachea. This interferes with swallowing and is a minor complication that can be rectified easily.

The persisting stoma can be treated by dissecting the epithelialized track to the trachea, trimming it, and then closing it with a fine subcuticular stitch. Muscle and skin are next sutured over the closure [31]. This method has been very successful. Jackson and Jackson [30] have also described a simple procedure for the plastic closure of a persisting trachea fistula, involving dissection in a tube-like form down to the trachea. Simple ligation is performed close to the trachea and the excess of the track is cut off. The short stump is then covered in layers by muscle, subcutaneous tissue, and skin.

In the case of an indurated and restricting scar, the following technique is applicable. The scar is excised and all tissue planes down to the trachea are freed by lateral dissection, taking care to identify and loosen the strap muscles. These are drawn over the trachea and sutured together in the midline with fine silk. The subcutaneous tissues and skin are then closed in separate layers without drainage. The development of the plane that includes the strap muscles is the most important step. The outcome is a soft scar that gives a good plastic result and does not interfere with swallowing.

REFERENCES

1. Abouav J, Finley TN: Prevention of tracheal injuries in prolonged ventilation. Chest 71:1, 1977
2. Avery EE, Mörch ET, Benson DW: Critically crushed chests. J Thorac Surg 32:291, 1956
3. Baronofsky ID, Dickman RW, Vanderhof ES: The treatment of acute chest injuries with especial reference to the use of tracheostomy. Minn Med 33:49, 1950
4. Bartlett RH, Niccole M, Travis H, et al: Acute management of the upper airway in facial burns and smoke inhalation. Arch Surg 111:744, 1976
5. Beatrous WP: Tracheostomy (tracheotomy): its expanded indications and its present status. Laryngoscope 78:3, 1968
6. Björk VO, Engström CG: The treatment of ventilatory insufficiency by tracheostomy and artificial ventilation. J Thorac Surg 34:228, 1957
7. Blair E, Topuzlu C, Deane RS: Major blunt chest trauma, Current Problems in Surgery. Chicago, Year Book, 1969
8. Brantigan CO, Grow JB: Cricothyroidotomy: elective use in respiratory problems requiring tracheotomy. J Thorac Cardiovasc Surg 71:72, 1976
9. Brewer LA, III, Burbank B, Samson PC, et al: The "wet lung" in war casualties. Ann Surg 123:343, 1946
10. Brewer LA, III: Discussion of Dugan DJ, Samson PC: Tracheostomy: Present Day Indications and Techniques. Am J Surg 106:303, 1963
11. Carter BN, Giuseffi J: Tracheostomy: a useful procedure in thoracic surgery with particular reference to its employment in crushing injuries of the thorax. J Thorac Surg 21:495, 1951
12. Carter BN, Giuseffi J: Further experience with tracheostomy in management of crushing injuries of the chest. Arch Surg 69:483, 1954
13. Committee on Therapy of the American Thoracic Society: Cleaning and sterilization of inhalation equipment: a statement. Am Rev Resp Dis 98:521, 1968

14. Cooper JD, Grillo HC: Experimental production and prevention of injury due to cuffed tracheal tubes. Surg Gynecol Obstet 129:1235, 1969
15. Dedo HH, Fishman NH: Laryngeal release and sleeve resection for tracheal stenosis. Ann Otol 78:285, 1969
16. DeMuth WE, Smith JM: Pulmonary contusion. Am J Surg 109:819, 1965
17. Dugan DJ, Samson PC: Tracheostomy: present day indications and techniques. Am J Surg 106:290, 1963
18. Eiseman B, Spencer FC: Tracheostomy, an underrated surgical procedure. JAMA 184:684, 1963
19. Feldman SA (ed.): A Review of Tracheostomy and Artificial Ventilation. London, E Arnold, 1967
20. Fishman NH, Dedo HH, Hamilton WK, et al: Postintubation tracheal stenosis. Ann Thorac Surg 8:47, 1969
21. Galloway TC: Tracheostomy in bulbar poliomyelitis. JAMA 128:1096, 1943
22. Garrison FHL: An Introduction to the History of Medicine. Fourth edition. Philadelphia, Saunders, 1929
23. Glas WW, King OJ, Lui A: Complications of tracheostomy. Arch Surg 85:56, 1962
24. Grillo HC: Circumferential resection and reconstruction of the mediastinal and cervical trachea. Ann Surg 162:374, 1965
25. Grillo HC: Surgery of the trachea, in Current Problems in Surgery. Chicago, Year Book, 1970
26. Guthrie D: Early records of tracheostomy. Bull Hist Med 15:59, 1944
27. Hardy KL: Tracheostomy: indications, techniques, and tubes. Am J Surg 126:300, 1973
28. Hardy KL, Fettel BE, Shiley DP: A new tracheostomy tube. Ann Thorac Surg 10:58, 1970
29. Jackson C: Laryngeal, bronchial and esophageal endoscopy. Laryngoscope 21:1183, 1911
30. Jackson C, Jackson CL: Diseases and Injuries of the Larynx. New York, MacMillan, 1942
31. Lawson DW, Grillo HC: Closure of persistent tracheal stomas. Surg Gynecol Obstet 130:995, 1970
32. Berry FB (ed.): Surgery in World War II: Thoracic Surgery. Vols 1 & 2. Washington DC, Office of the Surgeon General, 1963 & 1965
33. Moore FD, Lyons JH, Pierce EC: Post-traumatic Pulmonary Insufficiency. Philadelphia, Saunders, 1969
34. Office of the Surgeon General: Forward Surgery of the Severely Wounded: A History of the Activities of the Second Auxiliary Surgical Group, 1942-1945. Washington, 1945 (unpublished)
35. Plum F, Dunning MF: Techniques for minimizing trauma to the tracheobronchial tree after tracheostomy. N Engl J Med 254:193, 1956
36. Priest RE: History of tracheostomy. Ann Otol 61:1039, 1952
37. Pruitt BA, Flemma RJ, DiVincenti FC, et al: Pulmonary complications in burns. J Thorac Cardiovasc Surg 59:7, 1970
38. Sahn SA, Laksminarayan S, Petty TL: Weaning from mechanical ventilation. JAMA 235:2208, 1976
39. Shelly WM, Dawson RB, May IA: Cuffed tubes as a cause of tracheal stenosis. J. Thorac Cardiovasc Surg 57:623, 1969
40. Silen W, Spieker D: Fatal hemorrhage from the innominate artery after tracheostomy. Ann Surg 162:1005, 1965
41. Solliday NH, Shapiro BA, Gracey DR: Adult respiratory distress syndrome. Chest 69:2, 1976
42. Stone HH, Martin JD: Pulmonary injury associated with thermal burns. Surg Gynecol Obstet 129:1242, 1969
43. Thompson St.C: A patient who wore a tracheostomy tube for 50 years. Proc R Soc Med 5:158, 1911–1912
44. Watts J McK: Tracheostomy in modern practice. Br J Surg 50:954, 1963
45. Willerson JT, Fred HL: Delayed fatal hemorrhage after tracheostomy. Ann Intern Med 116:138, 1965

4. CHEST WALL TRAUMA

Paul C. Adkins
Paul J. Corso
J. Laurance Hill

At the present time, automobile accidents cause over 50,000 deaths each year in the United States and account for half the deaths in young people 15 to 25 years old. At least 25 percent of these vehicular deaths are the result of chest trauma alone; in another 50 percent there was an associated thoracic injury. The majority of the deaths follow blunt injury to the rib cage and its internal components [29, 35, 40]. In the management of this type of injury, a thorough understanding of the physiological derangements associated with blunt trauma to the chest is essential for early recognition and proper treatment.

PHYSIOLOGICAL CONSIDERATIONS

The rib cage may be considered a membranous shell supported by strong, but lightweight costal struts protecting its vital contents. Normal ventilatory function is dependent upon an intact chest wall. The other components of a properly functioning ventilatory mechanism are:

1. Normal action of the intercostal muscles and accessory muscles of respiration
2. Adequate elevation of the ribs and sternum
3. Sufficient movement of the diaphragm
4. Normal function of the abdominal musculature
5. A negative intrapleural pressure
6. Normal lung compliance
7. A patent upper airway
8. Normal amount of lung surfactant
9. Normal peripheral and central neurological reflexes
10. Normal cardiopulmonary hemodynamics

Blunt chest trauma may affect any or all of these essential components of ventilation. Nevertheless, a considerable reserve exists since the normal vital capacity is 4500 cc and the tidal volume is 500 cc. An adult who can only breathe with diaphragmatic excursion because of a cervical injury can still produce a vital capacity of 1000 cc. Furthermore, any effort that will depress a diaphragm just one centimeter will increase the tidal volume approximately 50 percent [11, 30, 37, 42]. Thus, it is obvious that the human body is capable of tolerating a considerable amount of injury to the respiratory mechanism without immediate death and that proper support may allow the individual to survive without a serious deficit.

Preexisting pulmonary disease is often not readily discerned at the time of injury and may significantly interfere with the ability of the individual to compensate for a relatively minor injury to the normal respiratory mechanism. Associated injuries elsewhere in the body can also significantly contribute to respiratory embarrassment. Injuries to the brain or spinal cord may impair normal reflexes and muscular function as well as interfere with the normal cough mechanism. Abdominal injuries also affect movement of the diaphragm. Shock and trauma to extrathoracic organ systems may seriously interfere with normal hemodynamics and result in secondary alterations within the lung itself [40].

MINOR TRAUMA—INJURY TO THE RIB CAGE

Even minor injury to the thoracic cage will cause some pain and subsequent depression of ventilatory function. The amount of interference with ventilation depends not only on the extent of the injury, but also on the age of the patient and the presence or absence of some degree of pulmonary disease. A simple contusion may cause muscle spasm as well as pain, resulting in immobilization of a segment of the thoracic cage. The underlying lung may also incur intrinsic pathological changes that compound the injury [37] (Fig 4-1). A young, robust individual with normal pulmonary function and a resilient chest wall can tolerate such a minor injury without any significant depression of ventilatory function and requires only mild

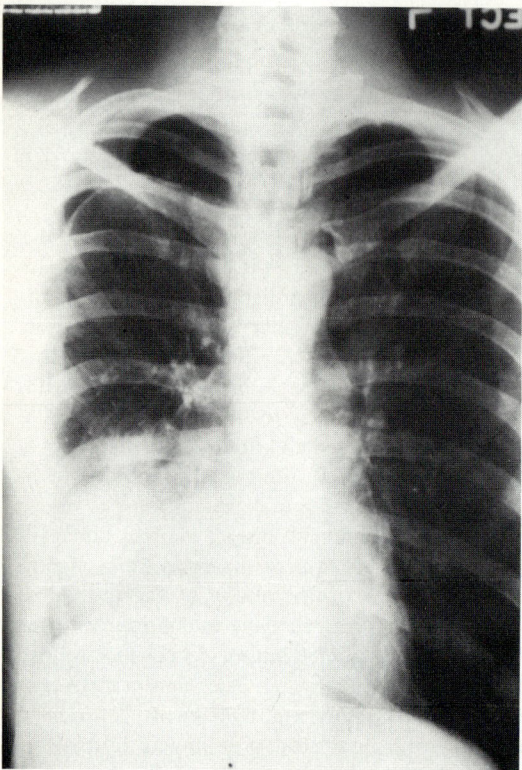

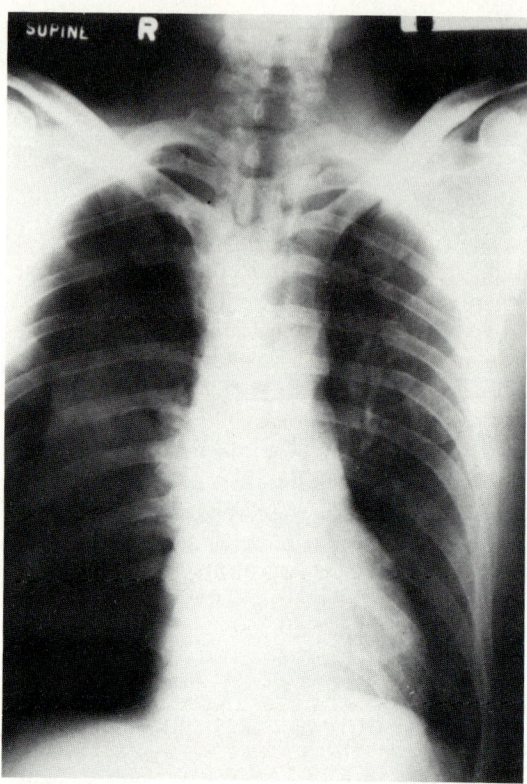

Fig 4-1. Pneumothorax and pulmonary contusion in a 60-year-old male after blunt chest wall injury.

Fig 4-2. Multiple rib fractures and a contralateral pneumothorax in a patient with preexisting pulmonary emphysema. Patient was treated by insertion of a chest tube on the right and multiple intercostal nerve blocks on the left. Recovery was satisfactory.

sedation for treatment. On the other hand, in an older individual with preexisting pulmonary emphysema or fibrosis and an inelastic chest wall suffering the same minor injury the consequences would be far more serious. Muscle spasm and fixation of that segment of the chest wall as well as pain result in an inability to ventilate the underlying lung adequately, with resultant atelectasis and subsequent pneumonia. In the presence of significant previous pulmonary disease, this impairment in ventilation may become lethal unless promptly recognized and treated.

Simple rib fracture is a common injury that can and should be diagnosed primarily by the clinical manifestations. The pain, tenderness, and muscle spasm associated with rib fracture may lead to the same inadequate ventilation as the contusion alone. In general, too many roentgenograms are ordered in emergency rooms to identify rib fractures. Approximately one-half of single rib fractures will be missed on initial roentgenograms. A chest film is

of value to rule out associated injuries such as hemothorax or pneumothorax (Fig 4-2), but initial treatment should not be predicated on the visualization of a fracture, but rather on the amount of pain and immobilization of the involved segment of the chest wall. If a film is desirable for medicolegal purposes, a roentgenogram taken 10 days later will suffice and generally clearly reveal the fracture site.

The danger of a simple rib fracture is not in the fracture itself, but rather the complications. Pneumothorax, hemothorax, widening of the mediastinum, or subcutaneous emphysema are signs of more serious and potentially lethal problems [34]. The jagged edge of a fractured rib can lacerate the lung, spleen, or liver [17]. The development of subcutaneous emphysema associated with a simple rib fracture may indicate more serious damage to the underlying lung or tracheobronchial tree. Rupture of a bronchus or the trachea may be suspected by a significant degree of pneumothorax or atelectasis. In the absence of a pneumothorax, a laceration of the lung with accompanying pleural symphysis may be the cause of the subcutaneous emphysema.

The initial objectives in the management of the acute rib fracture not accompanied by major damage to the intrathoracic structures are the relief of pain and promotion of adequate ventilation of the underlying lung. In the young, robust individual without a history of lung disease, mild sedation is generally sufficient. Although vigorous exercise should not be forced, ordinary activity may be allowed in order to encourage satisfactory ventilation. In older individuals, however, a simple fracture may become a significant threat if not adequately managed. Sedation should be given in appropriate amounts so that the pain is relieved and deep breathing and coughing can be carried out. Close observation is necessary to detect signs of impending atelectasis or respiratory embarrassment. Adhesive strapping or restrictive binding should not be used in the acute phase following the rib fracture. These tend to restrict motion of the chest and further the development of underaeration of the lung, atelectasis, and pneumonia.

A very effective anesthetic technique in the control of somatic thoracic pain following a chest wall injury is intercostal nerve block. With very limited experience, any physician can perform this procedure and produce immediate relief of the chest wall pain, thus allowing more adequate respiratory excursions of the involved segment and enabling the individual to cough and breathe deeply without significant discomfort. The procedure is performed with the patient sitting upright. The area of the injury is identified and 3 to 4 cc of a local anesthetic such as procaine or Xylocaine is injected into the intercostal nerves close to the rib's junction with the transverse process of the vertebral bodies. Injection should be made at the lower border of the rib in the region of the intercostal nerve (Fig 4-3). Care must be exercised not to inject the anesthetic into the intercostal vessels or to advance the needle too far and create a pneumothorax. The injection should be made into the intercostal nerves of the involved rib or ribs and, additionally, into one intercostal nerve above and below the site of injury. In those patients with severe pain or in whom coughing or ventilation is a problem, it may be necessary to repeat these injections at 6- or 8-hour intervals during the first few days following the injury. Recently it has been shown that intercostal nerve blocks performed with a mixture of Marcaine and low molecular weight dextran have resulted in pain relief for up to 48 hours.

An important dividend of this anesthetic technique is being able to differentiate between intra-abdominal injury and thoracic trauma alone. Particularly in those individuals with lower rib cage injuries, abdominal guarding and tenderness may ensue and the possibility of internal abdominal injuries must be entertained. The intercostal nerve block will frequently clarify the picture by alleviating the abdominal discomfort associated with an injury to the chest wall alone and produce an obvious "nonsurgical abdomen." In many instances an unnecessary laparotomy will be avoided as the clinical picture becomes clear.

COUGH

Following an injury to the rib cage, there is considerable pain and a natural reluctance or inability on the part of the patient to cough. The patency of the upper respiratory tract is essential for survival, and the accumulation of secretions in the trachea or main stem bronchi usually cleared by the normal cough mechanism can lead to serious interference with the respiratory system [44]. The use of adequate sedation or intercostal nerve block may relieve the pain sufficiently to allow the patient to cough at regular intervals. He should be instructed that one productive cough every hour is far more desirable than repeated ineffectual attempts that serve merely to tire him. The nursing staff may be very helpful in this respect by encouraging patients to cough and breathe deeply at regular intervals, particularly during the period following sedation or intercostal nerve block when they are relatively free from pain. Temporary local support of the injured area by the nurse's hands or a towel wrapped around the chest is often helpful in reducing the discomfort associated with a cough and a deep breath. In those individuals in whom the cough mechanism is not effective and who show evidence of retained secretions within the tracheobronchial tree, a more aggressive approach should be employed.

Nasotracheal suction (Haight maneuver [13])

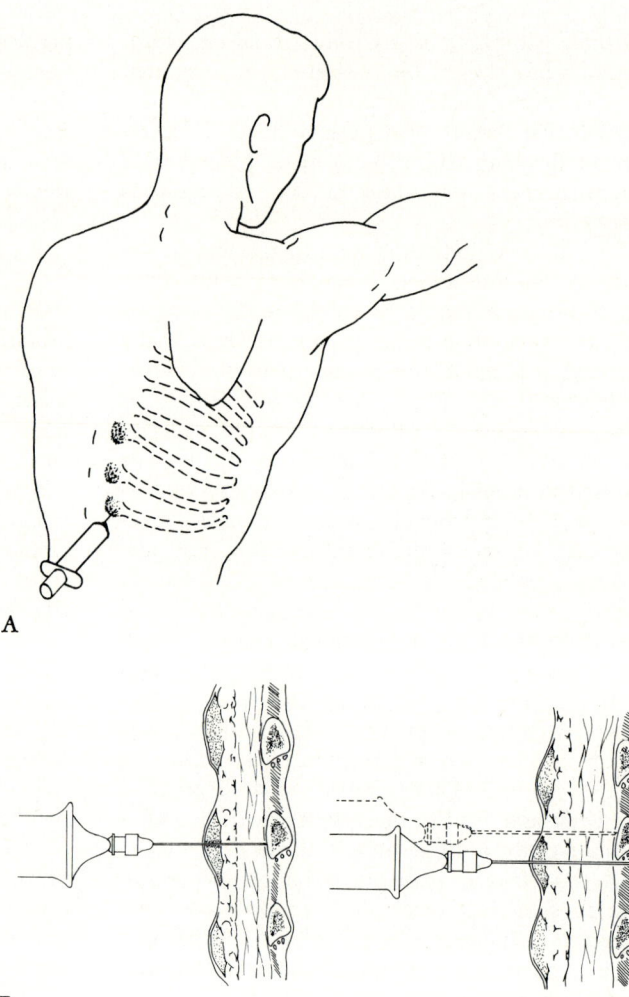

A

B

is extremely useful in producing a cough and suctioning the material within the trachea and main stem bronchi. This is performed preferably with the patient in a sitting position. The neck is hyperextended and the patient's tongue is grasped by a sponge and pulled forward. A rubber or soft plastic catheter is inserted through either nostril and passed down to the glottis (Fig 4-4). With practice the physician will learn to advance the catheter quickly into the trachea, which procedure immediately stimulates involuntary coughing. Suction may be applied for a few seconds to aspirate material from the trachea or main stem bronchi. This should be done with care since application of suction for longer than 4 or 5 seconds can seriously reduce the amount of oxygen within the tracheo-

Fig 4-3. Technique for intercostal nerve block. (A) Skin wheals are raised posteriorly at the inferior border of involved ribs. (B) A needle is advanced to the rib and then positioned immediately beneath the rib for injection of 3 to 5 cc local anesthetic. Care must be taken not to enter the pleural space or intercostal vessels.

bronchial tree. The maneuver may be repeated as necessary if secretions tend to accumulate. One of the major disadvantages of nasotracheal suction is its unpleasantness. To avoid repeated suctioning by this route, most patients will eventually cooperate and cough.

In the event that nasotracheal suction is not successful in clearing the tracheobronchial tree, or in

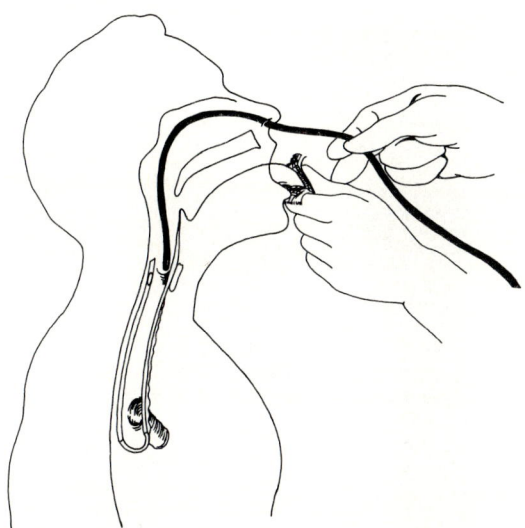

Fig 4-4. Haight technique for nasotracheal suction. When the rubber or soft plastic catheter advances into the trachea, involuntary coughing is stimulated. Suction can then be applied to aspirate secretions from the trachea or main stem bronchi.

the presence of obvious atelectasis, bronchoscopy should be carried out. This may be performed under topical anesthesia while the patient is in bed and is very effective for removal of viscid secretions from the main stem and segmental bronchi. Equipment for laryngoscopy and bronchoscopy should be available in every emergency room and intensive care unit.

With the advent of the fiberoptic bronchoscope, very complete evacuation of secretions has become possible, even from subsegmental bronchi. Endoscopy with this flexible instrument is relatively atraumatic for patient and doctor alike; it is used more frequently, which in turn may decrease the incidence of tracheostomy. Even with the fiberscope, however, the relative unpleasantness of the experience for the patient can be a major factor in encouraging him to cough in order to avoid repetition of the procedure.

In the event that the tracheobronchial tree cannot be cleared by the above maneuvers or when production of secretions continues to pose a problem in ventilation, a tracheostomy should be performed without hesitation [2, 4]. This simplifies suction of the tracheobronchial tree, reduces the resistance of the upper airway passages, and allows

repeated bronchoscopies, when necessary, through the tracheostomy stoma without undue stress to the patient. Suctioning through the tracheostomy should be performed with meticulous sterile technique since infection of the trachea and main stem bronchi is a significant hazard.

COSTOCHONDRAL SEPARATION

A blunt injury to the anterior chest wall may result in a separation of the anterior portion of the rib from its costal cartilage. This type of injury usually involves a single rib and cartilage, but on rare occasions multiple separations may occur with or without accompanying fractures. In the acute phase, the injury is similar to that of a fractured rib—with localized pain and tenderness. In contrast to simple rib fracture, however, the localized pain and tenderness may continue for some weeks because of the poor healing capacity of the cartilage at its junction with the rib. In addition, a "clicking" sensation may occur as a result of this injury and is particularly apparent on deep breathing or coughing. In the absence of other injuries to the bony thorax, there may be no significant change on the chest roentgenogram or films of the rib cage and sternum. The diagnosis is established on the basis of the clinical examination with localized pain, tenderness, and a sensation of crepitation when mild pressure is applied over the involved costochondral junction.

During the acute stage, the treatment consists primarily of the injection of local anesthetic in the region of the costochondral junction. In our experience of the chronic phase, a combination of local anesthetic and hydrocortisone acetate injected locally has afforded subjective relief. In some instances the pain and false motion or "clicking" at the costochondral junction may persist as a result of a nonhealing process. In such instances the discomfort is due primarily to the impingement of the cartilage on the anterior end of the rib, and simple resection of a centimeter or more of the cartilage will alleviate the problem.

FRACTURE OF THE CLAVICLE

One of the most common injuries from a blunt blow to the upper anterior chest is clavicular fracture. Because of its juxtaposition to the neurovascular structures supplying the upper limb, this fracture is rarely complicated by damage to the subclavian vessels or brachial plexus. Physical examination will determine neurovascular integrity in the ipsilateral upper extremity. The simple fractures are almost uniformly treated with conservative management, i.e., by the figure-eight shoulder dressings or belts. The professional sports' demands and pressures of the past decade have caused open reduction with intramedullary pins to be reintroduced as an adjunct to speedy recovery and improved stability. However, as Neer [26] has again demonstrated, nonunion is over forty times more prevalent with the open method (2 of 45 or 4.9 percent) as compared to the closed management (3 of 2235 or 0.1 percent). Thus, open reduction should be reserved for the rare complicated case with which the orthopedist, neurosurgeon, and vascular surgeon are more familiar.

FRACTURE OF THE STERNUM

Major blunt trauma to the anterior chest wall may cause a fracture of the sternum. With the frequency of steering wheel injuries, it is surprising that sternal fractures are not seen more often. They occur alone or in combination with multiple rib fractures. When sternal fracture occurs as an isolated lesion, the manubriogladiolar junction and first gladiolar segment are the most often involved. The injury is extremely painful and can usually be pinpointed by the conscious patient. The diagnosis should be made on physical examination and confirmed by lateral roentgenograms of the sternum (Fig 4-5). It should not be confused with the intrasternal cartilages in young persons where bony union has not yet taken place.

In evaluating patients with isolated sternal injuries, it is essential to rule out significant trauma to the underlying structures, especially cardiac injuries and tamponade. If no other significant injuries are present, the management of the fracture consists primarily of analgesics and observation for signs of respiratory embarrassment. In the aged and in patients with reduced pulmonary reserve or in the presence of obvious instability or underlying lung damage, treatment should consist of positive pressure ventilation by way of tracheostomy as in other flail chest injuries. If there is excessive motion of the fractured segments and stabilization is advisable, substernal struts or longi-

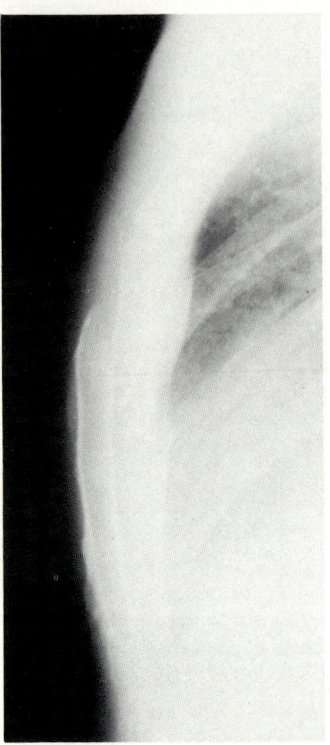

Fig 4-5. Lateral roentgenogram demonstrates sternal fracture.

tudinal intramedullary screws have been used for this purpose [6, 45].

MAJOR TRAUMA

Fracture of the First Rib

A fracture of the first rib is of special significance because of its anatomy. Structurally it is broad, flat, and relatively strong with a coronal rather than a vertical plane. Thus, it presents a stout edge to most of the traumatic forces applied to it. (Because it is formidably protected by the scapula, clavicle, humerus, and related soft tissues, any force capable of fracturing this rib must be of great magnitude and destructive impact. Invariably other bony structures in the immediate vicinity are also broken. When the examiner observes this fracture on roentgenogram, he should automatically search for other nearby osseous injuries. Also, when this fracture is fully appreciated, the traumatologist should anticipate other serious injuries to organs and soft tissues within and distal to the thorax.

The anatomical relationships of the first rib to adjacent structures make fractures of this rib unique and somewhat complicated. The subclavian vessels and brachial plexus lie immediately above it. These may be directly injured by the fracture or compressed between the clavicle and the first rib. Inferior to the rib are the pleura and lung. Injuries to these structures are common accompaniments of a first rib fracture.

Physiologically, the first rib acts as the main beam from which the other ribs are suspended by their respective intercostal muscles. Contraction of these muscles elevates each lower rib, whose gravity and function are therefore dependent upon an intact, stable first rib. The ends of these ribs are anchored, but the terminal joints can be considered mainly as hinges. When the auxiliary muscles of respiration are called into play, the strap muscles of the neck elevate the "main beam" further to enhance the expansion of the thorax.

The treatment of a fracture of the first rib entails the diagnosis and management of the complications discussed previously. Since neurological and vascular injuries are not uncommon, detailed neurological examination and arteriography may be necessary to delineate the location and extent of the trauma. Fractures of adjacent ribs frequently occur and may comprise a flail segment. When the upper ribs are involved, tracheostomy and positive pressure ventilation should be instituted without delay.

Flail Chest

One of the most common and potentially fatal injuries resulting from blunt chest trauma is the flail chest. This occurs when three or more ribs are fractured at two points, creating a "floating segment" of the chest wall. This segment loses its normal attachments to the remainder of the rib cage. It bulges outward with expiration when the rest of the thorax is moving inward and the intrapleural pressure rises; when the remainder of the rib cage is expanding on inspiration, this segment moves inwardly—the classic paradoxical motion that is the hallmark of the flail segment [22]. Obviously the more ribs broken, the greater the "flail" until with six or more ribs fractured there may be paradoxical motion of nearly the entire hemithorax, and to detect the paradox the examiner must compare the motion with the opposite,

intact chest wall. The mortality of patients with more than six ribs fractured is twice that of a flail segment involving six or less ribs. A flail segment involving the upper four ribs will be the most difficult to detect because of the very subtle paradoxical motion, which may be masked by the musculature of the chest wall. Yet injury to these ribs results in a far more dangerous situation than fractures of the lower ribs because of the greater dependence of respiration on the stability of the upper rib cage, especially the first rib [5, 15, 16].

A flail segment may be anterior, involving the rib cage on both sides of the sternum and in severe injuries may include a sternal fracture. However, the most common injury is lateral and most often involves the third to eighth ribs. The lateral thorax has the least amount of overlying soft tissue to cushion an injury and has neither the support of the pectoralis and rectus muscles of the anterior thorax nor of the trapezius and spinalis muscles of the posterior thorax. The tenth through the twelfth ribs are more elastic and a double fracture of these structures is uncommon even in the elderly individual.

The flail chest injury is usually the result of a significant amount of blunt trauma. Consequently, not only is there a derangement in the normal forces of the chest wall in ventilation, but almost invariably there is some degree of damage to the underlying structures. Lung contusion and its progressive interference with normal gas exchange is commonly associated with this type of injury. Damage to the heart and shearing or tearing of the great vessels is not uncommon and can be fatal. Rupture of the trachea or a bronchus and less commonly of the esophagus or diaphragm may occur in conjunction with this type of injury. Hence, the examiner who sees a patient with this type of injury should quickly search for and identify any possible injuries to the intrathoracic structures. Failure to recognize these major injuries can rapidly lead to castastrophic results.

PATHOPHYSIOLOGY. By its nature, the flail segment constitutes a number of physical factors adversely affecting ventilation.

1. The flail segment moves inward on inspiration and outward on expiration because of its lack of bony attachment to the remainder of the rib cage and the relative changes in intrathoracic pressure in relation to atmospheric pressure during the respiratory cycle (Fig 4-6).

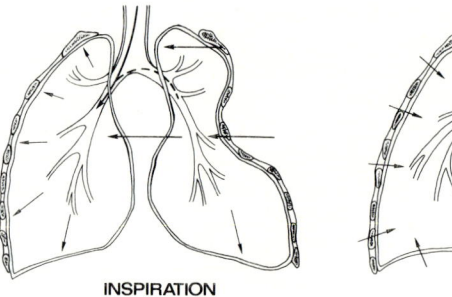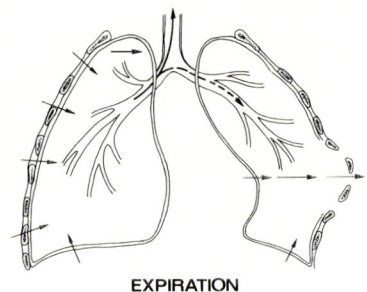

INSPIRATION   EXPIRATION

2. The inward pressure of the flail segment during inspiration compresses the ipsilateral lung and no decrease in intrathoracic pressure can take place on this side to promote lung expansion.
3. The mediastinum shifts toward the contralateral side on inspiration because of the greater negative pressure on that side and consequently restricts expansion of the "good" lung.
4. The flail segment bulges outward on expiration, thus impairing the thoracic force assisting this phase of the respiratory cycle.
5. The shift of the mediastinum may partially obstruct venous return to the heart.

Fig 4-6. Pathophysiology of paradoxical motion associated with a flail chest injury.

The consequences of these major alterations are a marked reduction of tidal volume and vital capacity, focal atelectasis, hypoxemia, pulmonary arteriovenous shunting, and diminution in cardiac output [37]. However, it is important to subsequent discussions to remember that the physiological alterations in these patients are related to changes in the pressure volume curve of the chest as well as possible underlying lung trauma. The patient with a large enough injury may lack the mechanical ability to produce adequate pulmonary ventilation. Some recent authors even question this as a significant factor in the respiratory distress. In any event, *pendelluft* or the pendulum-like movement of air from the involved lung to the other probably does not exist despite the widespread teaching and acceptance of such [22].

DIAGNOSIS. The diagnosis of a flail chest is initially based on clinical observation of the injured patient. Initial chest roentgenograms frequently will not demonstrate the double fractures. However, the fractures of three or more adjacent ribs should alert the physician to the possibility of additional fractures, which could in turn lead to the flail segment. Blair and Mills [3] report that 30 percent of flail segments were not recognized

in the first six hours of observation. Those involving the upper ribs require careful observation of the patient to detect the subtle paradoxical motion. Pain and muscle spasm may splint the segment temporarily until fatigue or analgesics intervene and the segments separate again.

Examination in good light in a tangential plane provides the observer with the maximum opportunity for detecting paradoxical motion. Tactile sensation is helpful in identifying fractures and false motion of a segment of the chest wall, especially under the anterior or posterior chest muscle groups. Subsequent roentgenograms may demonstrate the full extent of the fractures as well as trauma to the underlying lung, hemothorax, or pneumothorax (Fig 4-7). Nevertheless, the initial diagnosis of a flail chest is based upon careful, repetitive observations of the patient.

In addition to recognizing and defining the flail chest injury itself, additional studies may be necessary to rule out major associated injuries [5, 15, 29, 34]. Should there be any evidence of mediastinal widening or obliteration of a peripheral pulse, the possibility of a tear of the great vessels must be considered and immediate aortography should be performed [20, 21, 39, 41]. If physical signs suggest the possibility of cardiac tamponade, pericardiocentesis may be both diagnostic and therapeutic [7, 19, 24]. The presence of mediastinal air may give rise to a tentative diagnosis of tracheal or bronchial rupture or rupture of the esophagus [14, 23]. These can be confirmed by appropriate endoscopic studies or, in the case of the latter, a Gastrografin swallow. All of the above demand immediate diagnosis and definitive surgical intervention.

MANAGEMENT. The treatment of flail chest in-

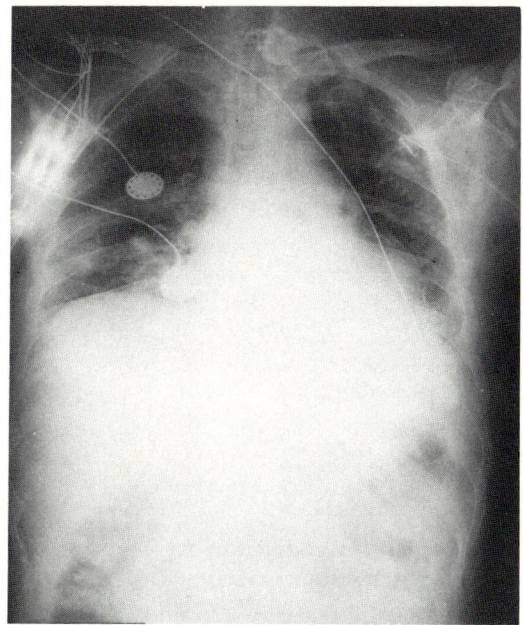

Fig 4-7. Roentgenogram following severe anterior chest wall injury with bilateral pneumothorax and pulmonary contusion. Management of the patient included bilateral chest tubes, tracheostomy, and CPPV with eventual recovery.

juries involves difficult clinical decisions. In general, the objective is stabilization of the involved segment of chest wall and maintenance of adequate ventilation of the underlying lung. Internal pneumatic stabilization with tracheal intubation and a volume-cycled ventilator has replaced external fixation. Despite this therapy, however, the mortality rate remains high and morbidity secondary to tracheostomy and long-term ventilatory support has been added to the picture. In recent years a more selective and objective method of management based on measurable variables has evolved.

There is some controversy over how or if the chest wall should be stabilized and over the indications for ventilatory support. In general, however, after a brief evaluation, establishment of a patent airway, and insertion of an intravenous line, temporary stabilization of the flail segment should be carried out to reduce excessive paradoxical movement during which time the ventilatory condition of the patient can be ascertained. Stabilization may be achieved with a pillow, sandbag, or noncircumferential taping. Care must be taken not

to restrict the contralateral side. The use of towel clips or wire sutures around the involved ribs attached to some form of traction (five pounds or more) [18] has been employed in the past but probably has no place except as a last resort in those patients whose deformity is massive and when a form of positive pressure ventilation is not available.

Several surgeons are currently using a variety of internal methods of fixation in order to decrease the duration of positive pressure ventilation and thereby negate the need for tracheostomy. With high-volume, low-pressure balloons used on oral or nasal endotracheal tubes, ventilation without tracheostomy may be carried out relatively safely for 5 to 7 days. Moore and Grillo [25] used intramedullary pin fixation in 50 *selected* patients and tracheostomy was required in only 8 patients. Hospital mortality was 22 percent. Paris and co-workers [27] recommend internal strut fixation and believe that this technique substantially reduces the need for positive pressure ventilation and tracheostomy.

Although there is wide availability of mechanical ventilators in the United States, occasionally the management of a patient with respiratory insufficiency and flail chest may, by necessity, be carried out without these devices. In these circumstances, a tracheostomy can be extremely beneficial, as pointed out by Carter and Guiseffi [4]. Tracheostomy reduces the anatomical dead space and thus increases the tidal volume available for gas exchange, reduces the degree of intrapleural pressure change needed to move a given volume of air, and hence decreases the amount of paradoxical movement. It must be noted, however, that with the currently available methods of respiratory care in intensive care units across the country, the need for tracheostomy has decreased.

Mechanical ventilators are the most widely used and accordingly may be the preferred method of management of flail chest injuries. The use of constant positive pressure ventilation (CPPV), with or without positive end-expiratory pressure (PEEP), should be instituted with either a nasotracheal or oral tracheal tube with a high-volume, low-pressure cuff. Using a minimal leak technique so that a small amount of air escapes around the cuff with each ventilatory cycle, these tubes may be left in place with relative safety for 5 to 7 days. If further CPPV is required, then a tracheostomy should be performed in a controlled situation with the endotracheal tube in place. In order to maintain adequate and uniform ventilation, a volume-controlled respirator should be used with a tidal volume of 10 to 15 cc per kilogram of body weight and a low-to-moderate flow rate (40 to 55 liters/min). Sankaran and Wilson [36] reported a 6.65 percent mortality rate in patients with flail chest injuries treated with this type of regimen compared to a mortality of 56.25 percent using tracheostomy and traction on the flail segment. This low mortality rate, however, must be compared with other reported series using similar methods in which death rates were 12 to 50 percent [8, 9, 12, 28, 31–33].

There is no unanimity of opinion regarding the optimum method of management of flail chest injuries, and this is appropriate since it seems reasonable that not all such injuries have to be treated in exactly the same manner. Obviously, positive pressure ventilation as a method of internal stabilization is effective, while operative stabilization with struts may play a significant role in certain cases. However, not all patients require either of these modalities. Trinkle and associates [43] have shown that if the underlying lung injury is aggressively treated, patients can do well in the presence of a significant flail without the need for intubation and mechanical ventilation. Shackford and associates [38] have demonstrated that there were a greater number of complications in those patients treated with mechanical ventilation than in those who were not ventilated. He believes that mechanical ventilation should be predicated on the extent of the pulmonary injury and the amount of ventilatory dysfunction rather than on the presence of the flail segment alone.

It is thus possible to individualize the management of flail chest injuries based upon readily available physiological data. The mere presence of a paradoxical segment of the chest wall should not be an indication for tracheostomy and CPPV. Obvious impairment to ventilation such as pain or hemopneumothorax should be corrected and the patient evaluated before a decision to initiate mechanical ventilation is made, since indiscriminate use of this treatment method may lead to increased morbidity and a longer hospital stay.

Although sound clinical judgment must always be exercised, the following guidelines are of considerable value in making the decision regarding initiation of mechanical ventilatory support:

	Normal Range	Indication for Intubation and Ventilation
Mechanics		
Respiratory rate	12–20	35
Vital capacity	65–75	15
Inspiratory force (cm H_2O)	75–100	20
Oxygenation		
PaO_2	75–100	70 on O_2
$P(A\text{-}a)O_2$ ($FiO_2 = 1.0$)	50–75	350
Ventilation		
$PaCO_2$	35–45	65 pH 7.25
V_D/V_T	0.3–0.4	0.6

Vital capacity and inspiratory force are indexes of a patient's respiratory reserve. This reserve is necessary for deep breathing, coughing, and overcoming airway obstruction. The measurements of these indexes will depend on the patient's state of consciousness, his cooperation, primary pulmonary process, and degree of fatigue. The $PaCO_2$ and alveolar-arterial O_2 difference $P(A\text{-}a)O_2$ must be interpreted with the physical and clinical judgment must be exercised. The patient's ability to perform the work necessary to ventilate is often the deciding factor in deciding whether or not to institute ventilatory support. This ability is closely related to V_D/V_T ratio and is interrelated with all other criteria. As a patient tires from the too great work of breathing, his tidal volume usually decreases, his respiratory rate increases, PaO_2 drops, and V_D/V_T and $PaCO_2$ increase.

Once the patient is on the ventilator, meticulous and aggressive pulmonary care must be exercised. Fluid balance (on the dehydrated side), blood volume, plasma oncotic pressure, and good nutrition must be maintained. Infection must be constantly checked for and aggressively treated. Regular tracheobronchial suction and, if necessary, bronchoscopy should be employed to prevent atelectasis. Drugs such as morphine and diazepam should be used judiciously to obviate pain and anxiety.

Mechanical respiratory support for 2 to 3 weeks may be necessary in patients with a significant flail and in some patients for as long as 6 weeks (Fig 4-8). Along with clinical judgment, however,

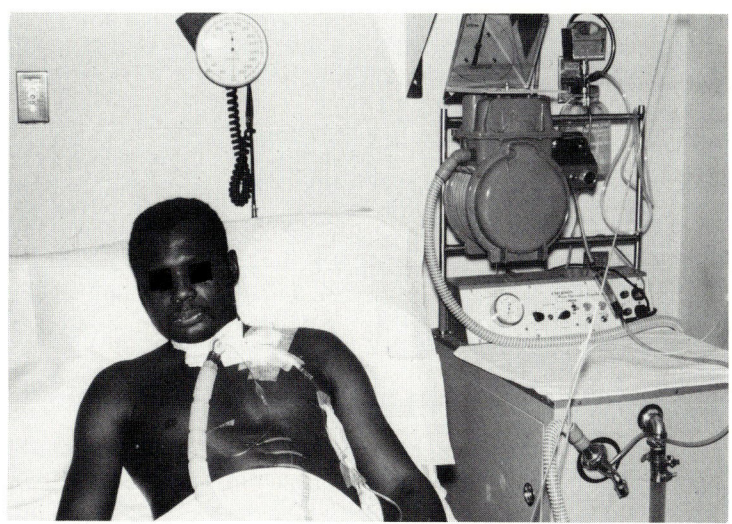

Fig 4-8. A 36-year-old male 5 days after severe blunt injury to left chest with multiple rib fractures and pneumothorax. Laparotomy was performed to remove lacerated spleen. Tracheostomy and CPPV were necessary for 3½ weeks.

weaning from the ventilator should depend more on objective criteria than on the mere presence of a flail segment. Respiratory physiological criteria for weaning would include the following:

Vital capacity	10–15 ml/kg
Inspiratory force	−20 cm H_2O
FEV_1	10 ml/kg
P (A-a)O_2 (FiO$_2$ = 1.0)	300–350 mm Hg
V_D/V_T	0.6

In addition to physiological improvement, there are a number of general factors that require at least consideration, if not correction, before weaning is initiated:

Anemia	Water balance
Cardiac output	State of consciousness
Arrhythmias	Pain
Fever	Renal function
Infection	Electrolyte abnormalities
Acid base balance	Nutrition
Sleep deprivation	Strength

In summary, flail chest injuries are complex problems usually associated with underlying parenchymal damage. Treatment should be based on objective evaluation of pathophysiology so that mortality due to the injury and morbidity of therapy is minimized.

Sucking and Avulsion Wounds of the Chest Wall

Armed with knowledge of pulmonary physiology, modern antibiotics, and good surgical debridement [10], some would contend that a "sucking" wound does not constitute major trauma. On the other hand, historically physicians have been fascinated with the chest wound in direct communication with the atmosphere and its characteristic sound. Ambroise Paré and other celebrated surgeons have remarked about the drama associated with this wound. Nevertheless, the immediate threat of inadequate ventilation and the eventual threat of empyema are serious enough to classify these wounds as major.

The most common cause of open, sucking wounds of the chest are close-range or high-velocity (over 1800 ft/sec) gunshot wounds [2]. Large tissue defects may also result from other unlikely incidents such as swipes of bear claws and slashes from a motor propeller.

The principles of management have been cited at the beginning of the section on major trauma. Because of the abundant collateral blood supply to the chest wall, a major tissue defect or laceration is always accompanied by considerable blood loss. Particularly troublesome when they are partially severed are the internal mammary, intercostal, and perforating arteries. The total volume lost may not be evident if the patient has been transported or has had a dressing change. Under these circumstances, recognition and anticipation of significant hemorrhage can prevent hypotension and its complications. Experience, if not instruction, readily recognizes the need for transfusion before and during debridement or reconstructive surgery.

Closure of the tissue defect to furnish negative intrathoracic pressure and promote lung expansion may be accomplished by almost any wet dressing. The uninitiated may place dry gauze over a defect only to discover that the air leak continues until petrolatum or another impervious dressing is added. If the hole is small, it can serve as the site for introduction of a thoracostomy tube. If the tissue gap is large, a flap of muscle, skin, or even rib and muscle together should be mobilized. After surgical debridement, an avulsion lesion may require split-thickness skin graft for eventual epithelial cover. The complications of pleural thickening with lung entrapment and overt empyema are treated in detail elsewhere.

REFERENCES

1. Ashbaugh DG, Peters GN, Halgrimson CG, et al: Chest trauma: analysis of 685 patients. Arch Surg 95:546, 1967
2. Berry FB (ed.): Surgery in World War II: Thoracic Surgery. Vols. 1 & 2. Washington D.C., Office of the Surgeon General, 1963 & 1965
3. Blair E, Mills E: Rationale of stabilization of the flail chest with intermittent positive pressure breathing. Am Surg 34:860, 1968
4. Carter GN, Giuseffi J: Tracheostomy: a useful operation in thoracic surgery with particular reference to its employment in crushing injuries of the thorax. J Thorac Surg 21:495, 1951
5. Conn JH, Hardy JD, Fain WR, et al: Thoracic trauma: analysis of 1072 cases. J Trauma 3:22, 1963
6. D'Abreau AL: Thoracic injuries. J Bone Joint Surg [Br] 46:581, 1964
7. DeMuth WE, Jr., Finsser HF, Jr.: Myocardial contusion. Arch Intern Med 115:434, 1965
8. Diethelm AG, Battle W: Management of flail chest injury: a review of 75 cases. Am Surg 37:667, 1971
9. Duff JH, Goldstein M, McLean APH, et al: Flail chest: a clinical review and physiological study. J Trauma 8:63, 1968
10. Edlich RF, Custer J, Madden J, et al: Studies in management of the contaminated wound. Am J Surg 118:21, 1969
11. Ferris BG, Jr., Whittenberger JL, Affeldt JE: Pulmonary function in poliomyelitic patients. N Engl J Med 246:919, 1952
12. Garzon AA, Gourin A, Seltzer B, et al: Severe blunt chest trauma. Ann Thorac Surg 2:629, 1966
13. Haight C: Intratracheal suction in the management of postoperative pulmonary complications. Am Surg 107:218, 1938
14. Hood RM, Sloan H: Injuries to the trachea and bronchi. J Thorac Cardiovasc Surg 38:458, 1959
15. Howell JF, Crawford ES, Jordan GF: The flail chest: analysis of 100 patients. Am J Surg 106:628, 1963
16. Hughes RK: Thoracic trauma. Ann Thorac surg 1:778, 1965
17. Johnson RS: Pulmonary laceration complicating closed chest injury. Br J Dis Chest 61:205, 1967
18. Jones TB, Richardson EP: Traction on the sternum in the treatment of multiple fractured ribs. Surg Gynecol Obstet 42:283, 1926
19. Kahn D: Myocardial contusion due to steering wheel injury. JAMA 200:255, 1967
20. Katz RI, Briggs JN: Traumatic ruptured bronchus and injury of major thoracic vessels. Ann Thorac Surg 3:325, 1967
21. Kirsh MM, Behrendt DM, Orringer MB, et al: Treatment of acute traumatic rupture of the aorta: a 10 year experience. Ann Surg 184:308, 1976
22. Maloney JV, Jr., Schmutzer KJ, Rajgke E: Paradoxical respiration and "pendelluft." J Thorac Cardiovasc Surg 41:291, 1961
23. Meade RH, Jr., Graham JB: Rupture of a primary bronchus from compression of the thorax without bone injury. Am Surg 92:154, 1930
24. Miller GE: Blunt thoracic trauma producing heart laceration. Am Surg 166:852, 1967
25. Moore B, Grillo H: Operative stabilization of nonpenetrating chest injuries. J Thorac Cardiovasc Surg 70:619, 1975
26. Neer CS, II: Nonunion of the clavicle. JAMA 172:1006, 1960
27. Paris F, Tarazona V, Tarazona F, et al: Surgical stabilization of traumatic flail chest. Thorax 30:521, 1975
28. Perry JF, McClellan RJ: Autopsy findings in 127 patients following fatal traffic accidents. Surg Gynecol Obstet 119:586, 1964
29. Perry JF, Galway CF: Factors influencing survival after flail chest injuries. Arch Surg 1:216, 1965
30. Rahn H: Respiration. Ann Rev Physiol 17:107, 1955
31. Ransdell HT: Treatment of flail chest injuries with a piston respirator. J Trauma 5:412, 1965
32. Rehlihan M, Litwin MS: Morbidity and mortality associated with flail chest injury: a review of 85 cases. J Trauma 13:663, 1973

33. Reid JM, Baird WLM: Crushed chest injury: some physiological disturbances and their correction. Br Med J 1:1105, 1965
34. Reynolds J, Davis JT: Injuries of the chest wall, pleura, pericardium, lungs, bronchi and esophagus. Radiol Clin North Am 4:383, 1966
35. Roberts JL: Experimental studies on thoracic and abdominal injuries, in The Prevention of Highway Injuries. Ann Arbor, Highway Safety Research Institute, 1967
36. Sankaran S, Wilson RF: Factors affecting prognosis in patients with flail chest. J Thorac Cardiovasc Surg 60:402, 1970
37. Schramel RJ, Tyler J, Kirkpatrick JL, et al: Studies of respiratory function after thoracic injuries. J Trauma 3:206, 1963
38. Shackford S, Smith D, et al: The management of flail chest—a comparison of ventilatory and nonventilatory treatment. Am J Surg 132:759, 1976
39. Shamblin JR, McGoon DC: Acute thoracic compression with traumatic asphyxia. Arch Surg 87:967, 1963
40. Stapp JP: Human tolerance to deceleration. Am J Surg 93:734, 1957
41. Stapp JP: Biomechanics of injury, in The Prevention of Highway Injuries. Ann Arbor, Highway Safety Research Institute, 1967
42. Starling EH, Evans L: Principles of human physiology. Chapter 19. Edited by H Davson and MG Eggleton. Philadelphia, Lea & Febiger, 1968
43. Trinkle J, Richardson J, et al: Management of flail chest without mechanical ventilation. Ann Thorac Surg 19:355, 1975
44. Whittenberger JL, Mead J: Respiratory dynamics during cough. Trans Nat Tuberc Assoc 48:414, 1952
45. Zuhdi N, Bynum E, Carey J, et al: Intramedullary fixation of sternum and corrective procedures for funnel chest. J Thorac Cardiovasc Surg 50:83, 1965

5. INJURIES TO THE PULMONARY PARENCHYMA AND VASCULATURE

Robert E. Carr

BASIC PRINCIPLES OF MANAGEMENT

The basic principles of thoracic trauma management in civilians evolved from the experience gained in treating combat casualties in World War II. The changes in the past 30 years include more frequent use of endotracheal intubation, tracheostomy, improved ventilatory assistance, better control of blood volume, greater use of antibiotics, use of blood gas studies to aid in monitoring the effectiveness of the treatment, and specialized nursing in intensive care units. The improvement in survival is therefore not due primarily to operative measures but rather to improved supportive measures.

The immediate objective in the management of injuries to the lung is restoration of cardiorespiratory function to as near normal as possible. With adequate treatment of shock, airway obstruction, hypoventilation, and hemopneumothorax, early deaths can be considerably reduced and mortality and morbidity from late complications minimized. Injury to the lung requires less surgical attention than the associated injuries. Bleeding from the pulmonary parenchyma usually ceases spontaneously with reexpansion of the lung, due to the low pressure in the pulmonary artery system (30/10 mm Hg). Operation, when necessary, is usually not for pulmonary injury but for continuous hemorrhage from systemic vessels.

PENETRATING WOUNDS

The classification of open chest wounds as penetrating or perforating is of some value in estimating the course of the wound tract but does not necessarily indicate the gravity of the injury. A wound of either variety in the hilar area or medial one-third of the lung may be fatal, but a peripheral wound caused by a similar weapon may produce minimal damage. The problems of management are similar.

The weapons or objects responsible for most penetrating wounds in civilians are knives, small-caliber bullets, ice picks and other sharp objects, shotguns, and miscellaneous flying objects. Stab wounds accounted for more than two-thirds of the injuries in several large series reported [4, 14, 18, 34]. Ice pick injuries have decreased in recent years but the extent of injury is deceiving as the wound may appear insignificant. The most lethal stab wounds are usually inflicted by a butcher's knife. The affluent society has produced a higher incidence of gunshot wounds; these were responsible for approximately two-thirds of the penetrating injuries seen in private practice by the author over the past 20 years. Due to a gunshot's depth of penetration, the mortality in patients with gunshot wounds is considerably higher than in those with stab wounds. Most civilian wounds are caused by low-velocity weapons, but hunting rifles produce serious damage to the lung and chest wall.

Initial Evaluation

In penetrating wounds the presenting symptoms are usually pain, dyspnea, cough, hemoptysis, and shock. A description of the wounding object and the position of the victim and assailant at the time of the attack aid in estimating the extent of damage to the lung and other viscera. Missiles may ricochet but the majority travel in a straight line, and even those from small arms are usually not deflected by ribs.

Trauma victims can have multiple problems, and complete examination on admission is desirable. Directing attention to the chest wound and overlooking more serious injuries to other areas may be disastrous. The wounds of entry and exit (if present) should be located, and the presence of multiple wounds should be determined. In severe injury with profound disturbance of cardiorespiratory function, the initial evaluation should be brief, priorities established, and therapy begun immediately. Shock and acute respiratory insufficiency are responsible for most early deaths.

Chest roentgenograms are necessary to ascertain the possible extent of the lung injury. Films taken with the patient erect or semierect should be obtained initially. In perforating injury of the chest the course of the missile through the lung can usually be determined by reconstructing the line between the entry and exit wounds. Occasionally frontal and lateral roentgenograms showing lead markers over the wounds of entry and exit are helpful. The path of the penetrating wound can be estimated only by location of the wound in relation to the missile, which requires frontal and lateral roentgenograms. Although initial roentgenograms may not reveal pneumothorax or hemothorax, one or both may develop within 24 hours or less. After thoracocentesis or tube thoracostomy, repeat films are necessary to be sure the pleural cavity has been properly evacuated. Frequent examinations are required as part of the total assessment of patients with continued blood loss or massive air leaks and those showing poor response to therapy. All hospitalized patients with proved or suspected pulmonary injury should have films done before discharge.

Emergency Treatment

The initial treatment should be directed toward resuscitation. Restoration of normal cardiorespiratory function as quickly as possible by establishing an airway and treating shock receive priority. Gray and associates [18] reported a 10 percent mortality when shock was present, as compared to 1.3 percent in its absence. Contributing causes of shock such as airway obstruction, tension pneumothorax, hemothorax, and sucking wound of the chest, must be treated simultaneously. Management of shock is discussed in Chapters 2 and 18.

AIRWAY AND VENTILATION. The type of ventilatory assistance required immediately is dictated by the severity of respiratory impairment. Oxygen should be administered to all patients with chest injury until an experienced attending physician deems it unnecessary. If dyspnea and cyanosis are not relieved by nasal oxygen or intermittent positive pressure breathing (IPPB), immediate endotracheal intubation is indicated. An endotracheal tube may be used for several days with relatively few laryngeal and tracheal complications, and emergency tracheostomy is seldom indicated.

DECOMPRESSION OF PLEURAL SPACE. Evacuation of air and blood from the pleural space is the procedure most frequently required in the management of lung and other chest injuries. Thoracocentesis may be lifesaving in tension pneumothorax or massive hemothorax. Tube thoracostomy can be accomplished rapidly under local anesthesia and is often the only definitive procedure required for pulmonary injuries. Subcutaneous emphysema is usually indicative of pulmonary parenchymal or bronchial injury. The presence of pneumothorax, hemothorax, or extensive subcutaneous emphysema is an indication for tube thoracostomy prior to a general anesthetic and operative intervention for associated extrathoracic injuries.

Definitive Therapy

The definitive treatment of most penetrating injuries of the lung is usually a continuation of the emergency measures and prevention of pulmonary and pleural complications. A booster dose of tetanus toxoid should be given. Broad spectrum antibiotics should be used and the need for specific antibiotics determined by cultures. Grover and colleagues [19] in a prospective double blind randomized study found that those receiving prophylactic antibiotics had a lower incidence of pneumonia, fever, empyema; required fewer operations; and had a shorter hospital stay. Corticosteroids may be beneficial for those in shock with a slow response to therapy.

MANAGEMENT OF TRACHEOBRONCHIAL SECRETIONS. Tracheobronchial secretions are greatly increased after trauma. Removal of secretions is difficult because of their increased viscosity and an impaired cough mechanism. Failure to maintain a clear airway ultimately leads to hypoxemia, atelectasis, and pneumonitis. Intratracheal suction is of great value in maintaining patent airways, which is necessary for proper respiratory function. Bronchoscopic tracheobronchial aspiration may be indicated for massive atelectasis. Narcotics or other depressant drugs should be kept to a minimum. Experience with Levo-Dromoran has convinced me that it has many advantages over the opiates. It provides adequate pain relief and produces minimal respiratory depression and less suppression of the cough reflex than does a comparable dosage of other narcotics, and it is not addictive.

Adequate hydration and the use of expectorants reduce the viscosity of secretions. The relief of bronchospasm by aminophylline is well known. I have been impressed with the increased productivity of cough and rapid clearing of atelectasis in many patients after they have been given intravenous aminophylline and sodium iodide.

COUGHING. Effective coughing depends on the cooperation of the patient, encouragement by nursing personnel, hand support of the chest wall, and relief of pain. Frequent changes of position and coughing while turned on each side and while upright aid in the removal of secretions from the lower airways.

INHALATION THERAPY. Since the introduction of intermittent positive pressure breathing in the treatment of chest trauma by Brewer and associates [6, 7] in 1944, specialized equipment and trained inhalation therapists have improved the results of this therapy. Adequate humidification of inspired gases is essential.

TRACHEOSTOMY. After the patient's condition has stabilized, tracheostomy is indicated when: (1) long-term assisted ventilation will be required; (2) the endotracheal tube is not well tolerated; (3) difficulty is encountered in the removal of secretions through the endotracheal tube; and (4) other methods of removal of secretions are not satisfactory. More details of tracheostomy are found in Chapter 3.

Hemothorax and Pneumothorax

Hemothorax, pneumothorax, or a combination of the two occur in most penetrating injuries of the lung. Hemothorax is usually an indication of a more serious injury to the lung than is an uncomplicated pneumothorax. Complete evacuation of the pleural space and reexpansion of the lung are now generally accepted as the best means of controlling bleeding and air leaks and the prevention of pleural complications. This is best accomplished by tube thoracostomy decompression, preferably using a No. 28 to 30F catheter.

ENZYMATIC DEBRIDEMENT. I have found Varidase (streptokinase and streptodornase combined) extremely valuable in preventing the organization of hemothorax or fibrothorax. Thoracotomy has not been required, either for evacuation of clots or pleural decortication, when patients were initially treated with tube thoracostomy and the instillation of a solution of Varidase into the pleural cavity when indicated.

Enzymes should be injected only through chest tubes so that immediate and complete release of the fluid, when indicated, can be accomplished by simply unclamping the tubes. Enzymes are effective when they remain in the pleural space for 4 hours, but do not allow Varidase to remain longer than 6 hours. It has been found safe to use

24 hours after injury, or as soon as massive air leaks have diminished.

Thoracotomy

Usually less than 10 percent of penetrating injuries in civilian practice require thoracotomy. With nonoperative management of most cases, a low mortality of 2 percent was reported by Garzon, Amer, and Karlson [17], 3.1 percent by Conn and associates [13], and 3.8 percent by Gray and co-workers [18]. In my experience thoracotomy has rarely been required for wounds of the lung parenchyma and their complications. Immediate thoracotomy *is* indicated for: (1) failure of blood pressure to rise after adequate ventilation and blood replacement; (2) rapid loss of 1500 cc of blood after initial removal of that amount by thoracocentesis or tube thoracostomy; (3) continued bleeding at an undiminished rate of 500 cc or more per hour for 3 hours; (4) blood loss at the rate of 1500 cc per 24 hours after tube thoracostomy and evacuation of the pleural cavity; (5) increased bleeding after removal of large objects upon which the patient had been impaled; (6) wounds in the sternal or parasternal area with possible injury to the hilar vessels; (7) large thoracotomy wounds with deep lacerations of the lung; (8) uncontrollable massive air leaks; (9) close-range shotgun wounds; (10) broken knife blades or other sharp objects in the pleural cavity or pulmonary parenchyma; and (11) when the supply in the blood bank is not enough to allow for observation to determine if bleeding will cease spontaneously.

If the hilar area is not involved, early exploration is seldom required except for close-range shotgun blasts and large thoracotomy wounds. A wound in the parasternal area should alert one to the possibility of injury to hilar vessels. If hemorrhage continues after tube thoracostomy and rapid reexpansion of the lung, immediate exploration of the wound is necessary, and if a lacerated internal mammary artery or intercostal vessel is not found, more extensive thoracotomy and exposure of the hilar vessels is mandatory. The incidence of hilar vessel injury reported has usually been less than 1 percent except for the reports of Rothman and co-workers [32] and Haller and associates [20]. Pulmonary resection for badly damaged vessels may be required (Fig 5-1A, B).

Extrapericardial laceration of the hilar vessels will result in rapid death if bleeding is not con-

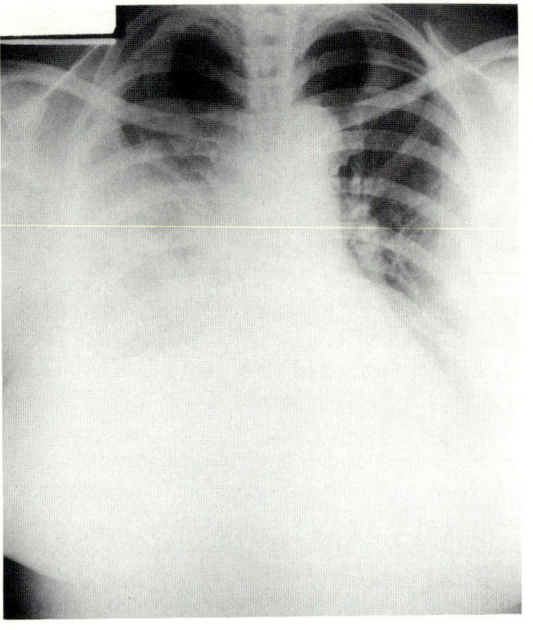

A

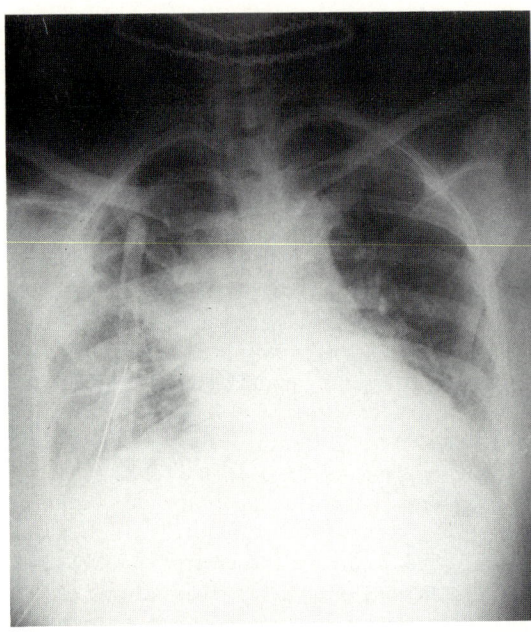

B

Fig 5-1. (A) Admission chest film of a 51-year-old obese black female in profound shock with nine stab wounds and three open sucking thoracotomy wounds on the right. Film shows hemorrhage into lung. Hemothorax is minimal due to partial obliteration of the pleural space from a previous thoracotomy. Immediate exploration through a long anterior traumatic thoracotomy wound revealed massive hemorrhage from the hilar area. Because old adhesions were present, intrapericardial occlusion of vessels was necessary to rapidly control bleeding. A laceration of the pulmonary artery was repaired and 3500 cc of whole blood was necessary. (B) Portable chest film 2 days later. Recovery was uneventful.

trolled by ligation or repair. If the hilar vessels are injured close to the pericardium or hematoma prevents the use of an occluding clamp, a long incision in the pericardium anterior to the phrenic nerves has provided access to the pulmonary vessels. This procedure has enabled immediate control of hemorrhage with occluding clamps or tapes in 4 patients in my experience. The lung has a remarkable recuperative ability and even severe damage heals rapidly if major vessels are successfully repaired. If ligation of a major pulmonary vessel is required, appropriate pulmonary resection is indicated as pulmonary infarction may occur.

Embedded objects, except in the parasternal area, can usually be removed safely and the wound treated as other penetrating wounds. Thoracotomy is indicated for broken knife blades or other sharp objects in the lung or pleural cavity and if massive hemorrhage ensues after the removal of embedded objects. Long, deep lacerations of the lung require ligation of major bleeding points and repair of the defect with continuous catgut suture. Small penetrating wounds do not usually require repair.

Close-range shotgun blasts can produce horrendous destruction of the chest wall and lung. Extension of the wound usually provides adequate exposure for exploration of the lung and the other thoracic structures. Following removal of clothing, cotton wadding, rib fragments, and other material, debridement of the lung and control of hemorrhage are mandatory, but one should not attempt to remove all palpable metallic foreign bodies from the lung parenchyma. What may appear at the outset to be irreparably damaged lung usually shows rapid clearing and returns to reasonably good function, if adequate pleural drainage and careful reconstruction of the chest wall have been accomplished (Fig 5-2A–C).

DELAYED THORACOTOMY. Clotted hemothorax has frequently been reported as an indication for delayed thoracotomy for evacuation of blood clots. This problem would be expected to occur more

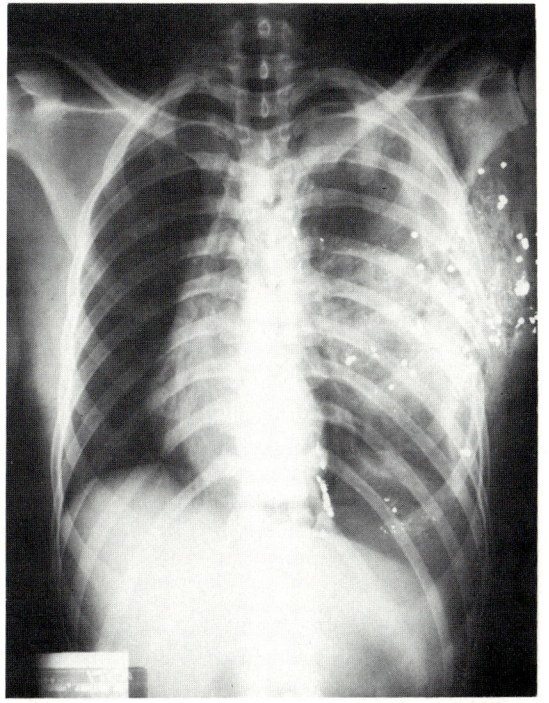

A

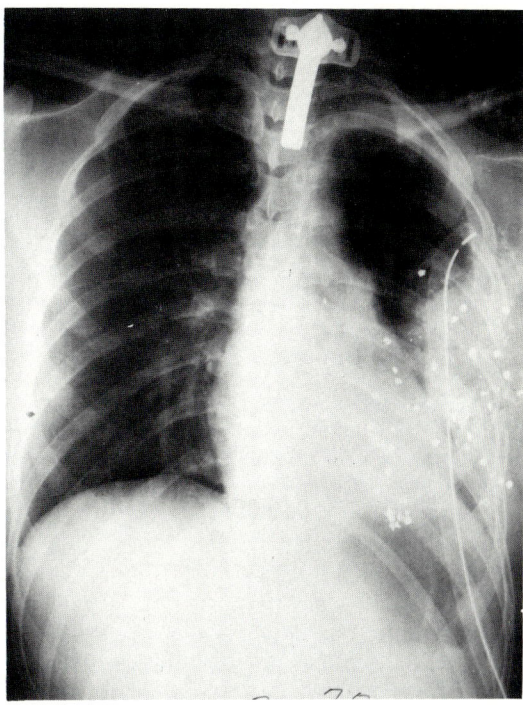

B

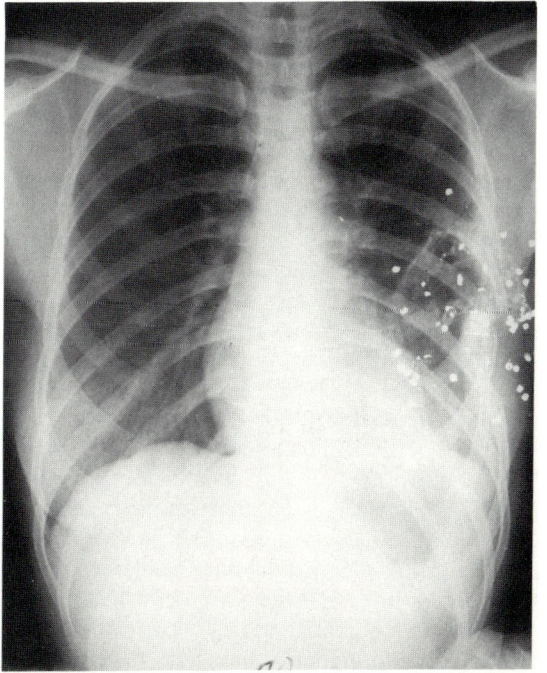

C

Fig 5-2. (A) Admission anteroposterior chest film of a 22-year-old white female who suffered a tangential wound of the left chest from a shotgun fired at close range. Film shows extensive injury to the left chest wall and lung with tension pneumothorax and displacement of the heart and mediastinum to the right. Debridement and closure of wound, tube thoracostomy (two tubes), and tracheostomy were carried out shortly after admission. (B) Anteroposterior chest film taken 4 days postinjury and after removal of one chest tube shows expansion of the lung but pulmonary hematoma is now evident. (C) Posteroanterior chest film taken more than 2 months after injury demonstrates clearing of the pulmonary hematoma. Multiple metallic fragments still remain in the lung and chest wall, but the patient was asymptomatic.

frequently in combat casualties if they are evacuated late, but in civilian injuries this complication can be virtually eliminated when adequate size chest tubes are properly placed, the patency of the tubes is maintained, and early enzymatic debridement is used when indicated.

Occasionally, late thoracotomy may be required for recurrent infections associated with foreign bodies; infected, persistent cavities; fibrothorax; or empyema. Traumatic lung cavities may be obscured initially by hemorrhage and atelectasis in the surrounding lung tissue. Cavity closure and absorption of hematoma may require weeks but are complete in most cases. Resection of asymptomatic uncomplicated cavities is not indicated even if closure appears slow. Arom and Lyons [1] reported a case of traumatic pulmonary arteriovenous fistula due to a stab wound.

RECOVERY OF PULMONARY FUNCTION. Clinical observations indicate excellent recovery of pulmonary function in 4 to 8 weeks after most penetrating injuries. Any prolonged disability has usually been due to associated injuries. Ventilatory function studies by Jolly and Thomas [25] in patients with penetrating or perforating wounds revealed a trend toward improvement in vital capacity through the third month, but a combination of severe chest wall and lung injury resulted in delayed recovery of ventilatory ability. The ultimate decrease in pulmonary function is usually related to pleural complications, e.g., fibrothorax or empyema, rather than the pulmonary injury itself.

BLUNT TRAUMA (NONPENETRATING)

Vehicular accidents are responsible for more serious blunt thoracic trauma than all other causes combined. The work of Zuckerman [43] in 1940 demonstrated that blast injuries to the lung resulted from high pressure waves transmitted through the chest wall to the underlying lung. Most civilian blast injuries are due to industrial accidents or gas explosions in the home. The damaging force of the blast wave dissipates rapidly in the atmosphere and rarely is the injury fatal if the person was more than 30 feet from the explosion.

Blunt trauma to the thorax frequently produces diffuse chest wall and pulmonary injuries that are usually more severe than a single penetrating wound. Management is usually more difficult, and

morbidity and mortality are higher. Severe damage to both lungs is not uncommon. Many victims are older and have preexisting cardiovascular or chronic bronchopulmonary disease, which may result in a more complicated course and require more involved therapy.

Initial Evaluation and Emergency Treatment

The clinical picture shortly after blunt thoracic trauma is often deceiving since the initial examination and roentgenograms may not reveal any evidence of pulmonary damage, rib fractures, or flail chest. The less severely injured may complain only of slight chest pain or minimal dyspnea. The extent of injury and possible complications cannot be predicted immediately, since pulmonary contusion and hemopneumothorax may not become apparent for several hours. In a crowded emergency room in the middle of the night, a serious error in judgment may be made with those with no apparent external injury. Patients with suspected pulmonary trauma should be kept in the hospital for 24 hours or more for observation and have another chest roentgenogram prior to discharge.

There is little doubt about the critical nature of the injury when dyspnea, cyanosis, and hypotension are present. Flail chest with paradoxical motion and subcutaneous emphysema are easily detected. Tension pneumothorax or massive hemothorax can usually be determined by auscultation. Resuscitative therapy as outlined under penetrating injuries must be instituted immediately. Most of the early deaths are due to shock and respiratory insufficiency. Initial and serial blood gas measurements are performed as indicated.

Shock is a grave prognostic sign in blunt chest trauma. When shock was present on admission, a mortality of 51 percent was reported by Harrison and colleagues [22] and 50 percent by Basset, Gibson, and Wilson [3]. Immediate endotracheal intubation with ventilatory assistance is indicated. Whole blood transfusions should be given for blood loss. For details of autotransfusion refer to Chapter 2. Initial roentgenograms are desirable, but tube thoracostomy should not be delayed when there is evidence of tension pneumothorax or massive hemothorax. Serial hematocrits, intravascular pressure monitoring, and continuous urine output measurements are aids in estimating adequate blood and fluid replacement. Follow-up roentgenograms after pleural drainage are advisable to determine the position of the tube and whether evacuation of the pleural space was adequate.

Pulmonary Contusion

Pulmonary contusion has long been known to be a complication of chest trauma. In 1909 Payne [30] described contusion of the lung without evidence of external injury. Westernak [40] in 1941 and Williams and Bonte [41] in 1961 reported pulmonary contusion to be the most common roentgenographic finding in nonpenetrating chest trauma, with occurrence in almost three-fourths of those examined; rib fractures, on the other hand, only occurred in approximately one-half of the cases.

Severe contusions are associated with considerable mortality [33, 38]. Roentgenographic evidence of contusions, frequently absent immediately after injury, usually becomes apparent within 6 hours and may show progression for 24 hours or more. A single, ill-defined parenchymal density may be seen, but, more often, multiple areas are present that may later coalesce. Irregular peribronchial infiltration occurs but is usually associated with patchy infiltrations.

Infiltrations that occasionally show clearing within 24 hours are usually due to blood or secretions in the bronchial tree and associated atelectasis and clear after adequate ventilation and removal of secretions. Resolution of contusions usually begins in 2 to 3 days unless complicated by pneumonia or atelectasis. Complete clearing has been reported to occur within 8 days, although large hematomas and cavities may require several weeks (Figs 5-3A–D).

Pulmonary Lacerations

Kemmerer and co-workers [26] found pulmonary lacerations in more than 10 percent of traffic deaths (60 of 585) and over 50 percent of these (34 of 60) died before arrival at a hospital. The classic roentgenographic features in cases described by Moghissi [29] were: (1) shallow apical pneumothorax; (2) hemothorax of not more than 500 to 700 cc; and (3) fairly well defined opacity in the lung substance with upward convexity. Hankins and associates [21] reported 13 cases of lacerations of the lung in 210 blunt trauma victims. Penetration of the lung by rib fractures occurred in 10 cases and in 3 there was a shearing-type pulmonary laceration (Fig 5-4).

Definitive Treatment

Even after successful resuscitation, the mortality in victims of blunt trauma is high. In most pulmonary injuries the treatment is nonoperative and is essentially a continuation of the resuscitative measures already instituted. Attention must be directed to ventilation, removal of tracheobronchial secretions, management of pulmonary and pleural complications, and prevention of sepsis. Thoracotomy is rarely required except for continuing hemorrhage or massive air leaks.

Since the damaged lung is susceptible to infection, broad spectrum antibiotics should be given to most patients. Cultures of tracheobronchial washings at least every 3 days should be routine. Specific antibiotics should be given as indicated by culture and sensitivity studies.

The beneficial effects of corticosteroids in trauma patients with preexisting chronic bronchopulmonary disease has been mentioned by Daughtry [15]. Steroids should not be used routinely, and the dosage should be rapidly reduced or discontinued as soon as improvement occurs because of the increased risk of gastrointestinal hemorrhage. Antacid therapy is indicated for all patients receiving steroids and positive pressure ventilation for more than 2 or 3 days, or who have a history of ulcer or previous gastrointestinal bleeding.

VENTILATORY ASSISTANCE. Impaired ventilation, the most frequent problem encountered in blunt thoracic trauma, should be anticipated even though it may not be apparent immediately following injury. Severe pulmonary contusions with intra-alveolar hemorrhage and edema affect not only the tidal volume but also diffusion and perfusion, often resulting in respiratory insufficiency with hypoxemia, hypercapnia, and acidosis. Complications of atelectasis, pneumonitis, and secondary infections greatly intensify the problem and further delay recovery (Fig 5-5A–C).

Hopkinson and associates [23] demonstrated in experimental closed chest trauma that atelectasis was the most frequent finding at postmortem examination. Marked disturbance in ventilation is obvious, but a lesser degree of hypoventilation may not be recognized and it may progress insidiously to respiratory insufficiency. Shallow breathing at an increased rate results in alveolar hypoventilation. Tidal volume can be determined at the bedside with a variety of ventilation meters; such

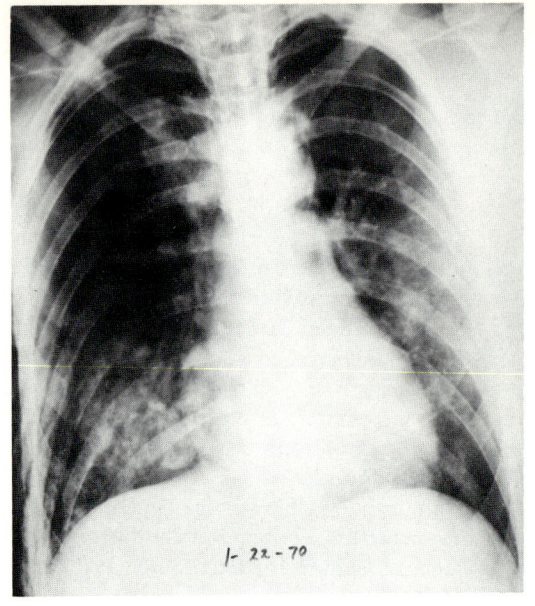

A

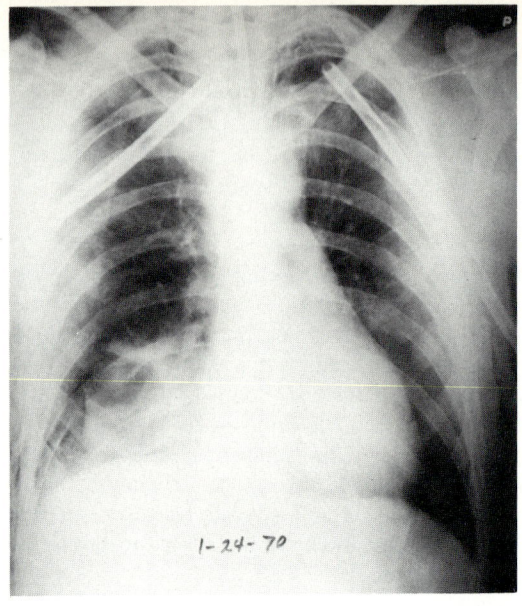

B

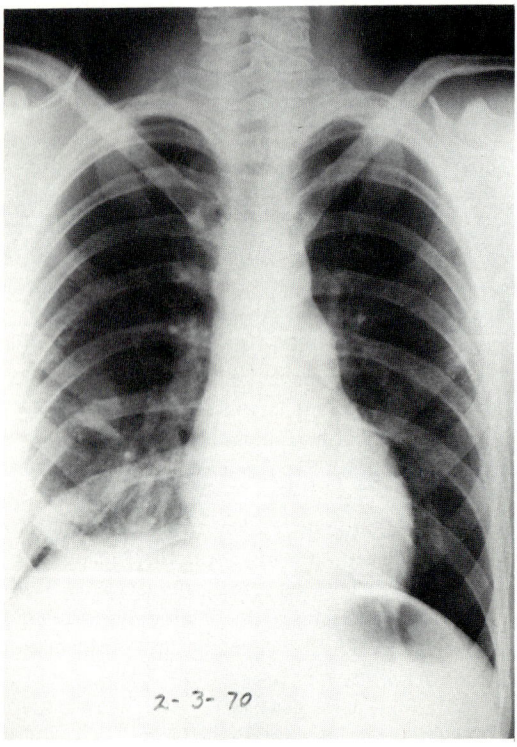

C

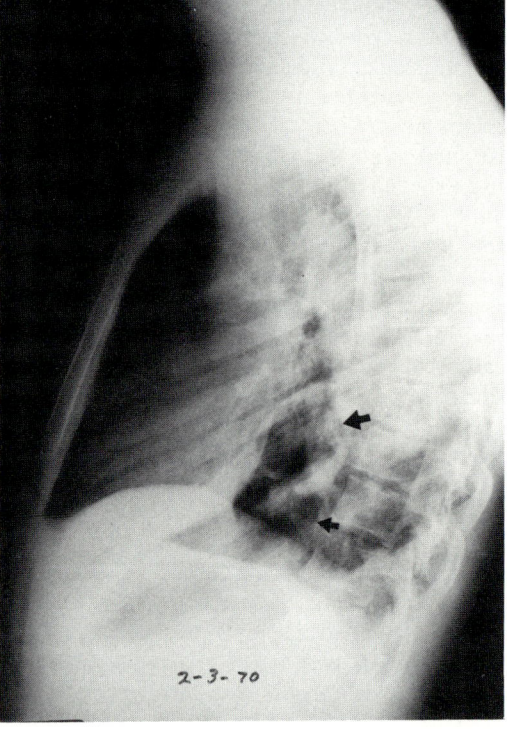

D

Fig 5-3. (A) Admission anteroposterior film of a 19-year-old white male injured in a motorcycle accident. Film shows subcutaneous emphysema on the right and bilateral pulmonary infiltrations that were interpreted as contusions. When the patient was seen 4 hours later, bilateral pneumothorax was present (B) Upright chest film taken 2 days later reveals traumatic cavity and pulmonary contusion in right lower lobe. The infiltrations in the left lung on the admission film were probably due to blood and secretion in the bronchial tree rather than hematoma since clearing occurred in 2 days. (C) Posteroanterior and (D) lateral chest films taken prior to discharge and 12 days after injury show two thin-walled cavities persisting in the right lower lobe. Subsequent films showed complete clearing within two months.

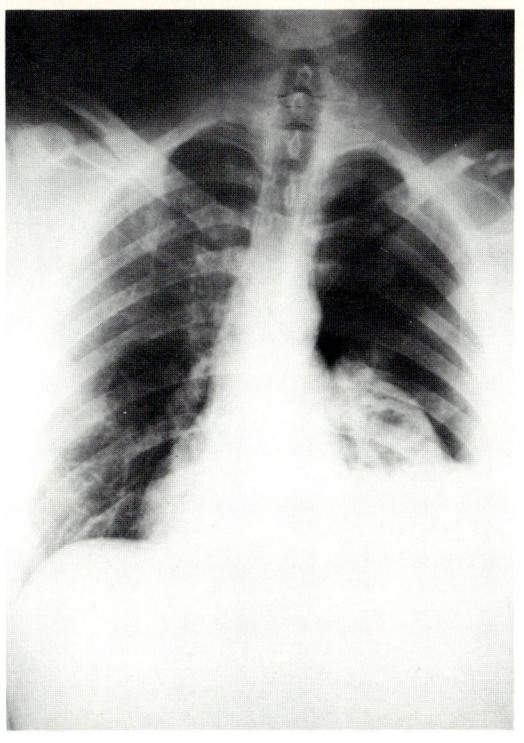

A

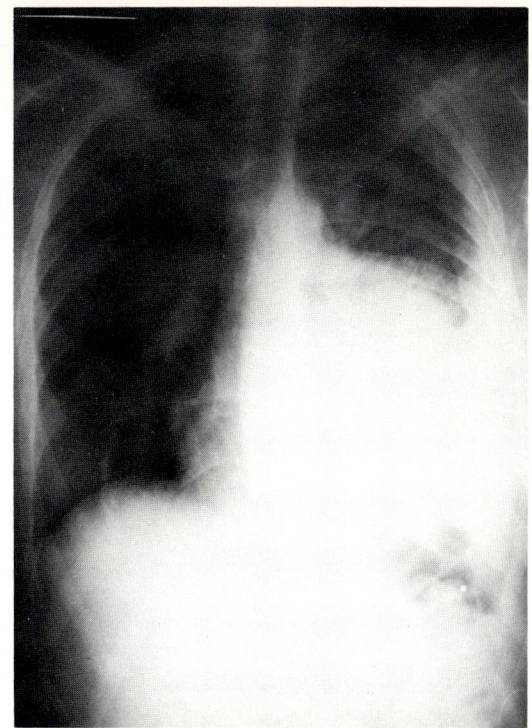

B

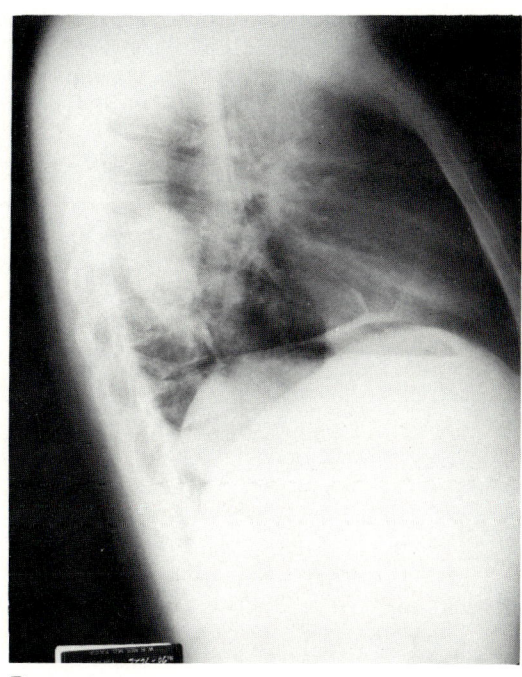

C

D

Fig 5-4. (A) Admission upright chest film of a 28-year-old white male rodeo performer who suffered multiple injuries when a horse fell on him. The film shows left hemopneumothorax, clavicular fracture, and rib fractures posteriorly on the left. (B) Over-exposed chest film taken 8 days after injury shows opacification of left lower chest due to contusion and hemorrhage in the lung. Two chest tubes, inserted after admission, were removed since there was no further drainage after the use of Varidase for 3 days. (C) Posteroanterior and (D) lateral views of the chest 1 month postinjury reveal a 7 × 8 cm hematoma in the left lower lobe and minimal residual pleural reaction. The hematoma was obscured on earlier films by severe lung contusion. Subsequent films show complete clearing of the pleural space and gradual resolution of the hematoma.

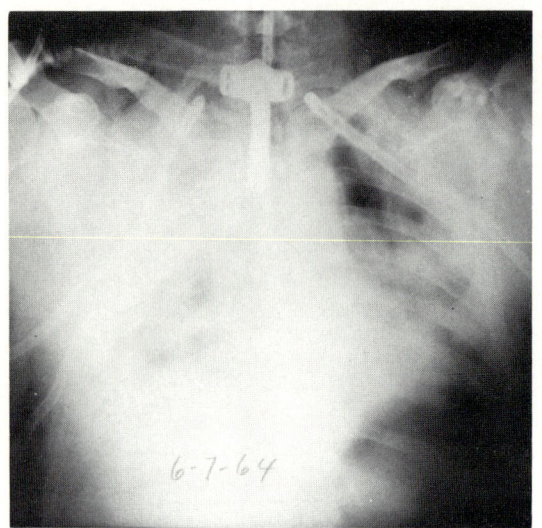

A

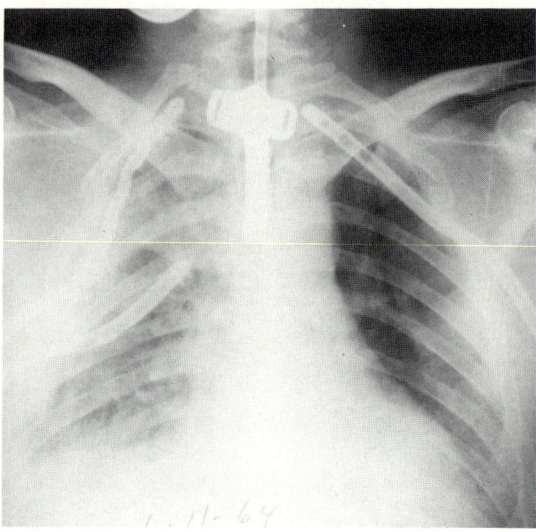

B

Fig 5-5. (A) Portable anteroposterior chest film of a 34-year-old white male taken 14 hours after he suffered severe bilateral chest trauma in an automobile collision. Film shows bilateral pulmonary contusions, rib fractures, and gastric dilatation with the tip of a Levin tube in the upper esophagus. (B) Portable chest film taken 4 days later shows marked clearing of the lung contusions on the left and considerable improvement on the right. (C) Portable chest film taken 10 days after injury reveals further clearing of both lungs. Ventilatory assistance was required for 14 days.

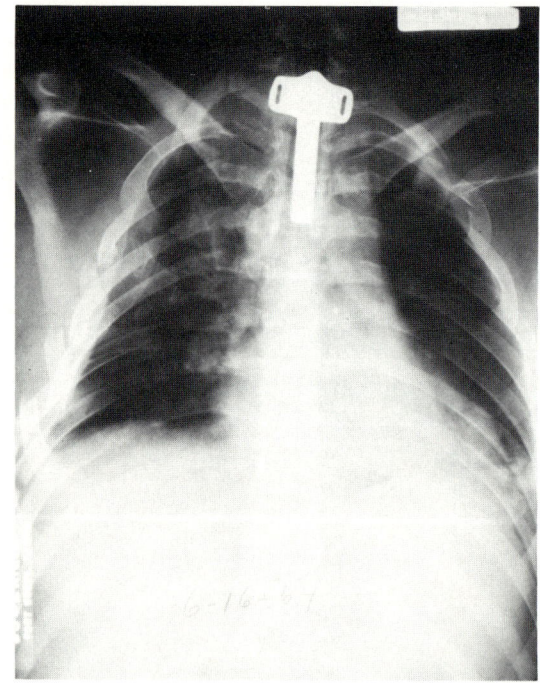

C

measurements are more reliable than the clinical observation of the patient. Restlessness, confusion, and belligerence are often due to hypoxia. Cyanosis, indicative of severe hypoxemia and oxygen desaturation, may be relieved temporarily by the administration of oxygen. Tachycardia and a rise in blood pressure are frequently due to ventilatory insufficiency and may progress rapidly to a dangerous state of hypoxemia, hypercapnia, and respiratory acidosis, cardiac arrhythmias, and cardiac arrest.

Arterial blood gas analysis (PCO_2, PO_2, PH, and oxygen saturation) frequently reveals derangements more severe than suspected clinically. These studies are necessary as part of the initial and subsequent evaluation of thoracic trauma and have contributed significantly to improved management.

PNEUMOTHORAX, HEMOTHORAX, AND TRACHEOSTOMY. These are managed as discussed under "Penetrating Wounds."

THORACOTOMY. For injuries of the lung, immediate thoracotomy is seldom required unless for massive hemorrhage or uncontrollable air leaks. Kish and associates [27] reported continued hemorrhage from torn apical adhesions. Severe lacerations of the lung may require repair of the lung or resection to control air leaks (Fig 5-6A–C). Rupture of the trachea or major bronchi may require immediate surgical repair as discussed in Chapter 7.

Lung Torsion and Hernia

Torsion of a lung due to thoracic trauma is extremely rare and the 3 cases in the literature were due to blunt trauma. Torsion of pulmonary tissue may be clockwise or counterclockwise, 180° or 360°, and may involve an entire lung or only a lobe. As a complication of blunt trauma, it is more likely to occur in children because of the compressibility and resiliency of the thoracic cage. Daughtry [16] postulated that sudden compression of the lower chest wall displaces the lower lobe upward, tearing the inferior pulmonary ligament, and when the pressure is released, the aerated upper lobe rotates to occupy the high vacuum space that was created in the lower thorax.

Stratmeier and Barry [37] reported that the initial chest roentgenogram shows peculiar striations in the midlung field extending from the hilus laterally and then sweeping upward toward the apex in a curving fashion. The initial roentgeno-graphic finding, however, may soon be obscured by atelectasis secondary to bronchial obstruction and pulmonary contusion. The development of venous engorgement occurs rapidly. Evidence of increasing opacification of the hemithorax after thoracocentesis or tube thoracostomy should increase the index of suspicion. Awareness of the possibility of pulmonary torsion following trauma and recognition of what appears to be a diagnostic sign on initial chest roentgenogram should result in diagnosis earlier and more frequently. Bronchoscopy will reveal a twisted or occluded bronchus.

In 1962 Brooks and Christie [8, 9] presented a case found at the time of thoracotomy for a shotgun wound and the results of a questionnaire on the subject to thoracic surgeons. The questionnaire revealed 82 unreported cases of torsion of pulmonary tissue. Of these, 9 were associated with trauma.

In the 3 cases reported in the literature and the 10 cases of Brooks and Christie contained in their unpublished report [9], 5 involved a whole lung and 8 a lobe. Only 2 of the 5 patients in whom the entire lung was involved survived and in both extensive resection was required. Of the 8 patients with only lobe involvement, 7 survived and in 3 of these only detorsion was required.

Early diagnosis and operation before irreversible damage occurs will allow detorsion as the definitive procedure and obviate resection. If there is delay, extensive resection due to infarction will usually be required. Flooding of the bronchial tree with bloody secretions when the torsion is corrected requires prompt aspiration by the anesthesiologist, and prolonged use of an endotracheal tube or tracheostomy postoperatively may be necessary to maintain a clear airway. Viable lung tissue should not be resected. In a patient reported by Daughtry [16] a single remaining segment expanded to almost completely fill the thorax and has remained functioning.

Intercostal pulmonary hernia may occur following blunt trauma but does not require immediate surgical intervention. Spontaneous healing may occur [36].

Pulmonary Fat Embolism

Zenker [42] in 1862 reported pulmonary fat emboli in a patient who died from thoracoabdominal trauma. Fat embolism occurs frequently as a complication of severe trauma but is often overlooked because attention is focused on the obvious injuries

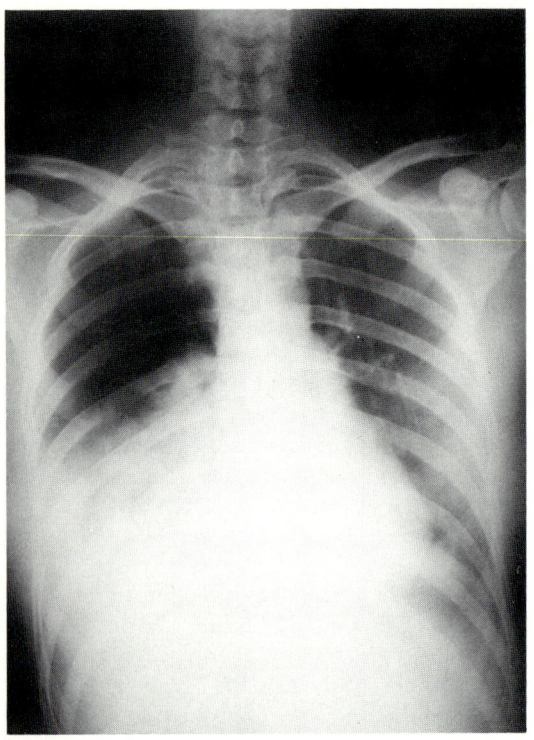

A

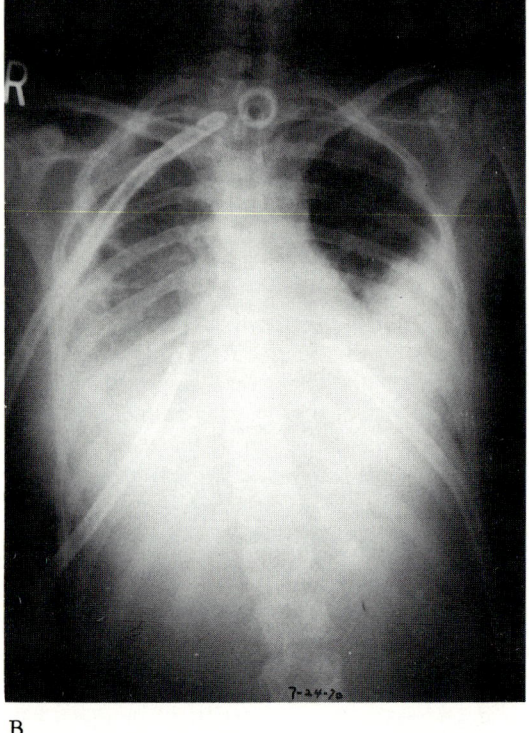

B

Fig 5-6. (A) Admission chest film of a 22-year-old white female who had suffered severe head injury and chest trauma after falling 30 feet. Film demonstrates right hemopneumothorax and pulmonary contusions. (B) Portable chest film taken 4 days later shows that pulmonary contusion persists on the right and has developed on the left. (C) A portable chest film taken 14 days after injury shows that contusions have not completely cleared. Right thoracotomy was necessary because uncontrollable air leaks prevented adequate ventilation with a volume ventilator. Pulmonary laceration extending from the diaphragmatic surface of the lower lobe to the hilar area required lobectomy.

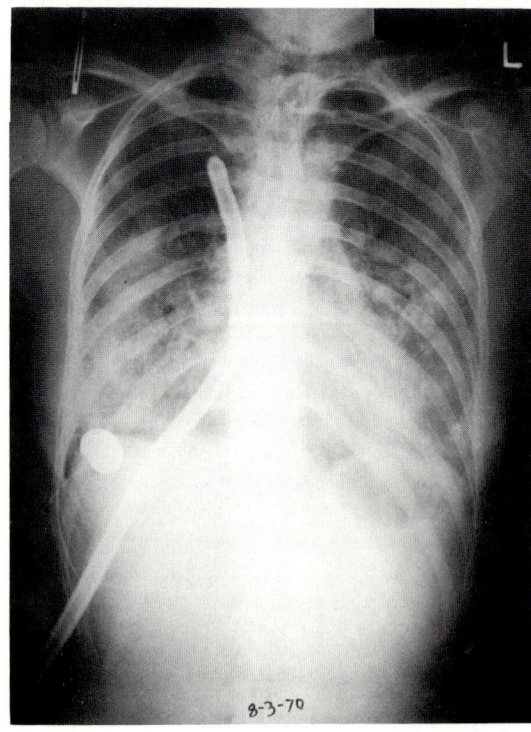

C

or complications. The highest incidence is associated with fractures of long bones and the pelvis but also occurs with fractures of ribs, the sternum, and vertebrae. Benoit, Hampson, and Burgess [5] found that almost 50 percent of patients with multiple fractures developed fat embolism, and an arterial PO_2 lower than 55 mm Hg was associated with a high incidence of embolization. Patients with multiple fractures, particularly when the femur is involved, should have arterial blood gases on admission and repeat studies if pulmonary symptoms increase.

Pulmonary fat emboli are found in trauma victims who die immediately, but most of the patients in whom the diagnosis is made clinically experience symptoms and clinical findings 24 or more hours after injury. Cobb and Hillman [12] found that fat injected intravenously is immediately arrested in the lung, thus usually protecting the brain and other organs. Analysis of fatty acids from the lipids of pulmonary emboli indicates a composition similar to that of bone marrow or adipose tissue [35].

Significant arterial oxygen desaturation may occur before tachypnea, tachycardia, and dyspnea are noted. Temperature elevation, diffuse rales, and cyanosis are usually present. Early chest roentgenograms are frequently not diagnostic but follow-up films may show diffuse bilateral infiltration if not obscured by severe pulmonary changes from trauma or complications (Fig 5-7). Petechiae are often found over the anterior axillary folds and pectoral areas and are occasionally seen in the conjunctivae or fundi. Fat may be found in the sputum or urine, and serum lipase is usually elevated after two or three days. Cyrostat sections of clotted blood may be positive for fat, and serum calcium is frequently lowered [11]. Onset of cerebral symptoms usually does not occur until after the pulmonary symptoms are noted. Restlessness, irritability, and confusion may progress to delirium and coma, and occasionally to decerebrate rigidity.

When this condition is suspected, therapy should be instituted immediately with the administration of oxygen, ventilatory assistance, and meticulous attention to tracheobronchial secretions. Endotracheal intubation or tracheostomy is frequently required, and periodic blood gas determinations aid in evaluating the effectiveness of ventilation.

Heparin therapy should be instituted unless

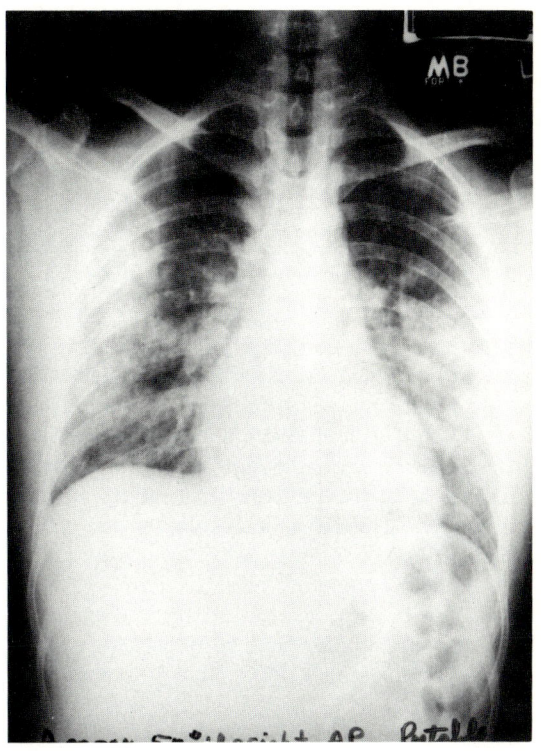

Fig 5-7. Portable anteroposterior chest film of a 22-year-old white male 2 days after blunt chest trauma and comminuted fracture of the femur. Admission chest film was negative. Fat embolism was proved, and patient recovered after therapy.

definitely contraindicated. Its lipemic clearing effect, inhibition of red cell agglutination, and its enhancement of the activity of lipase increase capillary blood flow in the lungs. Low molecular weight dextran has also been advocated to reduce blood viscosity and improve capillary blood flow. Ashbaugh and Petty [2] feel that corticosteroids aid in the alleviation of hypoxia. The hyperpyrexia is often unresponsive to usual measures and may require a hypothermia blanket to lower the temperature and reduce oxygen requirements. Whole blood or packed cells may be required for rapidly developing anemia but should be used cautiously to avoid right heart failure with aggravation of respiratory distress. If the condition of the patient deteriorates in spite of these measures, intravenous alcohol may be considered in place of heparin to inhibit hydrolysis of fat emboli and decrease reaction to fatty acids.

The mortality in patients with pulmonary fat

embolism has been estimated to be 10 to 20 percent but may reach as high as 85 percent in those with severe respiratory and cerebral symptoms [39]. The high mortality should be considerably reduced with early diagnosis, adequate ventilatory support with PEEP [28], administration of heparin and corticosteroids, and supportive therapy.

POSTTRAUMATIC PULMONARY INSUFFICIENCY

Hypercapnia (elevated PCO_2) is indicative of hypoventilation and can usually be corrected with the use of volume ventilators. Severe hypoxemia (low PO_2 and oxygen desaturation) is more difficult to reverse since the diffusibility of carbon dioxide is usually more than twenty times greater than oxygen. The large tidal volumes and pressure necessary to achieve adequate oxygenation often produce respiratory alkalosis (low PCO_2), but this can be remedied by adding dead space to the airway or bleeding in 1 to 3 percent carbon dioxide. Maintaining a PCO_2 above 30 mm Hg is desirable.

The possibility of further lung damage by prolonged ventilator delivery of high oxygen concentrations is well known and the lowest inspired oxygen concentrations that maintain arterial oxygen tension (PO_2) at an acceptable level should be used. In severe pulmonary contusions with intra-alveolar hemorrhage and edema, venous shunting, atelectasis, and secondary infection, however, oxygen concentrations of 50 percent or greater are often necessary for a week or more before resolution of the pulmonary lesions occurs. Petty and Ashbaugh [31] found that positive end-expiratory pressure (PEEP) breathing improved oxygen transport in severe respiratory insufficiency with lower inspired oxygen tension than is possible with IPPB. High-level PEEP is capable of aborting or reversing the pathophysiological process that produces respiratory failure. Frequent blood gas determinations should be obtained when volume ventilators are required. Additional discussion of ventilators is to be found in Chapter 8.

Traumatic Wet Lung

Burford and Burbank [10] introduced the term *traumatic wet lung* in 1944 to describe the changes in the lung associated with chest wall and lung trauma that were manifested by an increase in the amount of difficult-to-clear interstitial and intra-alveolar fluid. After further experience [7] the concept was broadened to include bloody mucus and alveolar transudates resulting from anoxia. The serious consequences of the condition were recognized as patients with wet lungs were difficult to resuscitate from shock and were poor operative risks, having frequent pulmonary complications. Therapy was directed toward controlling the production of moisture and promoting adequate bronchial drainage. Chest wall pain seriously impaired the cough mechanism and was considered a dominant factor in Wet Lung syndrome. Intercostal or paravertebral nerve blocks relieved the pain and improved the cough. Clearing of the tracheobronchial tree by coughing, tracheal aspiration, and bronchoscopy often produced dramatic improvement. Brewer and associates [6, 7] introduced the principle of IPPB treatment in chest trauma with the use of a portable anesthetic machine to treat the advanced stages of wet lung.

Congestive Atelectasis

Jenkins and co-workers [24] used the term *congestive atelectasis* in 1950 for the pulmonary changes noted in the traumatized or critically ill patient who received excessive amounts of intravenous fluids and blood. The symptoms of tachypnea and dyspnea may appear suddenly; findings on auscultation and chest roentgenograms are mimimal when the degree of respiratory distress and hypoxemia is considered. The condition may progress rapidly, with bloody, frothy secretion in the tracheobronchial tree, rales over both lungs, bilateral mottled densities, and severe cyanosis. Mortality is high, and the lungs at postmortem examination are congested and heavy.

Shock Lung

Shock lung is a term that originated during the Vietnam conflict for the pulmonary changes and complications that followed severe thoracic and nonthoracic trauma and resulted in progressive pulmonary insufficiency and high mortality. Significant hypoxia and the administration of large volumes of intravenous fluids appear to be common denominators. A period of hypotension occurs in some but is not a necessary factor to the development of the syndrome. The clinical course usually described is as follows: after resuscitation there is a period when the lungs are clear to auscultation; the findings on chest roentgenogram are insufficient to account for the hyperventilation that is followed by increasing respiratory difficulty. Pulmonary congestion is noted clinically and roentgenograms show progressive infiltration.

The terms *traumatic wet lung, congestive atelectasis,* and *shock lung* are often used interchangeably. Most cases of respiratory insufficiency following trauma previously covered by these terms are now classified as respiratory distress syndrome. Additional details of management are found in Chapters 8 and 18.

REFERENCES

1. Arom KV, Lyons GW: Traumatic arteriovenous fistula. J Thorac Cardiovasc Surg 70:918, 1975
2. Ashbaugh DG, Petty TL: The use of corticosteroids in the treatment of respiratory failure associated with massive fat embolism. Surg Gynecol Obstet 123:493, 1966
3. Bassett JS, Gibson RD, Wilson RF: Blunt injuries to the chest. J Trauma 8:418, 1968
4. Beall AC, Jr., et al: Surgical treatment of penetrating thoracic trauma. Dis Chest 49:568, 1966
5. Benoit PR, Hampson LG, Burgess JH: Value of arterial hypoxemia in the diagnosis of pulmonary fat embolism. Ann Surg 175:128, 1972
6. Brewer LA, III, et al: Wounds of the chest in war and peace, 1943–1968. Ann Thorac Surg 7:387, 1969
7. Brewer LA, III, et al: "Wet lung" in war casualties. Ann Surg 123:343, 1946
8. Brooks JW: Personal communication, 1972.
9. Brooks JW, Christie LG: Torsion of the Lung. Presented at the Southern Thoracic Surgical Association Meeting, Ochos Rios, Jamaica, November, 1962
10. Burford TH, Burbank B: Traumatic wet lung. Observation on certain physiologic fundamentals of thoracic trauma. J Thorac Surg 14:415, 1945
11. Burgher LW, Dines DE, Linscheid RL, et al: Fat embolism and the adult respiratory distress syndrome. Mayo Clinic Proc 49:107, 1974
12. Cobb CA, Hillman JW: Fat embolism. Instruc Course of Lect Am Acad of Orthop Surgeons 18:122, 1961
13. Conn JH, et al: Thoracic trauma: an analysis of 1022 cases. J Trauma 3:22, 1963
14. Cordice JWV, Jr., Cabezon J: Chest trauma with pneumothorax and hemothorax. Review of 502 cases. J. Thorac Cardiovasc Surg 50:316, 1965
15. Daughtry DC: Management of nonpenetrating thoracic injuries. Am Surg 23:462, 1957
16. Daughtry DC: Traumatic torsion of the lung. N Engl J Med 256:318, 1961
17. Garzon AA, Amer NL, Karlson KE: Treatment of penetrating wounds of the chest. Arch Surg 88:397, 1964
18. Gray AR, Harrison WH, Couves CM: Penetrating injuries to the chest: clinical results in the management of 769 patients. Am J Surg 100:709, 1960
19. Grover FL, Richardson JD, Fewel JG, et al: Prophylactic antibiotics in the treatment of penetrating chest wounds. A prospective double-blind study. J Thorac Cardiovasc Surg 74:528, 1977
20. Haller JA, Canan ED, Ransdell HT: The treatment of single gunshot wounds of the chest. J Trauma 2:560, 1962
21. Hankins JR, McAslan TC, Shin B, et al: Extensive pulmonary laceration caused by blunt trauma J Thorac Cardiovasc Surg 74:519, 1977
22. Harrison WH, et al: Severe nonpenetrating injuries to the chest: clinical results in the management of 216 patients. Am J Surg 100:715, 1960
23. Hopkinson BR, Border JR, Schenck WG, Jr.: Experimental closed chest trauma. J Thorac Cardiovasc Surg 55:580, 1968
24. Jenkins MT, et al: Congestive atelectasis: a complication of the intravenous infusion of fluids. Ann Surg 132:372, 1950
25. Jolly PC, Thomas PA: Recovery of pulmonary ventilation after thoracic wounds. Ann Thorac Surg 6:282, 1968
26. Kemmerer WT, Eckert WG, Gathright JB, et al: Patterns of thoracic injuries in fatal traffic accidents. J Trauma 1:595, 1961
27. Kish G, Kozloff L, Joseph WL, et al: Indications for early thoracotomy in the management of chest trauma. Ann Thorac Surg 22:23, 1976
28. Katsuyuki K, Webb WR, Parker FB, Jr., et al: Pulmonary response of unilateral positive end expiratory pressure (PEEP) on experimental fat embolism. Ann Surg 181:676, 1975
29. Moghissi K: Laceration of the lung following blunt trauma. Thorax 26:223, 1971
30. Payne EM: Contusion of the lung with external injuries. Br Med J 1:139, 1909
31. Petty JL, Ashbaugh DG: The adult respiratory distress syndrome: clinical features, factors influencing prognosis and principles of management. Chest 60:233, 1971
32. Rothman M, Maynard A, Carter R: Traumatic hemothorax. Harlem Hosp Bull 5:27, 1952
33. Schramel R, Kellum H, Creech O, Jr.: Analysis of factors affecting survival after chest injuries. J Trauma 1:600, 1961
34. Sherman RT: Experience with 472 civilian penetrating wounds of the chest. Milit Med 131:63, 1966
35. Sherr S, Montemurno R, Roffner P: Lipids of recovered pulmonary fat emboli following trauma. J Trauma 14:242, 1974

36. Soreide O, Stidjeberg JO: Traumatic intercostal hernia. Injury 7:61, 1975

37. Stratmeier EH, Barry JW: Torsion of the lung following thoracic trauma. Radiology 62:726, 1954

38. Tygart RL, Mitchell JA, Glas WW: Pulmonary contusion. J Mich Med Soc 62:882, 1963

39. Weisz GM, Steiner E: The cause of death in fat embolism. Chest 59:511, 1971

40. Westernak N: A roentgenological investigation into traumatic lung arisen through blunt violence to the thorax. Acta Radiol 22:331, 1941

41. Williams JR, Bonte FJ: The Roentgenological Aspects of Nonpenetrating Chest Injuries. Springfield, Ill, Thomas, 1961

42. Zenker FA: Fat Embolism. Quoted by S Sevitt. London, Buttersworth, 1962

43. Zuckerman S: Experimental study of blunt injury of the lungs. Lancet 2:219, 1940

6. THE INTRAPLEURAL SEQUELAE OF CHEST INJURY

Paul C. Samson

Hemothorax or pneumothorax, or both, constitute the most common sequels of thoracic wounds and injuries; posttraumatic chylothorax occurs much less often and is seldom the source of immediate concern. In the early management of major chest injury it has been necessary to recognize such causes of actual or potential cardiorespiratory imbalance. In addition, prompt reexpansion of the lung will obliterate the pleural space and is the best insurance against clotted hemothorax, hemoorganization, and hemothoracic infection.

POSTTRAUMATIC PNEUMOTHORAX

Pneumothorax may result from blunt injury or penetrating or sucking wounds. In a personal series, pure pneumothorax occurred in 23 percent of patients with thoracic injuries [19]. The lung parenchyma may be torn by external trauma; it may be punctured by fractured ribs, by a missile, or by an instrument. Physical examination usually detects depressed breath sounds. Chest roentgenograms taken during expiration show the amount of pneumothorax most accurately. If it is minimal (10 percent or less) no treatment is necessary, although the patient is carefully followed by serial examinations and roentgenograms. Progressive symptomatic pneumothorax or pressure pneumothorax, or both, demand immediate therapy. Usually waterseal tube thoracostomy is employed. If right-angled catheters are used (size No. 28 to 30F) a 1-cm incision is made in the second intercostal space anteriorly and the catheter threaded into the pleural space, the tip being pointed toward the apex. In many instances, approach through the anterior first intercostal space is satisfactory. Here the site is just lateral to the costochondral junction and Malecot catheters (No. 24 to 26F) can be used to advantage.

Pressure pneumothorax—from check-valve mechanisms with a torn lung, from fractures of the trachea or extrapulmonary bronchi, or from a ruptured esophagus—is serious. The patient is obviously dyspneic, and there is often extreme restlessness. The chest is hyperresonant, breath sounds are absent, and the heart is shifted toward the opposite side. In an extreme emergency, a large-bore needle (13 gauge) may be plunged into the pleural cavity without local anesthetic or syringe; the air will escape under pressure.

The most common cause of uncontrolled pneumothorax is a tear in a major airway. Such injury requires early thoracotomy. A ruptured esophagus may be suspected by history, the type of injury, a nasal twang to the voice, mediastinal and subcutaneous emphysema of the tissues of the neck, and the early onset of clinical shock. A chest film taken after the patient swallows a radiopaque medium usually establishes the diagnosis; again, immediate thoracotomy is necessary as part of the resuscitative process.

POSTTRAUMATIC HEMOTHORAX-HEMOPNEUMOTHORAX

Hemothorax varies from a minimal to a massive amount of bleeding into a pleural cavity. Prior to World War II, it was the rule to remove just enough blood to relieve dyspnea and to practice air replacement. This routine was discarded during the early days of the war, since there was not the slightest evidence that prompt reexpansion increased air leaks or bleeding. Hemothorax-hemopneumothorax has occurred in approximately 48 percent of our patients suffering thoracic injury [19].

A minimum of 500 cc of fluid is generally necessary to produce physical and roentgenographic signs of hemothorax. The treatment should be prompt removal of as much blood as possible from the pleural cavity. In recent years, most physicians have employed closed tube thoracostomy on moderate to massive hemothorax. In the usual case, Argyle, right-angled, or Malecot catheters (No. 30 to 36F) are inserted in the seventh or eighth intercostal space posterolaterally. From 1000 to 1500 cc of blood may be removed at one time without difficulty. If, however, the patient becomes faint, complains of increasing tightness and pain, or coughs severely during removal, the procedure should be discontinued forthwith. Such symptoms are most likely occurring from the creation of a highly negative intrapleural pressure due to a pulmonary atelectasis that has been produced by obstructing secretions in the bronchi. This, in turn, should be treated by immediate nasotracheal suction or bronchoscopy. In the event of shock or other evidence of massive bleeding the blood may be collected in a sterile citrate container and returned to the patient as an autotransfusion.

Severe, continuing hemorrhage usually requires an emergency thoracotomy for control. The rapid evacuation of from 2000 to 2500 cc does not, per se, indicate an immediate thoracotomy if the patient's condition is otherwise stable and the hemorrhage does not continue. But, there are a number of factors involving hemorrhage that can determine the necessity for immediate thoracotomy. In our experience the following criteria have been the most reliable guides to the type of hemorrhage that indicates thoracotomy for control: (1) persistent bleeding of more than 500 cc per hour; (2) blood pressure that fails to rise after a rapid blood transfusion; (3) a fall in the blood pressure that had risen to relatively normal levels; and (4) persistent, severe anemia demonstrated by serial hematocrit determinations. The most frequent source of severe hemorrhage has been from the great intrathoracic vessels. Continued bleeding from the internal mammary and intercostal arteries usually follows laceration and incomplete division of the vessel. It is important to evacuate air or blood, or both, from a pleural cavity to facilitate reexpansion of the lung as soon as possible. Two-tube thoracostomies are frequently used; one tube is placed anteriorly and high and the other posterolaterally and low.

In smaller hemothoraces, thoracocentesis may be performed every day or two as long as appreciable blood can be aspirated from a pleural cavity.

COMPLICATIONS OF HEMOTHORAX-CLOTTING AND HEMOORGANIZATION

It is now universally accepted that blood in the pleural cavity frequently clots. Prior to World War II it was thought that blood in the thorax either remained liquid or was almost promptly defibrinated by churning movements in the chest. However, the inability to aspirate obvious blood from a pleural cavity, even where using a large-bore needle (13 gauge), is the proof of this clotting. Early

thoracotomy merely for the evacuation of clots is seldom necessary, although it has been recommended by some [8]. "Early delayed" (meaning 10–14 days post trauma) thoracotomy has been practiced in 3 percent of a more recent series [3].

In many clotted hemothoraces, fibrinolysis may occur within 10 days. The intrapleural administration of enzymes (streptokinase and streptodornase combined) seems to have been largely discontinued both in civilian and military practice [17, 31]. The common failure of clot lysis and the almost universal frequency of fever and the generalized toxicity of the drug have made the use of Varidase unpopular. During the past 10 years there has been only minimal reference to the procedure . . . "enzymatic debridement can be used" [33]. Chapter 5, however, contains an enthusiastic report on the management of clotted hemothorax with Varidase. I must confess I have not used this technique, so I therefore cannot speak from personal experience.

HEMOORGANIZATION—GROSS AND MICROSCOPIC PATHOGENESIS

A process known as hemoorganization takes place in some clotted hemothoraces. Within a few days of injury a thin film of fibrin and blood cells are deposited on the pleural surfaces. A sac or envelope (closed hematoma) is shortly formed, the "inner" or "younger" surface of which is bathed by liquid and coagulated elements of the hemothorax; the "outer" or "older" surface is loosely adherent to visceral and parietal pleurae. Within 7 days there is microscopic evidence of angioblastic and fibroblastic proliferation in the thickening layers. The process first extends into the walls of the envelope from both pleural surfaces. The "peel" increases in thickness through the progressive organization of clotted blood and fibrin. The advancing inner border of active organization is composed of young cellular tissue and wandering fibroblasts can occasionally be seen. Within 5 weeks fibrous tissue cells form in the outer portion of the peel, arranging themselves roughly parallel to the surface. The capillaries extend into the peel perpendicular to the surface, having penetrated from the pleurae. The parietal segment of the peel is always thicker than the visceral segment, possibly due to the presence of the lymph vessels located in the subepithelial layer of the parietal pleura [4]. Within 7 weeks arterioles with smooth

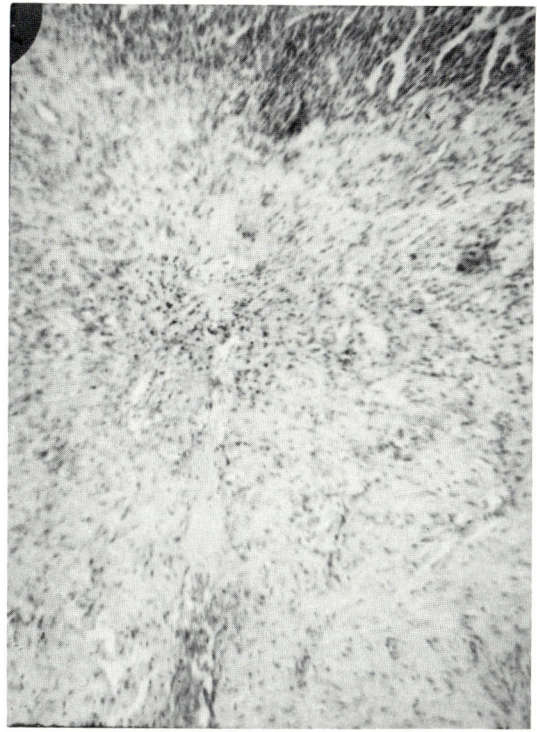

Fig 6-1. Cross section of peel in organizing hemothorax of 5 weeks' duration ($\times 250$). At the top is fibrin and fibroblastic tissue, the center of the closed hematoma. At the bottom is adult fibrous tissue near the older or pleural surface of the peel. The long axis of the young arteriole is at right angles to the surface. (From P. C. Samson and T. H. Burford, Total pulmonary decortication, J Thorac Surg 16:127, 1947. By permission.)

muscle and elastic fibrils can be identified in the older portion of the peel (Fig 6-1). In rare cases, layers of fat cells have developed in the peel along the older or pleural surface. This may be a regressive phenomenon, a forewarning of eventual degeneration or resorption of the peel [2, 25]. Microscopic calcium particles occasionally may be deposited within the peel during this time. Calcium has not always been in response to infection. When early infection does supervene, the peel matures more quickly. As hemoorganization progresses, the peel becomes a tough, inelastic fibrinofibrous membrane that effectively prevents pulmonary reexpansion.

That the visceral pleura itself remains a thin translucent membrane needs continuing reemphasis [25]. For instance, the wavy elastic fibers that are characteristically present just beneath the visceral pleura are never found in the resected peel unless the visceral pleura is taken with the peel and sectioned [23]. The parietal pleura likewise remains thin. The peel does not contain elastic fibers but is still relatively difficult to dissect. Knowledge of the endothoracic fascia, however, makes removal rapid and relatively avascular [11]. Dissection in the endothoracic fascial plane removes the parietal pleura. Elastic fibers are then found just deep to the pleural mesothelium, an observation previously described only twice [1, 2]. The sequel to chronic organizing hemothorax may be a crippling calcified fibrothorax.

INFECTED HEMOTHORAX— HEMOTHORACIC EMPYEMA

The onset of infection in a hemothorax is serious. It is heralded by increasing toxicity and positive cultures from the aspirate. If the hemothorax is still liquid, it may be handled by thoracocentesis, prompt tube thoracostomy, and administration of the appropriate antibiotic. Unfortunately, however, hemothoraces. The differentiation between infected hemothorax and frank empyma may not be easy, although gross pus is aspirated from the latter, infection has been present for a longer time, and the most infections develop in clotted and organizing patient may be more seriously ill.

PULMONARY DECORTICATION

Historical Aspects

In the past 75 years, pulmonary decortication was discovered, described, discarded, and once more rediscovered. Fowler [13] in 1893 described the first operation, followed closely by DeLorme [9]. DeLorme's contribution of the term *decortication* first appeared in 1896 [10]. With few exceptions, notably those of Lilienthal [22] and Ware [32], all of the early operations were attempted on patients with chronic pleural disease. The results were uniformly poor, if not disastrous. Eventually there was virtual abandonment of the operation as a planned procedure. This has happened to other major surgical advances discovered too far ahead of complementary specialties for a successful outcome.

In the early days of World War II, the fact of so many soldiers with organizing hemothorax and posttraumatic empyema once more focused attention on a possible means of preventing chronic invalidism. At this juncture, however, the time was right: blood replacement with blood was becoming routine; anesthesia had vastly improved; and thoracic surgeons were more intrepid, frequently opening the chest far earlier than before. (Although penicillin was soon to appear it was not available when the original pioneering decortications were performed.) It was during these days and in this atmosphere that pulmonary decortication was reborn.

The spark was first generated during discussions among the thoracic surgeons of the Second Auxiliary Surgical Group early in the North African campaign. In April 1943, Burford performed the first decortication for subacute, uninfected organizing hemothorax [25]. September 1943 saw primary decortication performed for infected hemothorax, and secondary decortication was first performed in a previously drained hemothoracic empyema; in March 1944, the first successful primary decortications in hemothoracic empyema were reported by Burford, Parker, and Samson [6] and Samson and Burford [25]. The most important contribution of thoracic surgeons in the North African theater of operations was their insistence that decortication be performed relatively early, long before chronic crippling sequelae appeared. Such was the success of those early experiences that others [16, 18, 21, 30] rapidly verified our results with their own experiences.

General Indications for the Timing of Operation

The timing of operation is also important. In uninfected organizing hemothorax, decortication is best performed in the period from 4 to 5 weeks from the time of injury. Waiting a month will insure that the operation is actually necessary; in many patients originally thought to be candidates for operation the condition will have cleared at least partially within 5 weeks. If decortication is performed earlier than 3 weeks, the peel is frequently thin and fragile, resulting in piecemeal decortication. Often, too, because of contusion the lung may not be satisfactorily expanded in less than 3 weeks.

Patients considered suitable candidates for decortication have some or all of the following signs and symptoms: thoracic discomfort, retraction and narrowing of the intercostal spaces, roentgeno-graphic evidence of a hazy chest, and pulmonary compression of at least 25 percent with the apex unexpanded.

The development of infection is manifested by increasing fever. Usually there is a rapid increase in the size of the pleural pocket, and multiple fluid levels become manifest. A wide variety of microorganisms have been reported, including clostridia. In general, decortication has been performed in these patients as soon as the infection is evident and the patient's general condition allows major surgery. Although this can be well within 10 days, the peel is usually firm enough to permit adequate removal. Posttraumatic empyema is not greatly different from infected hemothorax, but the patient has had his infection longer and may not be a candidate for major surgery. Adequate evacuation by airtight rib resection drainage is then advised, to be followed by secondary decortication as soon as the patient's condition permits. In the face of moderate to massive posttraumatic empyema, primary decortication is practiced whenever possible. This has several advantages, namely early reexpansion of the lung, prevention of chronic empyema, no prolonged discomfort from tubes and dressings, and a proportionately shortened disability time.

Techniques of Operation

A posterolateral incision is ordinarily used. Entrance is made directly into the organizing hemothorax or empyema (Fig 6-2). All clots and debris are evacuated, and the cavity is lavaged. The exposed tissue is usually brownish-red. The underlying lung is immobile. Sharp dissection is made through the peel to the visceral pleura while the lung is braced with moderate positive pressure by the anesthesiologist. As the visceral pleura is exposed, the lung will begin to herniate (Fig 6-3). By means of a small gauze dissector, finger, or scissors, the peel is gently separated from the visceral pleura. During separation the main pressure of the dissection is directed toward the peel. The peel is excised along its line of reflection onto the parietal membrane and the margins are smoothed. The fissures and apex are then freed and the lung is separated completely down to the hilum (Fig 6-4).

The diaphragm is decorticated if it can be done easily, and the costophrenic sinuses are reestablished. The costal segment of the peel is scrubbed with gauze to make the surface smooth. Routine parietal decortication is not practiced but is always

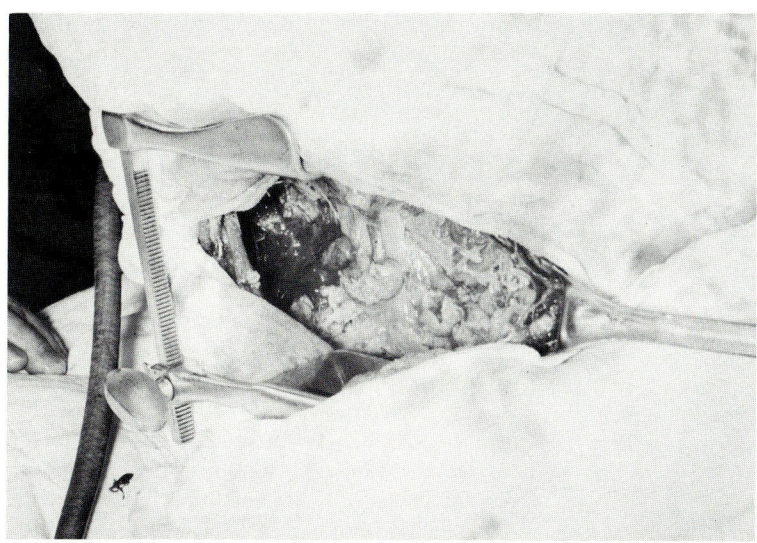

Fig 6-2. At operation entrance is made directly into this subacute posttraumatic empyema. The chest is filled with fibrin and purulent exudate. The lung is collapsed beneath the thickened peel and its outline is not discernible.

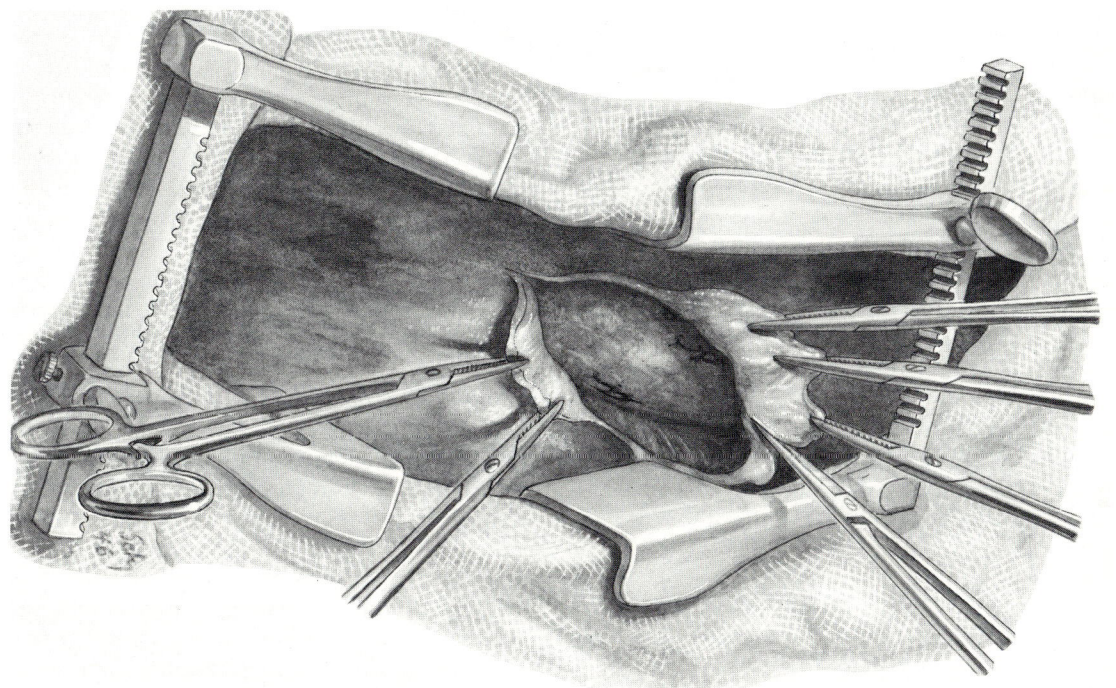

Fig 6-3. Normal visceral pleura is encountered after initial incision through the peel. The lung then herniates through the defect as gentle positive pressure anesthesia is given.

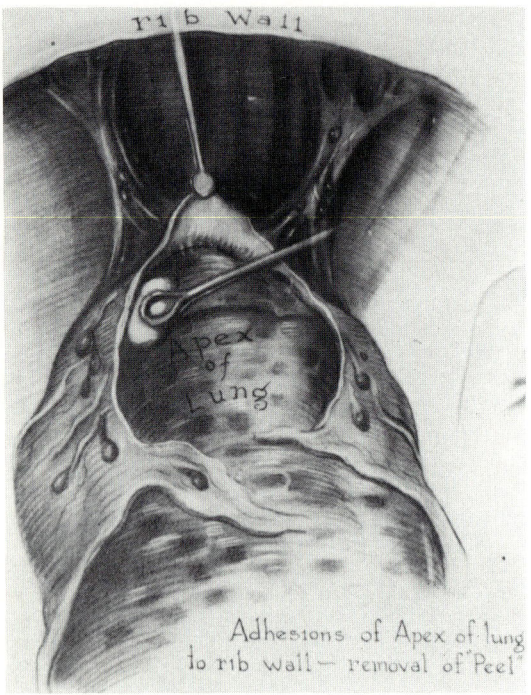

Fig 6-4. The technique used for freeing the apex of the lung is shown.

possible. In recent years we have frequently performed extraparietal pleural operations by dissection in the endothoracic fascial plane [11]. Following initial release of the lung, it should be expanded intermittently. Progressive reexpansion will aid in controlling ooze from the visceral pleura as well as giving a smoother, more circumferential silhouette.

Some 30 years ago we performed our first empyemectomy in a patient with tuberculosis [27]. Moderately localized hemothoracic empyema and other collections of clotted blood and calcified hematomas are similarly treated by closed total excision of the sac (Figs 6-5, 6-6). The thoracotomy is planned to remove a rib near the superior aspect of the pocket; careful dissection is performed, first incising the deep periosteal layer, then identifying the endothoracic fascia (Fig 6-7). Note that the line of cleavage established is outside the parietal pleura (Fig 6-8). Blunt dissection is carried out in the plane of the endothoracic fascia in all directions until the lung is visible. One can "turn the corner" (i.e., empyemectomy) (Fig 6-9), incise the parietal pleura and peel just beyond the sac,

and finally perform true decortication on the visceral pleural side. If the envelope is tense, it may be aspirated.

POSTTRAUMATIC CHYLOTHORAX

The thoracic duct may be ruptured or torn during blunt injury to the chest as well as during injury from penetrating wounds. In the past 30 years or so, intrathoracic surgical procedures have accounted for a substantial increase—now estimated to be at least 50 percent—in all chylous effusions (i.e., iatrogenic chylothorax). Thus, chylothorax has been described following pulmonary and esophageal surgery, excision of mediastinal tumors, and cardiovascular surgery. Maloney and Spencer reported iatrogenic chylothorax in 0.5 percent of 2660 patients undergoing cardiovascular operations over 20 years ago. Bower [5] noted 0.24 percent chylothorax among 2468 patients undergoing operations in the following decade. Through 1955, three excellent reviews described 90 cases of posttraumatic chylothorax; these reviews also showed that there has been a decrease in mortality from well over 50 percent to approximately 10 percent [14, 20, 29]. The first successful intrathoracic ligation of the thoracic duct was recorded in 1948 [20]. Since 1971, at least three articles about successful ligation have been recorded in the English literature [7, 12, 28].

The physical signs and symptoms of posttraumatic chylothorax are nonspecific. Diagnosis is made by the aspiration of typical milky fluid that is fat stain positive by Sudan III. The treatment of appreciable, symptomatic chylous effusion consists of repeated thoracocenteses or tube thoracostomy and occasionally delayed thoracotomy and ligation of the thoracic duct. Early open surgery to control chylothorax may be performed when it is due to a penetrating wound of the mediastinum. Early thoracotomy may be indicated to determine the extent of injury. As a rule, repeated thoracocenteses or tube thoracostomy, or both, may be required for 2 to 3 weeks. Additional supplementary measures advocated by Williams and Burford [34] are as follows: restricted lower extremity motion, abatement of increased intra-abdominal pressure (cough and so on), elimination of drug-induced vasodilatation, restriction of oral intake, and nasogastric suction. Persistence in conservatism can, however, be carried to an extreme [15].

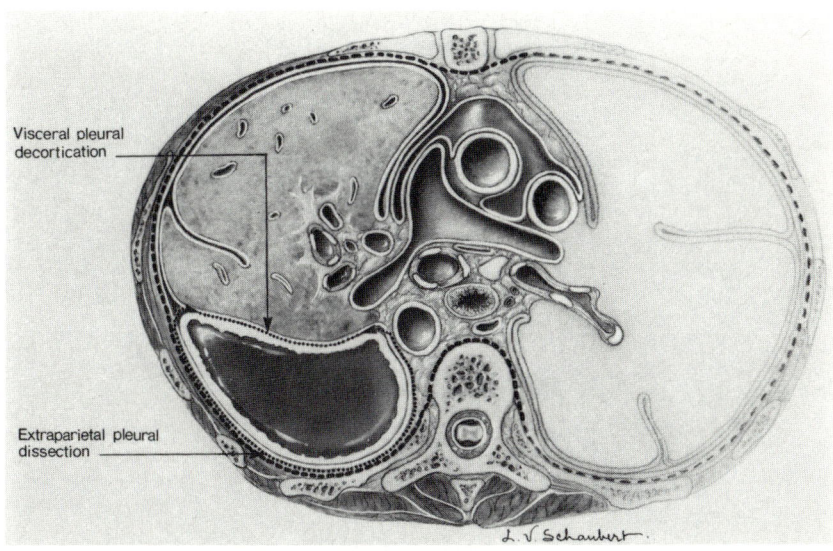

Visceral pleural
decortication

Extraparietal pleural
dissection

L. V. Schaubert.

Fig 6-5. Cross section of localized posttraumatic
empyema indicates proper planes of closed exenteration: dissection in the endothoracic fascial plane externally and decortication of the peel, leaving the
visceral pleura intact.

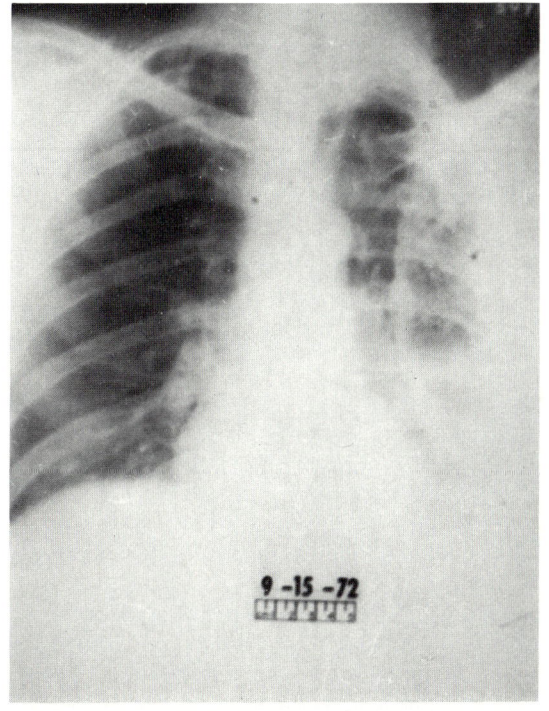

A

B

Fig 6-6. (A) Preoperative roentgenogram of a
chronic traumatic calcified fibrothorax. (B) A
closed exenteration, hemothorectomy, shown postoperatively.

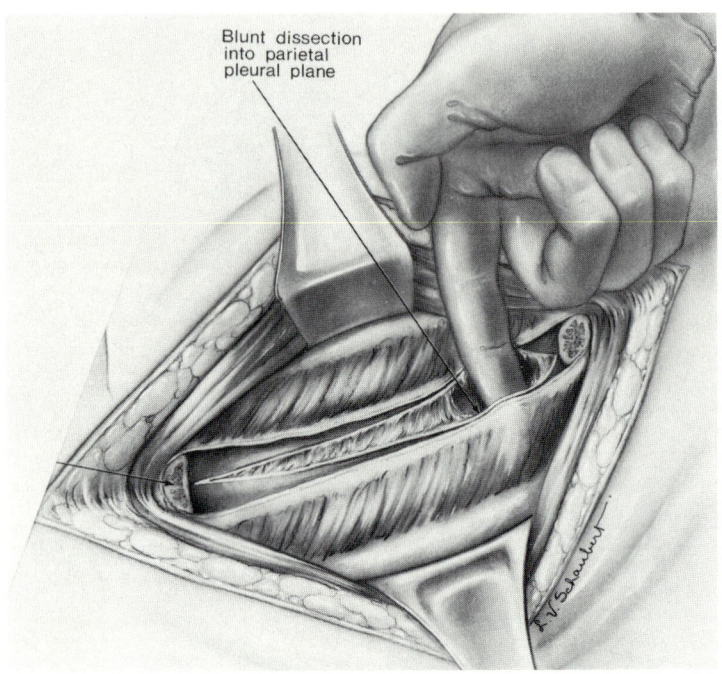

Fig 6-7. *The deep periosteum has been incised, exposing the endothoracic fascia. The finger is in the fascial plane* external *to the parietal pleura.*

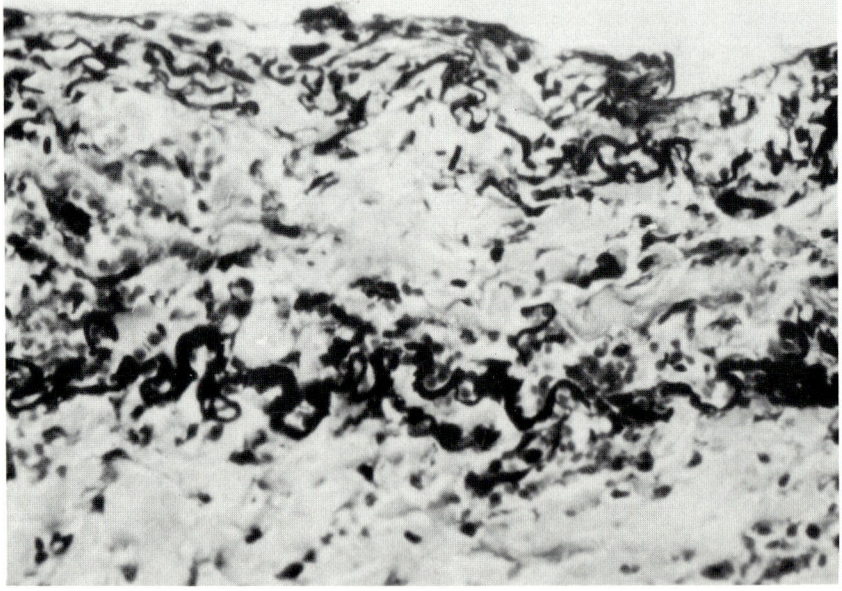

Fig 6-8. *Photomicrograph of the parietal peel and adjacent endothoracic fascia in empyema; special elastic tissue stain was used. The endothoracic fascial layer is at the top* (×400).

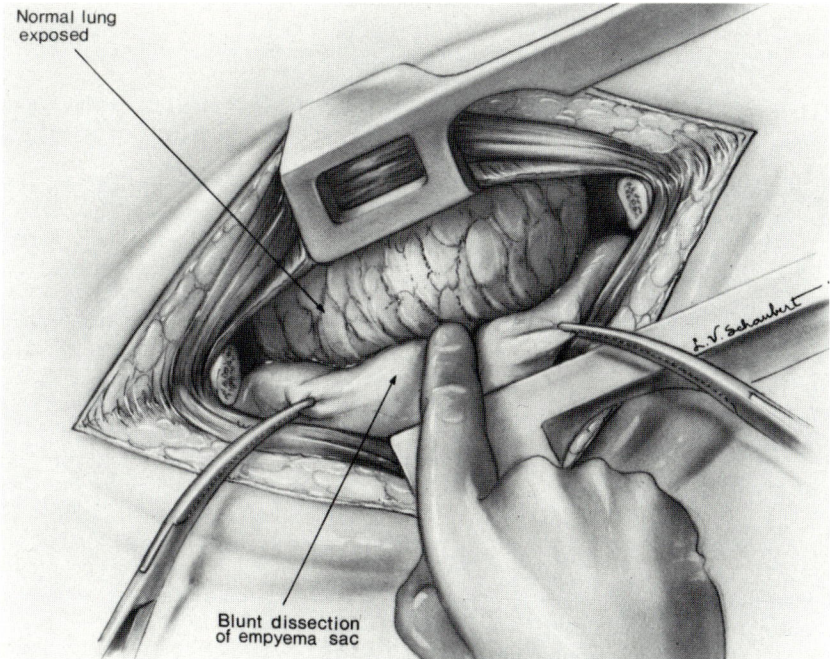

Normal lung
exposed

Blunt dissection
of empyema sac

Fig 6-9. After turning the corner, true viscera pleural decortication—empyemectomy—is then effected.

One of the main reasons for persistent flow is incomplete laceration of the duct. Among the indications for thoracotomy are: drainage in excess of 1500 cc for 24 hours, or 100 cc for every year of a child's age during a 5-day period; a flow of chyle that has not ceased after 14 days, or if the flow has ceased, but there is obvious loculation; or if the patient begins to exhibit plasma-protein and fat deficiencies. Small children may well suffer metabolic disturbances within 3 weeks.

A few hours prior to operation, the patient should ingest a few ounces of thick cream or have aqueous methylene blue introduced through a nasogastric tube. If the duct has been torn recently, a direct approach is indicated. If the tear cannot be found, it is best to dissect 2 or 3 centimeters above the diaphragm. In this location the thoracic duct lies anterior to the vertebrae, deep to the esophagus and just to the right of the aorta, and usually in front of the right intercostal arteries. Operation ordinarily is on the side of the chylothorax. In bilateral effusions, thoracotomy can be done on the right side with confidence. Complete division and double ligation with nonabsorbable sutures is usually successful.

ACKNOWLEDGEMENTS

I am indebted to Livia Ross, M.D., Anatomic Pathologist, Department of Pathology, Highland General Hospital, Oakland, California, for her expert assistance in developing some of the histopathological aspects of hemoorganization. In particular she has demonstrated, by special elastic staining, the existence of elastic tissue fibers just beneath the parietal pleural mesothelium; this has been especially valuable.

I am further indebted to Mr. Carl Stevenson, Medical Photographer, Audio Visual Department, Highland General Hospital, for the excellence of the reproductions of the photographs and art work.

REFERENCES

1. Arom KV, Grover FL, Richardson JD, et al: Posttraumatic empyema. Ann Thorac Surg 23: 254, 1977
2. Barrett NR: The pleura. Thorax 25:515, 1970
3. Beall AC, Crawford HW, DeBakey ME: Considerations in the management of acute traumatic hemothorax. J Thorac Surg 52:351, 1966
4. Black LF: The pleural space and pleural fluid. Mayo Clin Proc 47:493, 1972
5. Bower GC: Chylothorax. Dis Chest 46:464, 1964

6. Burford TH, Parker EF, Samson PC: Early pulmonary decortication in the treatment of posttraumatic empyema. Ann Surg 122:163, 1945

7. Bessone LN, Ferguson TB, Burford TH: Chylothorax (collective review). Ann Thorac Surg 12:527, 1971

8. Culliner MM, Roe BB, Grimes OF: The early elective surgical approach to the treatment of traumatic hemothorax. J Thorac Surg 38:780, 1959

9. DeLorme E: Nouveau traitement des empyemes chroniques. Gaz Hop (Paris) 67:94, 1894

10. DeLorme E: Du traitement des empyemes chroniques par la decortication du poumon. Dixieme Congres Francais de Chirurgie, 1896, p 379

11. Dugan DJ, Samson PC: Surgical significance of the endothoracic fascia. Am J Surg 130:151, 1975

12. Engevik L: Traumatic chylothorax. Scand J Thorac Cardiovasc Surg 10:77, 1976

13. Fowler GR: A case of thoracoplasty for the removal of a large cicatricial fibrous growth from the interior of the chest, the result of an old empyema. Med Rec 44:838, 1893

14. Goorwitch J: Traumatic chylothorax and thoracic duct ligation. J Thorac Surg 29:467, 1955

15. Gotsman MS: Chylothorax after closure of a patent ductus arteriosus. Thorax 21:129, 1966

16. Harken DE: A review of the activities of the thoracic center for the III and IV hospital groups. 160th General Hospital, ETO June 10, 1944 to January 1, 1945. J Thorac Surg 15:31, 1946

17. Hughes RK: Thoracic trauma (collective review). Ann Thorac Surg 1:778, 1965

18. Johnson J: Battle wounds of the thoracic cavity. Ann Surg 123:321, 1946

19. Jones RJ, Samson PC, Dugan DJ: Current management of civilian thoracic trauma. Am J Surg 114:289, 1967

20. Lampson RS: Traumatic chylothorax. J Thorac Surg 17:778, 1948

21. Langston HT, Tuttle WM: The pathology of chronic traumatic hemothorax. J Thorac Surg 16:99, 1947

22. Lilienthal H: Empyema. Ann Surg 62:309, 1915

23. Lindskog GE, Liebow AA, Glenn WWL (eds.): Thoracic and Cardiovascular Surgery, Vol 2. New York, Appleton-Century-Crofts, 1962, p 8

24. Maloney JV, Spencer FC: The nonoperative treatment of traumatic chylothorax. Surgery 40:121, 1956

25. Samson PC, Burford TH: Total pulmonary decortication. J Thorac Surg 16:127, 1947

26. Samson PC, Burford TH, Brewer LA, III, et al: The management of war wounds of the chest in a base center. J Thorac Surg 15:1, 1946

27. Samson PC, Merrill DL, Dugan DJ, et al: Technical considerations in decortication for the pleural complications of pulmonary tuberculosis. J Thorac Surg 36:431, 1958

28. Selle JG, Snyder WH, Schreiber JT: Chylothorax—indications for surgery. Ann Surg 177:245, 1973

29. Shackelford RT, Fisher AM: Traumatic chylothorax. South Med J 31:766, 1938

30. Tuttle WM, Langston HT, Crowley RT: The treatment of organizing hemothorax by pulmonary decortication. J Thorac Surg 16:117, 1947

31. Valle AR: Management of war wounds of the chest. J Thorac Surg 24:457, 1952

32. Ware MW: The trend of surgery in empyema of the thorax. Ann Surg 65:320, 1917

33. Webb WR: Thoracic trauma. Surg Clin North Am 54:1185, 1974

34. Williams KR, Burford TH: The management of chylothorax related to trauma. J Trauma 3:317, 1963

7. INJURIES OF THE TRACHEA AND MAJOR BRONCHI

Harold C. Urschel, Jr.
Maruf A. Razzuk

Traumatic injury of the trachea and major bronchi mainly results from blunt trauma and penetrating wounds of the thorax. The occurrence of this injury offers a challenge in management in the patient with serious multiple injuries because of the added derangement in the cardiorespiratory dynamics. The priorities for treatment of the various injuries must be directed toward the correction of coexisting impaired ventilation and reduction of cardiac output [14, 24, 46, 53]. The immediate diagnosis and accurate assessment of the site and extent of the tracheobronchial injury and early treatment of it greatly reduce morbidity and permanent loss of pulmonary function.

Small tears can be effectively treated by means of tracheostomy, which reduces the air leak by preventing an increase of the intraluminal pressure. Rupture separation or large tears require early surgical repair and restoration of the integrity of the airway. Failure to perform early repair of such major injuries will result in the delayed sequelae of stenosis or atresia and in pulmonary disability. The process of healing by extensive fibrosis adds to the difficulty when surgical correction of the stenosis is delayed [39, 45].

MODES OF TRAUMA AND MECHANISM OF INJURY

Injury to the trachea and major bronchi is caused by a variety of traumatic mechanisms. Stab wounds and gunshot wounds produce penetrating injuries of the tracheobronchial tree and other adjacent organs that add to the complexity of the clinical condition [28, 49]. Blunt trauma [26] to the anterior chest wall causes injury to the trachea and bronchi as a result of associated rib injuries, secondary to a sudden high intraluminal pressure developing in the tracheobronchial tree when expiration occurs with the glottis closed [42] or from a shearing force generated by sudden compression and release of the resilient anterior chest wall, which compresses the trachea and main bronchi against the spine [44]. A sharp blow to the neck may cause avulsion of the larynx and cricoid cartilage from the trachea [1]. Other modes of injury include the violent backward fling of the head during an extremely strong cough to expel a foreign body [36], sudden overstretch of the trachea [36], explosion of anesthetic gases within the tracheobronchial lumen [45], overinflation of the balloon cuff of an intratracheal tube [13, 27], and direct blows to the cervical trachea [5, 9, 50]. It is of importance to determine the mode of trauma, because the site and extent of the injury to the tracheobronchial tree and associated structures are related to this mechanism. Multiple fractures or serious concomitant injuries to the head, great vessels, heart, or esophagus may also occur in association with injuries of the trachea and bronchi.

SURGICAL PATHOLOGY

The site and extent of injury of the trachea and bronchi are related to the nature of the trauma. In penetrating wounds, any part of the tracheobronchial tree can be involved by a single, tangential, or coupled wound, depending on the trajectory [49]. In closed trauma, the points most likely to be injured are the main bronchi or trachea at or within a few centimeters of the carina. The character of the lesion in closed injuries varies from small lacerations to extensive linear tears involving the trachea, main bronchi, and branch bronchi or to complete rupture separation. When frank rupture and separation of trachea or bronchus occur, continuity is often maintained by the loose peritracheal or peribronchial tissue [2]. Associated ruptures of parenchyma of the lung, large vessels of the hilus, or esophagus are less frequent complications of this type of injury.

Fewer than 50 cases of traumatic, nonpenetrating tracheoesophageal fistulas have been reported [4, 8, 29]. Most such injuries were of the "steering wheel type." The mechanism of injury is thought to be a compression of the trachea and esophagus between the sternum and the vertebral body. As a result, the trachea is partially lacerated but usually heals rapidly. The esophagus is damaged anteriorly, with impairment of its blood supply and subsequent necrosis of the contused area [26]. The site of injury is usually at the level of the carina in 57 percent, and in the cervical area of about 10 percent [4].

The late sequelae of partial rupture of a main bronchus are eventual chronic fibrous stricture, bronchopulmonary suppuration with saccular bronchiectasis, atelectasis, and fibrosis. In complete rupture separation with complete obstruction of a main bronchus, the tributary lung is totally atelectatic and unaffected. This favorable pathological condition offers the possibility of late reconstruction of the bronchus and reaeration of the lung. After a period of collapse as long as 15 years, some lungs have reexpanded after reconstruction, although others did not [7].

CLINICAL MANIFESTATIONS AND DIAGNOSIS

Injury to the trachea and major bronchi should be suspected in the patient who is seen with subcutaneous emphysema and cough, with or without airway difficulty, and with a penetrating wound or blunt trauma to the neck or chest. Hemoptysis, pneumothorax, and fractured rib may be present. The site of injury of the tracheobronchial tree, leakage of air, and amount of blood loss are the main factors that determine the characteristics of the early symptoms. The degree of respiratory distress and shock varies with the rate and amount of air and blood loss [42]. With small tears, the cough is hacking and nonproductive and subcutaneous emphysema is delayed. With extensive lacerations, severe cough with hemoptysis and massive mediastinal and cervical emphysema develops rapidly. In these instances dyspnea and cyanosis occur and are not relieved by oxygen treatment [45].

Rupture of the cervical trachea is attended by subcutaneous emphysema appearing in and spreading from the anterior aspect of the neck at any interval after local injury. Pain on swallowing, hoarseness, and hemoptysis are other characteristic features. Airway obstruction may or may not be present. Fractures of the larynx are likely to result in suffocation. Associated injuries to the cervical spine must be considered when the mode of injury is secondary to a direct blow to or violent extension of the neck, and concomitant esophageal injury must be ruled out [48]. Its recognition might not be possible until the third or fifth day following injury, however, where violent episodes of

coughing and choking occur when the patient drinks liquids. The sudden appearance of these symptoms should arouse suspicion of an existing tracheoesophageal fistula. Diagnosis is established by a barium swallow, and bronchoscopy and esophagoscopy should be performed to outline the location and extent of the fistula [26].

Mediastinal and suprasternal emphysema appear in the majority of patients with injuries of the thoracic trachea and major bronchi. The emphysema spreads rapidly into the neck and face and down the shoulders and chest. Xiphisternal crunch or Hamman's sign may be elicited [7]. If the mediastinal pleura ruptures either directly from the injury, as in gunshot wounds, or from its inability to withstand the pressure of leaking air, as in instances of blunt trauma, pneumothorax is immediately produced, tension pneumothorax develops, and dyspnea and respiratory distress follow. Occasionally the pneumothorax is bilateral. Rib fractures may not be present, particularly if the patient is under 20 years old. A progressive and uncontrollable tension pneumothorax is a cardinal sign of tracheal or bronchial rupture. Bleeding occurs in varying degrees; a tear of the bronchus may only result in mild to moderate hemoptysis and a cough with frothy sputum. Blood clots gravitating distally into the bronchial tree may contribute to atelectasis. Bleeding may occasionally be severe, particularly if one of the major pulmonary vessels is injured. As a result, a massive hemothorax and a varying degree of hemodynamic disturbance complicate the tension pneumothorax and the attending respiratory distress [42]. In closed trauma to the chest, the pulmonary vessels usually escape injury because of their resilience and low intraluminal pressure [7].

If the patient survives the initial stage of the acute injury without surgical treatment, symptoms of respiratory distress follow the tracheal injury in 7 to 10 days. This is due to the ingrowth of granulation tissue, displacement of tracheal wall segment, and surrounding hematoma. Reconstructive operation, rather than local excision of the granulation tissues, is indicated at this stage. If the lesion is in the main stem bronchus, atelectasis and mediastinal shift to the ipsilateral side occur. Simple dilatation is ineffective, and corrective surgery is indicated [42], otherwise stenosis will develop at the site of injury.

Partial rupture of a main stem bronchus will lead to bronchopulmonary suppuration, atelectasis, and fibrosis if the rupture goes untreated. In complete bronchial rupture, the tributary lung is atelectatic and uninfected and often is capable of circulatory and ventilatory function after being reexpanded. This has been observed experimentally and clinically for periods of time ranging from 2 months to 15 years [22, 23, 52]. The reexpanded lung seems to function better and physiological results are better if reconstruction is carried out earlier. Normal pulmonary function has been observed when reconstruction was performed 2 months after the initial injury [7]. Patients in whom reconstruction of the bronchus was performed 11 [41] or 15 years [43] later had less favorable results. Occasionally, the chronically atelectatic lung fails to reexpand after reconstruction and causes left-to-right intrapulmonary shunt. Under such circumstances, pneumonectomy is recommended [7].

FACTORS AFFECTING IMMEDIATE SURVIVAL

A crucial site of injury in the tracheobronchial tree, the development of severe tension pneumothorax, and massive bleeding and associated injuries significantly influence an early mortality rate. A higher early mortality rate has been reported in patients with injuries of the thoracic trachea than among those in whom the cervical trachea is injured. Patients who were alive on arrival at the hospital predominantly had cervical tracheal injuries, while among those who were dead on arrival the thoracic trachea was most frequently injured. Associated injuries tend to be less severe in more proximally located injuries of the tracheobronchial tree, with the esophagus being most commonly involved. When the thoracic trachea or main stem bronchi are injured, the aorta is the most commonly associated injured structure. When secondary or tertiary bronchi are involved, the heart is the most commonly associated injured organ. Patients with gunshot wounds accounted for the highest percentage of patients dead on arrival [16].

TREATMENT

It is of prime importance when serious injury occurs that prompt and careful assessment of the various injuries and a decision as to the priority for treatment be made. Immediate evaluation is made to determine the existence of airway obstruction, tension pneumothorax, massive bleeding, or open wounds of the chest. Diagnosis of these life-endangering conditions complicating the injury can usually be made from the history, physical examination, and roentgenograms of the chest. However, the presence of acute respiratory distress should preclude investigation and demand immediate tracheostomy. Ventilation should be assured and existing shock corrected. Tension pneumothorax should be treated by chest tube drainage into a waterseal bottle. If tension pneumothorax continues despite active suction, immediate bronchoscopy and thoracotomy should be performed, since continued pneumothorax usually denotes injury to the thoracic trachea and major bronchi. The ability to correct the pneumothorax and expand the lung with closed intercostal chest tube drainage does not rule out injury to the tracheobronchial tree, however [47]. Bronchoscopy is of paramount importance in establishing the site and extent of the injury. It should be performed in the operating room prior to thoracotomy.

In all patients requiring surgical reconstruction, excellent anesthesia is the sine qua non of success. Each operation requires the close cooperation of surgeon and anesthesiologist, and each technical maneuver and innovation should be a joint effort.

The management of tracheobronchial trauma varies with the extent of the injury. In patients with a small tear of the membranous or the cartilaginous portions, a tracheostomy without suture repair is usually sufficient, provided the lumen is not compromised. Tracheostomy helps prevent the increase of intraluminal positive pressure and minimizes the leakage of air through the tear. The tracheostomy tube can usually be removed in 4 to 6 days [47].

Large tears or rupture separation of the trachea and bronchi require surgical treatment. If the lesion is in the cervical trachea, varying degrees of airway obstruction may be present and may require urgent treatment and possibly tracheostomy. Airway obstruction is often absent, however, even in complete rupture, because the surrounding structures form a sufficiently rigid tube for ventilation to take place unless severe hemorrhage occurs. In this type of injury, it is desirable, if possible, to evaluate cord movements and the function of the recurrent laryngeal nerves before operation. In the absence of airway obstruction requiring immediate tracheostomy, bronchoscopy allows accurate assessment of the injury and aspiration of the air passages, and it should be performed when suspicion of rupture of the trachea exists. It may also be wise to perform an esophagoscopy [48]. Exposure of the injury can be made through a transverse cervical incision that can be extended down over the sternum to expose the superior mediastinum by an inverted T sternotomy [47]. If the tear is incomplete, it is repaired and tracheostomy performed. In instances of complete rupture separation, the distal portion of the severed trachea may retract into the mediastinum. The retracted segment is pulled up, the two ends of the trachea are anastomosed, and tracheostomy is performed [40].

Rupture separations and large tears of the thoracic trachea and major bronchi also require surgical reconstruction. These are approached through a right thoracotomy exposure by way of the fourth interspace or the bed of the resected fifth rib. When the left bronchus is injured, a left thoracotomy is required. Tracheostomy should be performed before the removal of the endotracheal tube and maintained for a minimum of 4 days [47].

The management of the late sequelae of untreated injuries poses a more difficult problem because of resultant fibrosis and the entrapment of vital structures such as the recurrent laryngeal nerves. An increasing number of late repairs are being successfully done.

Bronchial lesions are relatively easy to repair. The stenotic segment can be excised and the continuity of the airway reinstituted by end-to-end or end-to-side anastomosis, depending on the bronchus involved. If an infection is superimposed on the atelectatic lung, a lobectomy or pneumonectomy may be necessary [42].

Among the chronic sequelae of traumatic rupture of the cervical trachea is the development of subglottic stenosis. In the treatment of this condition, it is extremely important to accurately assess the function of the larynx. If the vocal cords are paralyzed in the median position, arytenoidopexy [10, 12, 25] is required to establish an adequate airway [39]. Reconstruction of the stenotic segment should be performed as a separate procedure. In subglottic stenosis, tomograms and posteroanterior projections of the larynx and adjacent trachea should be taken to delineate the relationship between the upper edge of the stenosis and the cricoid and thyroid cartilages.

If the cricoid cartilage is involved by the stenosis, it must be partially excised, leaving the signet ring portion behind the larynx [15]. Otherwise, it can be widened, after excision of the stenotic segment, by partial resection of the cricoid cartilage, a median incision in the thyroid cartilage, and suture of a wedge of the cricoid cartilage into the gap thus produced in the larynx. If the cricoid cartilage has been lost because of injury or infection, a piece of hyoid bone may be used. The larynx thus widened at the cricoid area is an excellent aperture for anastomosis to the lower tracheal segment [39].

A more recent approach described by Pearson [40] for cricoid stricture is to transect the airway obliquely, the incision starting at the inferior border of the thyroid cartilage in front and passing posteriorly and inferiorly to cross the lower margin of the cricoid plate below the already exposed recurrent laryngeal nerves (Figs 7-1, 7-2). This results in resection of the cricoid arch and portions of its posterior plate. In order to transect the airway at a higher level posteriorly, a rim of the cricoid subjacent to the posterior and lateral aspects of the submucosa and high superiorly almost to the vocal cords, if necessary, can be rongeured. Although this results in loss of external support to the mucous membrane, skeletal support can be provided in another way as discussed below. That

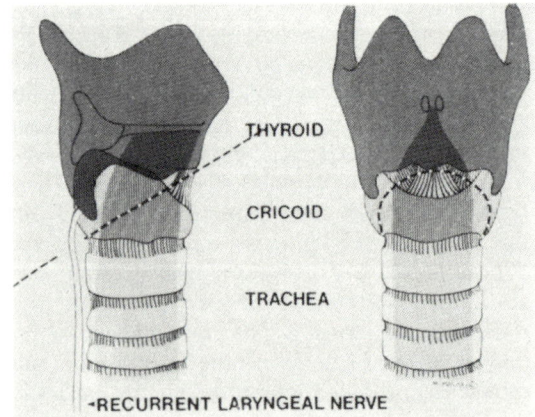

Fig 7-1. Diagram showing oblique resection line. The line begins anteriorly at the inferior border of thyroid cartilage in front and extends posteriorly and inferiorly to cross the lower border of the cricoid plate below the point of entry of the recurrent laryngeal nerves, which are already exposed. (From F. G. Pearson, Primary tracheal anastomosis after resection of the cricoid cartilage with preservation of recurrent laryngeal nerves, J Thorac Cardiovasc Surg 70:808, 1975. By permission.)

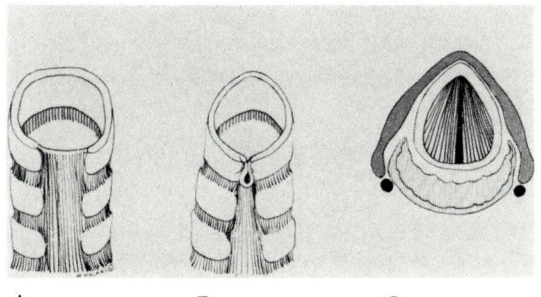

A   B   C

Fig 7-2. (A) Diagrammatic appearance of the distal tracheal resection line. The lumen is relatively larger than the subglottic lumen seen in (C). (B) Technique of plication of the membranous trachea at the distal resection line. This procedure approximates the ends of the uppermost tracheal ring and produces a complete circle of cartilage to replace the resected cricoid ring. The luminal diameter at the distal line is also reduced. (C) Diagrammatic appearance of the completed subglottic resection line seen in cross section. The vocal cords lie within 1 cm of the resection line. (From F. G. Pearson, Primary tracheal anastomosis after resection of the cricoid cartilage with preservation of recurrent laryngeal nerves, J Thorac Cardiovasc Surg 70:808, 1975. By permission.)

degree of cricoid resection makes it possible to divide the mucous membrane posteriorly at the level of the inferior border of the thyroid cartilage within 1 cm of the vocal cords. When reconstructing the continuity of the airway, the discrepancy of the distal trachea, which is larger than the proximal subglottic resection line, is corrected by plication of the membranous trachea. This maneuver decreases the luminal diameter of the trachea so that it will more readily fit the subglottic diameter. Furthermore, a complete cartilaginous ring has been created at the distal resection line. When anastomosed to the cuff of the mucous membrane at the proximal resection line, this ring restores the skeletal support previously provided by the cricoid cartilage.

If the inferior extent of the stenosis is above the sternal notch, a cervical approach through a collar incision will provide good exposure. Circumferential dissection is done only at, and immediately above and below, the stenotic segment to be excised. Care should be taken to avoid injury to the esophagus and the recurrent laryngeal nerves. In reestablishing the continuity of the trachea with a primary end-to-end anastomosis, excessive tension on the suture line should be avoided, since this is the major cause of recurrence of stricture [6, 17]. This can be overcome by mobilizing the trachea and carina through a median sternotomy, if needed, and performing laryngeal release with division of the thyrohyoid muscles, the superior horn of the thyroid cartilage, and the thyrohyoid membrane (Fig 7-3). The division of these major attachments of the larynx permits it to drop 2.5 cm; the technique is feasible if the resected segment does not exceed 4 cm in length [15]. If the stenotic segment extends below the sternal notch or access through the cervical exposure is difficult, the sternum should be divided to avoid injury to the innominate artery or compromise of a meticulous anastomosis [19] (Fig 7-4).

Loss of length may result when there is rupture separation of the trachea with chronic retraction. Length may be gained by mobilizing the trachea and performing laryngeal release. If the loss of length is marked, however, a staged procedure to promote lengthening of the retracted intercartilaginous ligaments can be performed, or when the disparity is marked, an airtight prosthesis to reconstitute the continuity of the trachea can be used [30, 39]. The Neville prosthesis [37, 38] (Figs 7-5, 7-6) has been used in patients with tracheal strictures and carcinoma, with a five-year survival in some cases being reported.

In cases of cervicomediastinal reconstruction, the innominate artery invariably traverses the graft. It is recommended that a cuff of Dacron and pericardium be interposed between the graft and the innominate artery to prevent erosion of the latter [39]. We have found that this technique is not totally adequate in preventing this complication. An alternate preventive measure is to divide the innominate artery from the aorta and reimplant it, with prosthetic vascular extension, on the ascending aorta.

In other cases of tracheal stenosis in which resection and reconstruction are contraindicated because of cardiorespiratory failure or in which surgical dissection is hazardous, a Montgomery tracheal T-tube can be used [3, 32] (Fig 7-7). A Montgomery tube is a good alternative for maintaining adequate airway [30–35]. The tube has a side arm and comes in a number of sizes. It is inserted through the tracheostomy opening or the site of the disrupted anastomosis and is positioned endotracheally with the upper arm below the vocal cords and the side arm protruding to the outside through the skin.

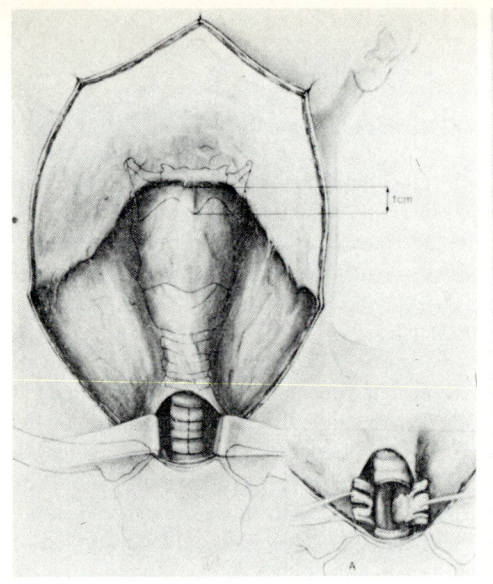

A

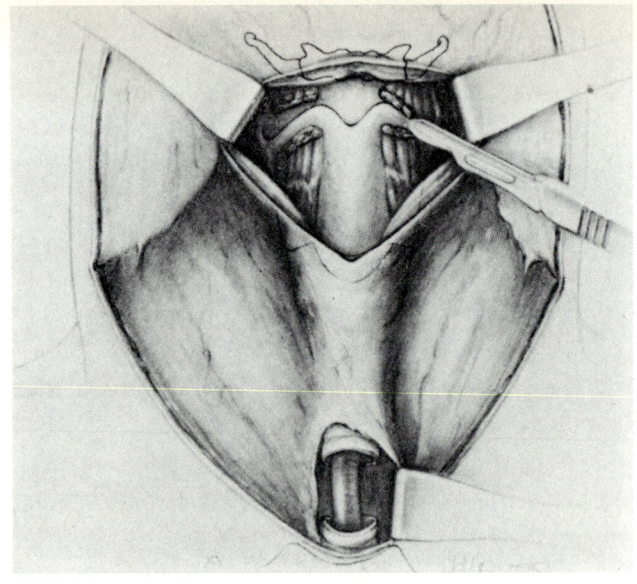

B

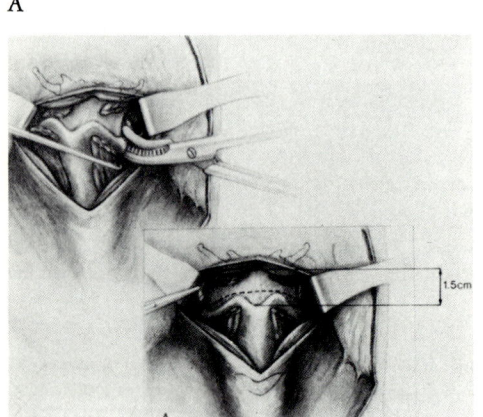

C

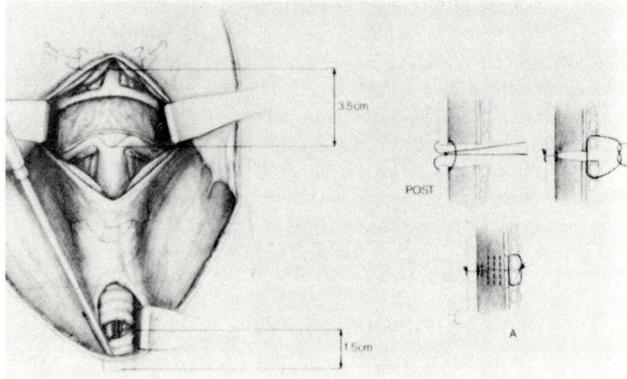

D

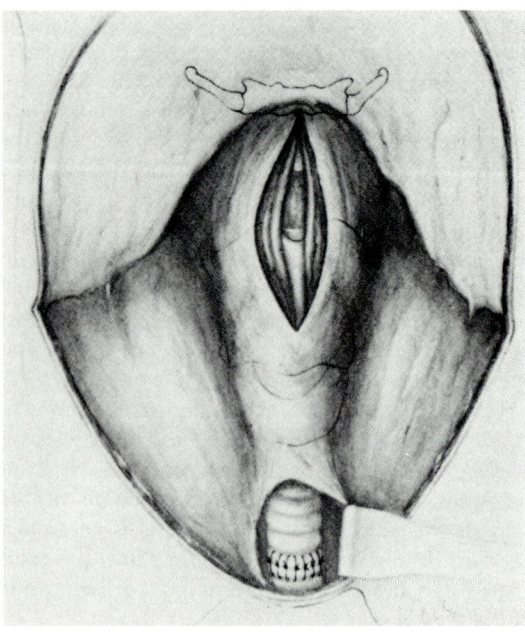

E

Fig 7-3. *Reestablishing continuity of the trachea.
(A) The tracheal stenosis is exposed through a collar incision and the upper flap of the incision is developed to expose the hyoid-thyroid area.* Inset A *shows resection of stenosed segment. (B) Division of thyrohyoid muscles. The sternohyoid and omohyoid muscles are retracted and preserved because of their downward pull on the hyoid bone. (C) Division of superior cornua. In* Inset A *division of thyrohyoid muscle and superior cornua drops larynx 0.5 cm. (D) Division of thyrohyoid membrane drops larynx an additional 2 cm. Mediastinal dissection of distal trachea had mobilized the distal segment for about 1.5 cm.* Inset A *shows details of suturing. (E) Completed tracheal anastomosis.
(From H. H. Dedo,* Laryngeal release and sleeve resection for tracheal stenosis, *Ann Otol Rhinol Laryngol 78:285, 1969. By permission.)*

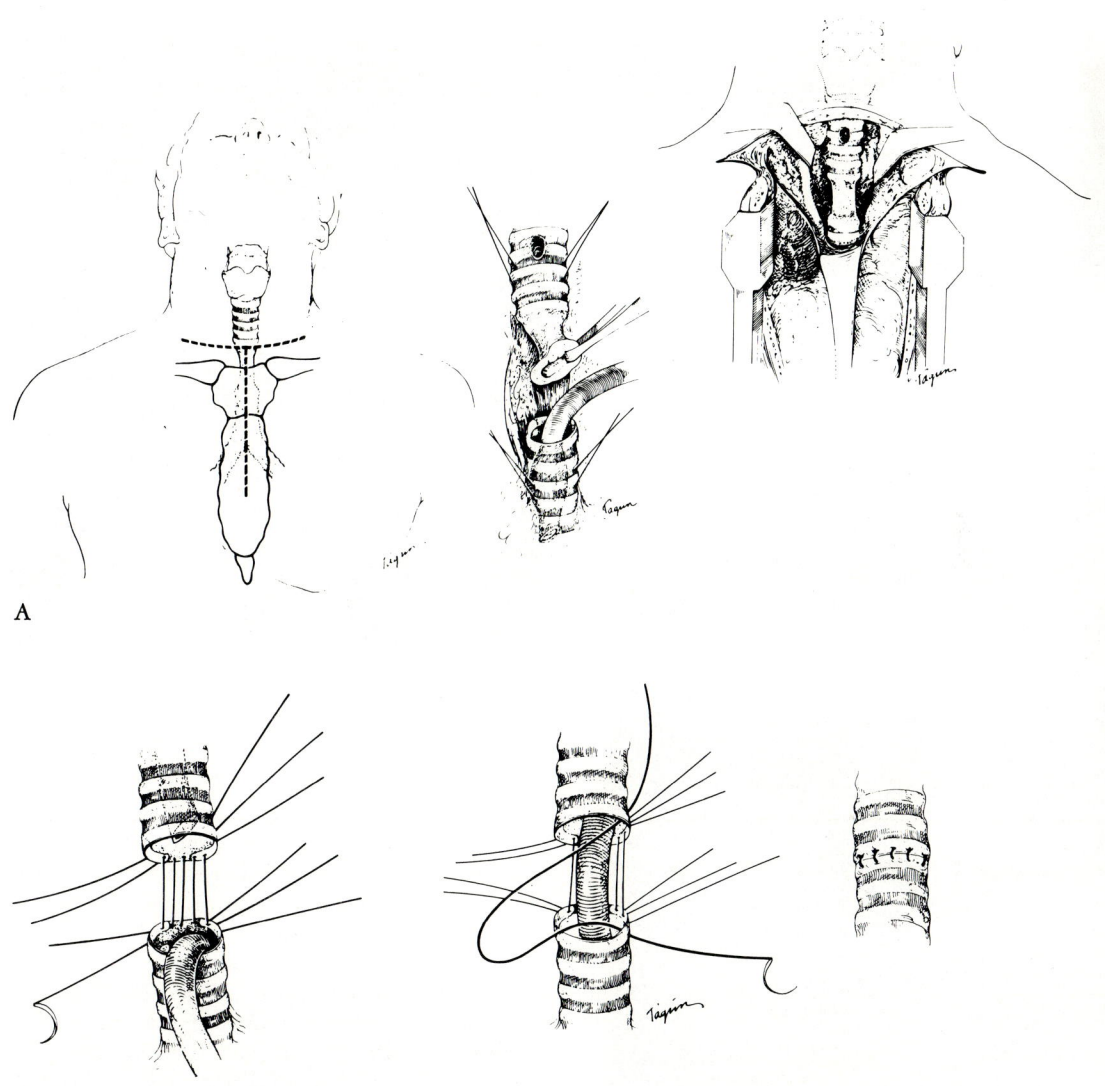

Fig 7-4. (A) Exposure of the tracheal stenosis through a collar incision permits exploration and, in many cases, reconstruction. Division of the sternum widens the access for lower or more difficult lesions. The trachea is divided below the stenosis and a sterile endotracheal tube is inserted in the distal segment for ventilation. (B) Technique of anastomosis. (From H. C. Grillo, Surgery of the Trachea. In Current Problems in Surgery. Copyright © 1970, Year Book Medical Publishers, Inc. Used by permission.)

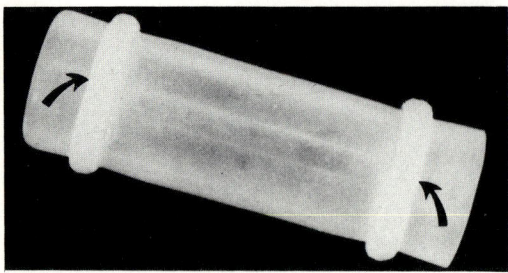

Fig 7-5. Neville silicone prosthesis with sewing rims (arrows).

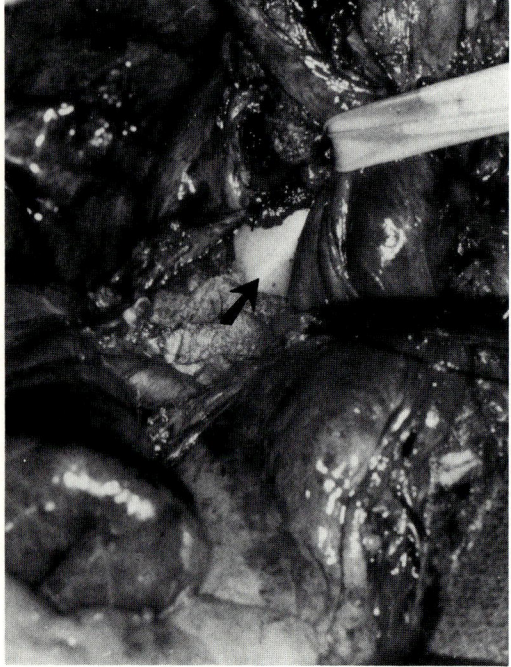

Fig 7-6. Neville prosthesis sutured to the thoracic trachea (arrow).

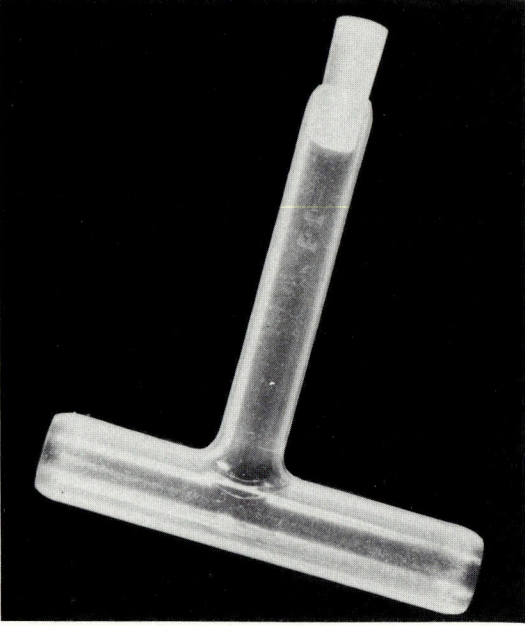

Fig 7-7. Montgomery endotracheal stent with side arm.

In late stenosis of the thoracic trachea, the lesion is usually located close to the carina and extends over a distance of 1 to 2 cm. Resection of the stenotic area and end-to-end anastomosis can be achieved through a right thoracotomy with the patient in the lateral or prone position. Length can be gained by mobilizing the trachea, the hilus of the right lung, and the pulmonary vessels from the pericardium and by dividing the right pulmonary ligament [21].

The anesthetic management of patients during tracheal resection requires certain technical maneuvers for the purpose of maintaining the patient in a continuous physiological balance, thus avoiding compromised reconstruction because of undue urgency. Dissection of the distal end of the stenotic segment should be performed first so that control of the airway can be secured safely at any moment. The trachea is divided just below the stenosis, and the distal segment is then intubated through the operative field with a sterile cuffed endotracheal tube. This establishes a circuit that bypasses the original endotracheal tube. Following excision of the affected segment, the anastomosis is reconstructed; ventilation is maintained through the bypass circuit until its endotracheal tube begins to hamper suturing. At this point, the latter endotracheal tube is removed, and the operation is completed with ventilation through the original oral tracheal tube after it is advanced in the trachea across the anastomosis. In lower tracheal lesions, the distal tracheal stump may be too short to hold an endotracheal tube. In such instances, the endotracheal tube of the bypass circuit is advanced into the left main stem bronchus, since lesions in this area are approached through a right thoracotomy. Ventilation is carried out with the

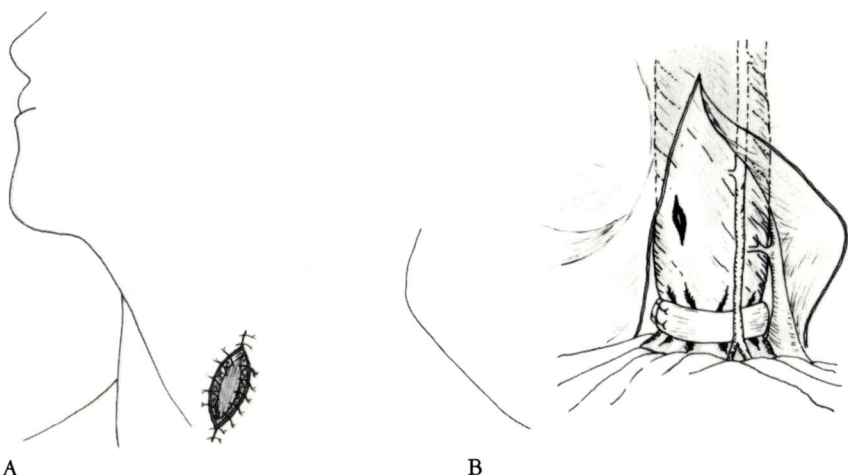

A   B

Fig 7-8. (A) Cervical esophagostomy in continuity sutured to subcutaneous tissue and skin. (B) Ligature is placed on the esophagus above the cardia, below the perforation, and deep to the vagus nerve.

left lung, and the principles of reconstruction remain unchanged [18, 20].

MANAGEMENT OF TRACHEOESOPHAGEAL FISTULA

Operative closure of the fistula should be carried out once the diagnosis is made and the patient's condition permits surgical intervention. Fistulas above the clavicle are repaired through a cervical approach, while intrathoracic fistulas are corrected through a right thoracotomy. The fistula is divided and suture closures of the esophageal and tracheal defects are affected. A pleural flap or pedicle of intercostal muscle should be interposed between the esophagus and trachea [26]. If severe mediastinal infection is present, a primary suture repair is precluded, and esophageal exclusion and diversion in continuity with chest drainage and gastrostomy for feeding should be performed [51] (Fig 7-8).

SUMMARY

Injuries to the trachea and bronchi are sustained as a result of blunt trauma to the neck or chest. These injuries should be suspected in patients who are first seen with subcutaneous emphysema and cough, with or without airway difficulty. Hemop-

tysis, pneumothorax, and fractured ribs may be present. In general, the characteristics of the early symptoms are determined by the degree of air leak and the amount of blood loss. Diagnosis can be established by history, physical examination, and roentgenograms of the chest.

The early recognition and prompt institution of therapeutic measures greatly reduce mortality and morbidity rates. Initial management is intended to correct the cardiorespiratory derangements, which should preclude any delaying diagnostic procedures. Tracheostomy is often life-saving and should be utilized early rather than late. Treatment of the tracheobronchial injuries varies with the nature of the lesion. Small tears can be treated by tracheostomy. On the other hand, rupture separation or large tears require early surgical treatment. Failure to perform early reconstruction of major injuries results in stenosis and loss of pulmonary function.

The management of chronic sequelae is a difficult problem due to entrapment of vital structures by the fibrosis. Lesions of the cervical trachea are approached through a collar incision, and, if better exposure is necessary, the sternum should be divided. Lesions of the thoracic trachea and right bronchi are approached through a right thoracotomy, whereas a left thoracotomy is performed for left bronchial lesions. In reestablishing the continuity of the air passages by primary anastomosis, tension on the suture line should be avoided. Length can be obtained by (1) performing a laryngeal release; (2) mobilizing the trachea, the hilus of the lung, and the pulmonary vessels, and (3) dividing the pulmonary ligament.

Good anesthetic management is of prime importance in a successful reconstruction. After interrupting the airway in the process of removing the stenosis, intubation with a second, sterile endotracheal tube ensures continuous ventilation and anesthesia.

REFERENCES

1. Ashbaugh D, Gordon J: Traumatic occlusion of the trachea associated with cricoid fracture. J Thorac Cardiovasc Surg 69:800, 1975
2. Battersby JS, Kilman JW: Traumatic injuries of the tracheobronchial tree. Arch Surg 88:644, 1964
3. Bergstrom B, Ollman B, Lindholm CE: Endotracheal excision of fibrous tracheal stenosis and subsequent prolonged stenting. Chest 71:6, 1977
4. Braun RA, Goldwater RR, Flores LM: Cervical tracheal transection with esophageal fistula. Arch Otolaryngol 96:67, 1972
5. Butler RM, Moser F: The padded dash syndrome: blunt trauma to the larynx and trachea. Laryngoscope 78:1172, 1968
6. Cantrell JR, Folse JR: The repair of circumferential defects of the trachea by direct anastomosis: experimental evaluation. J Thorac Cardiovasc Surg 42:589, 1961
7. Carter R, Wareham EE, Brewer LA, III: Rupture of the bronchus following closed chest trauma. Am J Surg 104:177, 1962
8. Chapman W, Braun R: The management of traumatic tracheo-esophageal fistula caused by blunt chest trauma. Arch Surg 100:681, 1970
9. Chavez CM, Anas P, Conn JH: Surgical approach to the injuries of the cervical trachea. South Med J 65:659, 1972
10. Clerf LH: The surgical treatment of bilateral posticus paralysis of the larynx. Laryngoscope 60:142, 1950
11. Clerf LH: Paralysis of the larynx of peripheral origin. Acta Otolaryngol 43:108, 1953
12. Clerf LH: Unilateral vocal cord paralysis. JAMA 151:900, 1955
13. Counot J, Santy P: Rupture of the trachea during anesthesia with intubation by balloon tube. Lyon Chir 50:104, 1955
14. Creech O Jr., Pearce C: Stab and gunshot wounds of the chest: diagnosis and treatment. Am J Surg 105:469, 1963
15. Dedo HH, Fishman NH: Laryngeal release and sleeve resection for tracheal stenosis. Ann Otol Rhinol Laryngol 78:287, 1969
16. Ecker RR, Libertini RV, Rea WJ, et al: Injuries of the trachea and bronchi. Ann Thorac Surg 11:289, 1971
17. Ekestrom S, Carlens E: Teflon prosthesis in tracheal defects in man. Acta Chir Scand 245:71, 1959
18. Geffin B, Bland J, Grillo HC: Anesthetic management of tracheal resection and reconstruction. Anesth Analg (Paris) 48:884, 1969
19. Grillo HC: Circumferential resection and reconstruction of the mediastinal and cervical trachea. Ann Surg 162:374, 1965
20. Grillo HC: Surgery of the trachea, in Current Problems in Surgery. Chicago, Year Book, 1971
21. Grillo HC, Bendixen HH, Gephart T: Resection of the carina and lower trachea. Ann Surg 158:889, 1963
22. Hodes PJ, Johnson J, Atkins JP: Traumatic bronchial rupture with occlusion. Am J Roentgenol 60:448, 1948
23. Holinger PH, Zoss AR, Johnston KC: Rupture of bronchus due to external chest trauma. Laryngoscope 53:817, 1948
24. Hopkins RW, Simeone FA: Early management of the patient with multiple injuries. Ohio State Med J 55:1094, 1959
25. King BT: New and function-restoring operation for bilateral abductor cord paralysis. JAMA 112:814, 1939
26. Kirsh MM, Orringer MB, Behrendt DM, et al: Management of tracheobronchial disruption secondary to nonpenetrating trauma. Ann Thorac Surg 22:93, 1976
27. Konig G, Hackel H: Tracheal rupture by an inflated rubber cuff. Arch Ohren- Nasen- Kehlkopfh 17:251, 1958
28. May M, Chadaratana P, West JW, et al: Penetrating neck wounds: selective exploration. Laryngoscope 85:57, 1975
29. Michelson E, Rogue AH: Cervical tracheoesophageal fistula due to steering wheel injury. Ann Thorac Surg 5:178, 1968
30. Montgomery WW: Reconstruction of the cervical trachea. Ann Otol Rhinol Laryngol 73:5, 1964
31. Montgomery WW: T-tube tracheal stent. Arch Otolaryngol 82:320, 1965
32. Montgomery WW: The surgical management of supraglottic and subglottic stenosis. Ann Otol Rhinol Laryngol 77:534, 1968
33. Montgomery WW: Surgery of the Upper Respiratory System, Vol 2. Philadelphia, Lea & Febiger, 1973
34. Montgomery WW: Posterior and complete laryngeal (glottic) stenosis. Arch Otolaryngol, 98:170–5, 1973
35. Montgomery WW: Silicone tracheal T-tube. Ann Otol Rhinol Laryngol 83:71, 1974

36. Nach RL, Rothman M: Injuries to larynx and trachea. Surg Gynecol Obstet 76:614, 1943
37. Neville WE, Bolanowski PJP, Soltanzadeh H: Prosthetic reconstruction of the trachea and carina. J Thorac Cardiovasc Surg 72:525, 1976
38. Neville WE, Hamouda F, Andersen J, et al: Replacement of the intrathoracic trachea and both stem bronchi with a molded silastic prosthesis. J Thorac Cardiovasc Surg 63:569, 1972
39. Paulson DL, Shaw RR: Injuries of the trachea and bronchi, in The Craft of Surgery. Boston, Little, Brown and Co., 1964. Pp. 311–319.
40. Pearson FG, Goldberg M, DaSilva AJ: A prospective study of tracheal injury complicating tracheostomy with a cuffed tube. Ann Otol Rhinol Laryngol 77:867, 1968
41. Peters RM, Loring WE, Sprunt WH, et al: Traumatic rupture of the bronchus: clinical and experimental study. Ann Surg 148:871, 1958
42. Richards V, Cohn RB: Rupture of the thoracic trachea and major bronchi following closed injury to the chest. Am J Surg 90:253, 1955
43. Samson PC, Brewster PA, Burbank B: Immediate care of the wounded thorax. JAMA 129:607, 1945
44. Schonberg S: Bronchial rupturen bei Thorax-Kompression. Berl Klin Wochenschr 49:2218, 1912
45. Shaw RR, Paulson DL, Kee JL: Traumatic tracheal rupture. J Thorac Cardiovasc Surg 42:281, 1961
46. Shires GT: Care of the Trauma Patient. New York, McGraw-Hill, 1966. Pp. 312–353.
47. Simeone FA: Shock and its treatment. Conn Med 27:79, 1963
48. Soothill EF: Closed traumatic rupture of the cervical trachea. Thorax 15:89, 1960
49. Symbas PN, Hatcher CR, Boehm GAW: Acute penetrating tracheal trauma. Ann Thorac Surg 22:473, 1976
50. Thomas RJ: Rupture of the cervical trachea. Med J Aust 1:415, 1972
51. Urschel HC Jr., Razzuk MA, Wood RE, et al: Improved management of esophageal perforation: exclusion and diversion in continuity. Ann Surg 179:587, May, 1974
52. Webb WR: Initial management of the patient with a chest injury. J La State Med Soc 116:1, 1964
53. Webb WR, Burford TH: Studies of the reexpanded lung after prolonged atelectasis. Arch Surg 54:801, 1952

8. MECHANICAL AIDS FOR MANAGEMENT

T. J. Gallagher
J. M. Civetta

Chest-related trauma may involve mechanical as well as specific organ dysfunction. Numerous technical devices are available to aid thoracic trauma management. Appropriate selection and skillful use of these devices can markedly influence morbidity, mortality, and recovery time. The etiology and appropriate treatment of hypoxemia related to chest trauma will be discussed, followed by a discussion of mechanical ventilation, including ventilator flow patterns and various ventilator types. The final section is devoted to specialized mechanical problems such as bronchopleural fistula and independent lung ventilation.

AIRWAY MAINTENANCE

Airway integrity is always a primary concern. Major chest trauma may involve the extrathoracic airway.

A fractured larynx or trachea often results from blunt traumas such as steering wheel injuries. Although uncommon, mainstem bronchus disruption can occur from this type of accident. Occlusion secondary to soft tissue swelling or hematoma formation may also result after blunt or penetrating trauma.

Airway maintenance cannot be left to chance; if there is any doubt, intubation should be carried out immediately. The choice of oral or nasal intubation is usually at the discretion of the person performing the procedure. Nasal intubation should be avoided if there are maxillary fractures, since the risk of sinusitis is increased. Mandibular fractures may be further disrupted or the mandibular artery damaged during oral intubation. Obviously, securing the airway takes precedence over all other considerations.

Fiberoptic bronchoscopy can be beneficial if intubation is especially difficult [33]. Once the larynx is identified, the endotracheal tube can be passed over the bronchoscope and into position. Transtracheal cannulation with a 14-gauge catheter can be lifesaving if obstruction precludes intubation. Ventilation can then be effectively carried out by jet insufflation [25].

Tracheostomy is indicated only if intubation is impossible. The major problem associated with endotracheal intubation is laryngeal injury [36]. Most damage occurs during the first 48 hours of intubation; thereafter, tracheostomy has no advantage and many disadvantages. Tracheostomy is by no means a minor procedure. Like any operation, it has a very definite mortality and morbidity [8]. Associated complications include infection, profound bleeding, nerve injury, pneumothorax, and tracheal stenosis. Hyperalimentation is now common therapy for critically ill patients [1]. The majority of hyperalimentation line placements are through the subclavian or internal jugular vein. These sites are then prone to contamination by continued tracheal secretions. For all these reasons, tracheostomy is usually reserved until late in the patient's course.

Evidence suggests that nasal or oral endotracheal tube placement is safe for 10 to 14 days without any increase in laryngeal injuries [9]. Tracheal wall injuries, including stenosis, fistula, and malacia, are cuff-related injuries. Therefore tracheostomy offers no greater protection than do endotracheal tubes.

The introduction of low-pressure, high-volume cuffs has significantly lowered the incidence of tracheal wall injuries [18]. Provided the tube is of proper size, cuff overdistention is not necessary. Lateral tracheal wall pressures above 20 mm Hg have been associated with injury. Increased cuff pressure is possible during nitrous oxide administration, and this should be considered after general anesthesia.

Extubation is performed only after all the conditions that require initial intubation have resolved. These include gastric distention or comatose states.

OXYGENATION

Trauma-induced respiratory failure has two components: failure of oxygenation and failure of ventilation. These two distinct entities each require specific treatment. If these differences are not recognized, treatment may not only be inappropriate but also detrimental.

Failure of oxygenation is common after chest trauma. Its clinical manifestations include cyanosis, tachypnea, and nasal flaring. Blood gas analysis provides the most sensitive discrimination. PaO_2 is low ($PaO_2 < 60$ mm Hg; $FIO_2 > 0.21$) and does not respond to increased inspired oxygen concentrations [2]. Hypercapnea is rare until the later stages of the disease. There may be few or no roentgenographic changes in the early stages.

The causes of respiratory failure include direct lung contusion as well as other associated major injuries. Aspiration of gastric contents, blood, or water can also precipitate respiratory failure. There is little evidence that hypovolemic shock alone can cause respiratory insufficiency; but the associated injuries responsible for the hemorrhage are the more likely culprits. There is no substantiation for the proposition that massive blood transfusion without micropore blood filters contributes to respiratory failure [14]. Available evidence does not support the presumption that balanced electrolyte infusions cause pulmonary dysfunction [40]. However, fluid overload is possible in patients with already compromised myocardial function.

The underlying pathological changes of acute respiratory failure (ARF) involve the alveolar capillary membrane and the interstitial space. Normally the Starling forces are balanced at the alveolar capillary membrane [31]. The capillary hydrostatic pressure and the interstitial fluid oncotic pressure act to direct fluid into the interstitial space. The capillary oncotic pressure and the interstitial hydrostatic pressure oppose that movement. The net result is a slight fluid flux through the junctional endothelial clefts that line the capillary. Once in the interstitium, the water moves to the central interstitial space, is drained by the lymphatics, and eventually returns to the central circulation [38].

While not completely understood, respiratory failure may result from disruption of these forces [34]. Either capillary pressure increases or alterations of pore size (increased permeability) can occur. The rate of water and protein flux across the alveolar capillary membrane then accelerates. Lymphatic flow can respond with a tenfold to twentyfold flow increase above baseline levels. However, if fluid flux rate is greater than can be removed by lymphatics, water and protein will soon accumulate in the interstitium.

Direct lung trauma causes hemorrhage and edema formation, also primarily in the interstitial space. The localized accumulation can affect gas exchange in the same manner as previously described.

A second possible safety mechanism is the interstitial space itself. Normally a potential rather than real space, there can be an 800 percent volume increase in the isolated dog-limb interstitial space without any elevation of hydrostatic pressure [19]. This may explain 30 percent lung water increases without any accompanying blood gas derangement.

Continued fluid accumulation can finally cause increased interstitial hydrostatic pressure. This pressure elevation can alter normal ventilation-perfusion relationship by narrowing or collapsing terminal airway units. Affected alveoli are relatively hypoventilated, yet perfusion remains intact. Blood coming from these units is poorly or incompletely oxygenated. When that blood combines with blood from other areas with normal oxygenation, the dilution decreases overall oxygen content. PaO_2 decreases and venous admixture (Qsp/Qt) or intrapulmonary shunt increases.

If the process continues unabated, alveolar flooding eventually results. It proceeds rapidly through interalveolar channels such as the pores of Kohn [35]. Surfactant is inactivated and the type II epithelial cells that manufacture it are destroyed. The increased surface tension forces, after surfactant destruction, contribute to alveolar instability. Alveolar volume decreases as documented by reduced functional residual capacity (FRC) [28]. Shunt and blood gas exchange further deteriorate.

When elevated, interstitial pressures prevent a transpulmonary pressure gradient during spontaneous ventilation sufficient to reexpand the narrowed or collapsed terminal airway segments. Instead, airway pressures above atmospheric pressure are required.

Positive pressure mechanical ventilation alone is unable to restore oxygenation. During a positive pressure breath the airway pressure exceeds the terminal airway unit's critical opening pressures. Gas can then flow to the previously poorly or nonventilated areas [26]. However, during exhalation, airway pressure returns to ambient pressure, falling below critical closing pressure, and hypoventilation and desaturation recur. Since the time of reexpansion is less than half of the entire inspiratory expiratory cycle, no lasting improvement in blood gas exchange can be expected.

If airway pressure remains positive during exhalation, then, conceivably, closing pressure will not be reached. This is precisely the role of positive end expiratory pressure (PEEP). It prevents terminal airway collapse after reexpansion and maintains patency. Oxygenation improves and venous admixture decreases [3].

Selection of a therapeutic end point is implied by PEEP usage. Varying with the practitioner, the goal may be oxygenation to a PaO_2 above 70 mm Hg while the patient is breathing less than toxic oxygen concentrations. Some advocate treating to the best compliance [32]. We prefer utilizing levels that restore or maintain intrapulmonary shunt at 15 percent or less [15]. Most authors have termed shunts higher than 15 percent as the onset of ARF [2]. Reduction to that level therefore seems reasonable. If mixed venous blood is not available for shunt calculation, the PaO_2/FIO_2 ratio can be used [20]. A ratio above 300 corresponds to a shunt of less than 15 percent. During periods of cardiovascular instability, this ratio is not reliable and should not be used.

Blood gas analysis provides the most reliable indication of respiratory failure. Therefore all chest trauma patients should be closely monitored. Treatment begins when the PaO_2 is less than 60 mm Hg ($FIO_2 > 0.21$). Obviously, other causes for a low PaO_2 have first been ruled out. These include reduced FIO_2, ventilator malfunction, pneumothorax, secretions, reduced cardiac output, and increased O_2 consumption.

When instituted, PEEP is added incrementally (3 to 5 cm H_2O) until the selected end point is reached. After each PEEP increase, equilibration should occur within 15 to 20 minutes; PEEP must be titrated just as any drug. Patient response is variable and not easily predictable. Minimal levels may be sufficient in some patients, while others may require significantly higher levels to attain the identical end point [23]. Resolution time does not seem related to eventual levels of PEEP employed.

After the appropriate PEEP level is instituted, that level should be maintained an arbitrary length of time. Again, this is variable and may be as short as 6 hours or as long as 24. In general, the longer

the time to optimal PEEP the longer the patient will remain at that level. Reduction occurs by the same incremental method, provided the shunt remains between 15 and 17 percent. Extubation is considered when spontaneous ventilation and an end expiratory pressure of 5 cm result in a shunt of 15 percent. Other extubation criteria, including airway maintenance, must also be considered.

The terms *PEEP* and *CPAP* often create confusion; the latter is applicable only during totally spontaneous ventilation. The baseline airway pressure is determined by expiratory positive airway pressure (EPAP). During spontaneous breathing, the baseline airway pressure has a negative deflection. However, that pressure never reaches ambient or subambient levels. The lowest inspiratory pressure is called the inspiratory positive airway pressure (IPAP) [39] (Fig 8-1). Airway pressure is positive during the entire respiratory cycle; hence the term *continuous positive airway pressure* [27].

PEEP is associated with both mechanical and spontaneous ventilation and means positive end expiratory pressure. During spontaneous breathing, at end inspiration, IPAP is ambient or subambient. When used during mechanical ventilation, PEEP refers to all positive expiratory pressures.

Fig 8-1. During continuous positive airway pressure (CPAP), airway pressure never reaches ambient. Hence inspiratory airway pressure is positive (IPAP). Positive end expiratory pressure (PEEP) implies positive pressure only during exhalation.

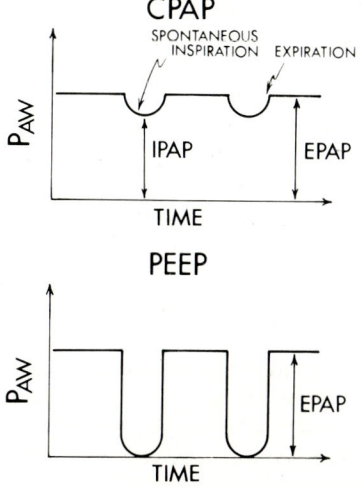

Cardiovascular insufficiency requiring hemodynamic monitoring is often present in patients with ARF. Additionally, the therapeutic interventions may contribute to cardiac depression. Then the intrapulmonary shunt (Qsp/Qt) determination best indicates respiratory function. A low or inadequate cardiac output results in a reduced mixed venous PO_2. This in turn causes lowering of the arterial PO_2 [21]. Increasing PEEP in these circumstances may further lower PaO_2. A pulmonary artery catheter provides access for mixed venous blood gas analysis, necessary for calculation of Qsp/Qt [5]; Qsp/Qt refers strictly to pulmonary function (ventilation-perfusion defects), and cardiovascular dynamics do not influence shunt determination. The catheter also permits accurate assessment of interrelated variables including preload, afterload, and contractibility.

ALVEOLAR VENTILATION

Ventilation is the physical movement of gas into and out of the lungs. Alveolar ventilation is the phase actually responsible for blood gas exchange. Arterial PCO_2 measurement clinically evaluates alveolar ventilation. The carboxyhemoglobin dissociation curve, unlike the oxyhemoglobin curve, is a straight line. Therefore arterial PCO_2 directly reflects alveolar ventilation. As ventilation decreases, PCO_2 increases; the converse is also true.

Alveolar hypoventilation is manifested by hypercapnea. The usual causes include airway obstruction, muscle relaxants, sedatives, head injuries, and cervical cord damage. Tension pneumothorax, hemothorax, or various combinations of these conditions can all result in increased PCO_2. Carbon dioxide retention is not present in early ARF, but can develop in the late terminal stages, concurrent with marked radiographic deterioration.

Appropriate therapy for alveolar hypoventilation includes intubation and mechanical ventilatory support. Central nervous system stimulants that increase minute ventilation have no role in this problem.

Mechanical Ventilators

After intubation, an appropriate ventilator and ventilatory pattern must be selected. Mechanical ventilators are classified according to the cycling mechanism as pressure-cycled, time-cycled, or volume-cycled ventilators.

A pressure-cycled machine delivers a mechanical breath until airway pressure reaches a predetermined level [22]. Inspiration then terminates and exhalation begins. The Bird Mark 7 is an example of a pressure-cycled ventilator.

Pressure-cycled ventilators are not suited for critically ill patients. As airway pressure increases, the machine gas flow rate decreases. The pressure-cycling mechanism operates at relatively low airway pressures, i.e., no more than 40 cm H_2O. Bucking, coughing, and decreased compliance all require high airway pressures to deliver the desired mechanical tidal volume. Therefore pressure-cycled mechanical machines may terminate inspiration before the desired tidal volume has been delivered to the patient. Since gas flow also decreases, breath-to-breath tidal volume may vary greatly. There is no guarantee of tidal volume consistency.

Most physicians have some knowledge of volume-cycled ventilators. A volume ventilator begins the exhalation mode after delivery of a preselected tidal volume [22]. Examples include the MA-1 and 2 and the Bear ventilator.

Despite changes in compliance or airway resistance the machine will deliver the desired tidal volume. The cost is an increase in peak airway inflation pressure. If compliance is a normal 100 ml/cm H_2O, then airway pressure will be 5 cm H_2O when the machine delivers 500 ml. If compliance worsened to 10 ml/cm H_2O, then the same tidal volume will generate a pressure of 50 cm/H_2O. In both cases the ventilator does deliver the 500 ml. However, the volume the patient actually receives may be less than that coming from the machine. Circuit compliance must be considered. Circuit compliance is usually 3 ml/cm H_2O. This means that a tidal volume of 15 ml will be lost whenever peak inflation pressure is 5 cm H_2O, whereas tidal volume is diminished by 150 ml whenever airway pressure is 50 cm/H_2O. Spirometers added to the exhalation limb do not detect this problem. Their measurement includes the volume lost in the circuit as well as that exhaled by the patient. Therefore alveolar volume is overestimated. Actual patient exhaled tidal volume must be measured at the airway.

At high airway pressures, gross performance alterations of volume ventilators may occur. Elevated back pressures much above 80 cm H_2O result in markedly decreased gas flow rates. Actual patient tidal volumes decrease, and eventually the machine may stall and fail altogether [17].

This discussion helps illustrate the overemphasis of tidal volume during mechanical ventilation. Even with a volume ventilator, the breath-to-breath patient volume, because of circuit compliance, will vary. Yet, despite these changes, there are usually no deleterious effects on the patient.

All volume ventilators have a secondary pressure-limiting feature. An overpressure governor is incorporated into the proximal circuit between patient and machine. This prevents the exceedingly high airway pressures that can result in barotrauma. When airway pressure reaches a preselected level, the valve opens, venting gas and preventing any further rise in airway pressure. Obviously, gas flow is no longer directed to the airway, and tidal volume will be affected.

Volume ventilators are popular for several reasons. Within the limits outlined, they are reliable, and the patient receives a tidal volume close to that indicated by the control settings. The controls are usually easy to understand. Once the ventilator is connected to a patient, very little readjustment is necessary unless lung mechanics markedly change [22].

Time-cycled, pressure-limited machines are the newest type of critical care ventilators. After a preselected interval, gas delivery is terminated and exhalation begins. Gas flow rate is also variable. Tidal volume is then a function of both inspiratory time and flow rate. For example, if gas flow is 250 ml per second and inspiratory time is 2 seconds, then after 2 seconds, when the ventilator cycles to exhalation, the tidal volume is 500 ml. If gas flow is 500 ml per second and inspiratory time is 1 second, tidal volume is still 500 ml. Most models have a wide performance spectrum. Flow rates are sufficiently high so that stalling will not occur at inflation pressures up to 180 cm H_2O. Tidal volume will be delivered despite markedly decreased compliance. In operation their performance is very similar to the volume ventilator.

Time-cycled and volume-cycled ventilators can usually be used interchangeably. However, in the 10 or 15 percent of patients with severe lung disease, the high performance characteristics of time-cycled equipment is preferred.

Recent work seems to indicate that gas flow rate and length of inspiratory time may also be important mechanical ventilatory factors. Evidence is accumulating that both alveolar ventilation and blood gas exchange can be affected by the ventilatory pattern [29]. Time-cycled ventilators are especially suited to altering these characteristics.

Ventilatory Modes

Once ventilation is indicated, an appropriate mode must be selected. Choices include controlled, assisted, or intermittent mandatory ventilation (IMV).

Controlled ventilation provides all the patient's minute ventilation. Tidal volume and rate are machine determined. There is no fresh gas flow; spontaneous breathing between mechanical breaths is not possible. (Spontaneous breaths are unsuccessful and result in breathing expired gases.) PCO_2 increases and the patient fights (bucks) the machine.

Sedation, paralysis, or hyperventilation in various combinations can usually eliminate spontaneous respiration. Hyperventilation to a PCO_2 of 30 to 32 mm Hg abolishes the ventilatory drive. However, the resultant respiratory alkalosis has several undesirable features. The incidence of cardiac arrhythmias increases and oxygen consumption rises markedly. The increased oxygen consumption combined with a low cardiac output can result in arterial desaturation. Also, alkalosis shifts the oxyhemoglobin dissociation curve to the left. The increased hemoglobin affinity for oxygen means less oxygen available for cellular uptake and utilization.

Paralysis and sedation have other practical and theoretical disadvantages. Neurological evaluation may be difficult or impossible. If accidental disconnection occurs, the patient will have no immediate means of ventilation. Also, without spontaneous respiration, respiratory muscle tone can be lost and weaning inordinately prolonged.

Assisted ventilation means that each spontaneous breathing effort triggers the ventilator to deliver a preselected mechanical tidal volume. As breathing rate increases, the number of breaths delivered by positive pressure also increases, and vice versa. When PCO_2 is low, the breathing slows until CO_2 reaccumulates. The result can be an alternating breathing pattern continued indefinitely.

Most assist mechanisms are difficult to use. They are either so sensitive that the slightest patient movement triggers the machine, or else so insensitive that a marked inspiratory effort is required. One theoretical benefit from assisted ventilation is that the spontaneous breathing activity preserves respiratory muscle tone.

CONTINUOUS FLOW IMV SYSTEM

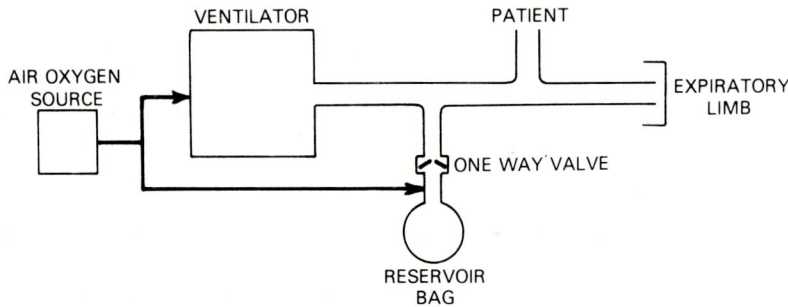

Fig 8-2. Fresh gas at same FIO_2 as to the ventilator flows continuously through the circuit at up to 15 liters per minute. The 5-liter anesthesia bag is a res- ervoir if spontaneous minute volume exceeds gas flow rate. The unidirectional valve closes during mechanical ventilation.

DEMAND VALVE IMV SYSTEM

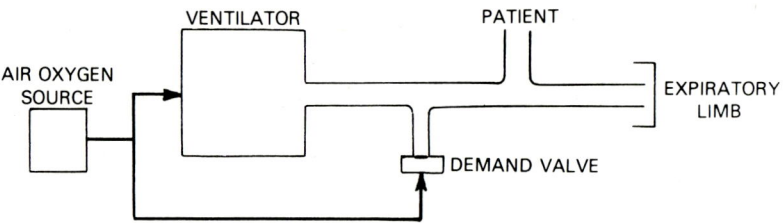

Fig 8-3. In demand valve circuitry there is no con- tinuous gas flow. When the patient initiates a spon- taneous breath, the valve opens and supplies fresh gas at up to 40 liters per minute for as long as the patient continues to breathe.

During assist-control ventilation the pattern is exactly as previously described for assisted ventila- tion. However, at predetermined intervals, a con- trolled positive pressure breath is also delivered. This provides a fail-safe system should spontane- ous breathing cease altogether.

Intermittent mandatory ventilation (IMV) is the newest ventilatory mode [11]. Originally pro- posed as a weaning technique, it is perhaps the most physiological method. The IMV circuit pro- vides for spontaneous ventilation between me- chanical breaths from the ventilator. Fresh gas with the same FIO_2 as the ventilator is delivered by one of two systems into the circuitry. One method utilizes continuous gas flow through a uni- directional valve (Fig 8-2). An anesthesia bag acts as a fresh gas reservoir if patient demand markedly increases. When the mechanical breath is delivered, the unidirectional valve isolates the alternate gas source. The second system employs a demand valve (Fig 8-3). Spontaneous breathing efforts open the valve, and fresh gas is supplied at up to 40 liters per minute. The patient utilizes whatever volume desired. The valve can be sensi- tized so that inspiratory effort can vary from mini- mal to maximal (Fig 8-4).

The patient on IMV usually provides most of the alveolar ventilation; the ventilator supplies the remainder. The mechanical rate employed is suffi- cient to maintain normal alveolar ventilation. The spontaneous ventilation eliminates fighting or buck- ing. Sedation and paralysis are usually not neces- sary. Similarly, hyperventilation with its attendant physiological derangements is not required. Spon- taneous respiration minimizes the danger to the patient if disconnection inadvertently occurs.

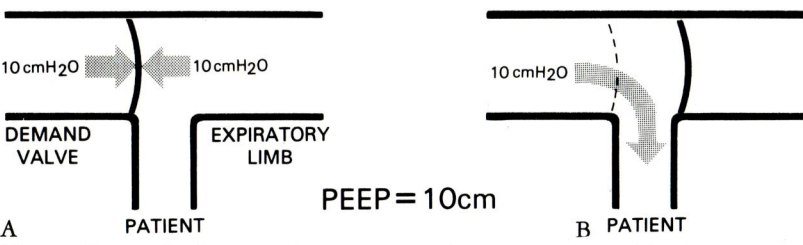

Fig 8-4. Demand valve operation. In part A the system has 10 cm H_2O pressure generated by PEEP. The valve is sensitized with 10 cm H_2O pressure. If spontaneous breathing lowers airway pressure by 1 cm, the value is no longer balanced and moves to the new position in B. Gas now flows to the patient. If the valve is pressurized to 6 cm H_2O, airway pressure would have to decrease to 5 cm H_2O before the valve opened.

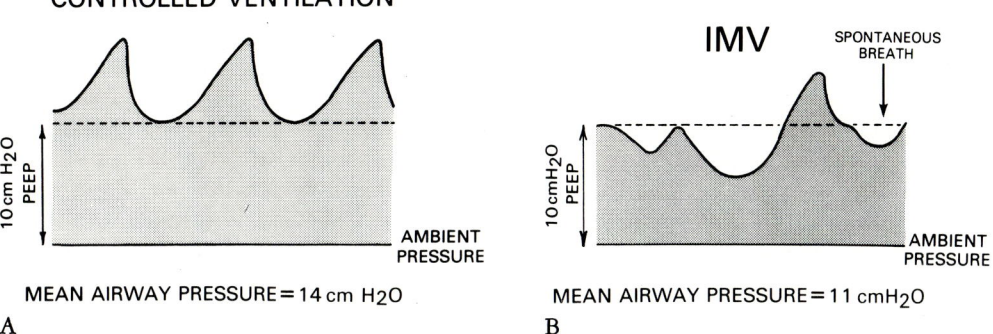

Fig 8-5. (A) During controlled ventilation with 10 cm H_2O, positive pressure ventilation results in a mean airway pressure of 14 cm H_2O. (B) Since IMV has fewer positive pressure breaths and more spontaneous breaths, mean pressure is less.

Intermittent mandatory ventilation can also promote optimal matching of ventilation and perfusion, thereby maximizing oxygenation. The low pressure pulmonary circulation distributes blood mainly to dependent lung areas. Both blood and lung tissue compress dependent alveoli. Their decreased volume shifts these regions lower on their compliance curve. Therefore they require less transpulmonary distending pressure than do their nondependent counterparts. They are thus preferentially filled first during spontaneous ventilation. The mixing of gas and blood in the same lung areas results in optimal matching of ventilation and perfusion.

During spontaneous breathing in the supine patient, the posterior or dependent diaphragm's radius of curvature is shortened. Therefore greater pressure changes and hence greater movement occur in that portion. This further promotes preferential filling of the dependent or posterior alveoli.

Paralysis has a different effect. The abdominal contents push up against the posterior diaphragm. Resistance to passive movement is increased in the dependent areas. Positive pressure ventilation will move the anterior, nondependent diaphragm more effectively. Ventilation is directed to the nondependent, relatively hypoperfused areas. The result is a ventilation-perfusion mismatch [12]. Intermittent mandatory ventilation optimizes ventilation and perfusion because most of the patient's breathing is spontaneous.

Mechanical ventilation can also cause cardiovascular depression. Figure 8-5 illustrates the airway pressure during controlled positive pressure ventilation with PEEP and during IMV. The mean airway pressure is the area under each curve. Note the differences between the two ventilatory modes. Compared with controlled ventilation, IMV with spontaneous breathing has a lower mean airway pressure. This reduction improves venous return to the heart, and stroke volume increases.

The pulmonary barotrauma incidence during

IMV and PEEP is the same as during controlled ventilation [4]. The same rationale that explains cardiac output enhancement applies. Pneumothorax during mechanical ventilation seems more related to mean airway and peak inflation pressure than to PEEP levels. Intermittent mandatory ventilation exposes the pulmonary parenchyma less often to the high inflation pressures that seemingly cause lung rupture.

The introduction of IMV and PEEP drastically altered the management of flail chest injuries. In flail chest the unstable chest wall moves inward during inspiration, preventing lung expansion. Hypoxia and arterial desaturation supposedly result. In the past, therefore, paralysis and controlled mechanical ventilation were utilized to prevent the flailing motion, thereby improving gas exchange. Treatment continued until the chest wall stabilized, usually in about 3 weeks.

The usual, slow mechanical ventilatory rate during IMV helped delineate the problem. As hypoxia developed after flail chest injury, PEEP was increased. Concurrently, the IMV rate was decreased, following the usual criteria. As long as PEEP prevented hypoxia, the flail motion was minimal [7]. Increasing or lowering the IMV rate had no effect on the flail motion. It became clear that hypoxia was due to the accompanying lung contusion and not to the flail itself. The paradoxical motion became markedly exaggerated during the hypoxia-induced hyperventilation. When PEEP restored oxygenation, hyperventilation and flailing stopped. Obviously, Trinkle et al. [37] were able to treat flail chest injuries without mechanical ventilation because there were no accompanying direct lung injuries.

Although originally proposed as a weaning modality, IMV has still not been shown to be any more effective than other conventional weaning methods. However, IMV simplifies nursing care during graduated removal from the ventilator.

Usually, discontinuation of controlled ventilation begins after various measurements are satisfactory. These may include vital capacity, negative inspiratory force, PaO_2, and the like. Conventional weaning maneuvers include short-term removal from the ventilator that has been supplying 100 percent of the ventilatory support. After a short time on a T-tube with no mechanical support, the patient is reattached to the machine. If all goes well, weaning proceeds, with continued intermittent removal from the ventilator for progressively longer periods. Eventually, weaning is completed. However, much valuable nursing time has been required.

Intermittent mandatory ventilation permits a smoother transition than does PEEP. The patient gradually assumes more of his or her own ventilatory support as the ventilator rate is incrementally decreased one to two breaths per minute each change. Criteria for IMV rate reduction include a $PaCO_2$ of 35 to 45 mm Hg, a pH > 7.35, and a spontaneous breathing rate less than 30 breaths per minute [15]. The selected PCO_2 range implies normal alveolar ventilation. A pH > 7.35 accounts for patients with chronic compensated hypercapnea. Despite elevated PCO_2 the normal pH implies adequate renal compensation. A respiratory rate greater than 30 breaths per minute indicates an increased work of breathing to normalize the other factors. The work of breathing is increased partly because exhalation changes from a passive to an active maneuver. In our experience with ARF, early treatment intervention with PEEP and IMV results in minimal mechanical ventilatory requirements. The IMV rate can usually be reduced within 24 hours to between 2 and 4 breaths per minute. Concomitantly, PEEP may still be increasing if oxygenation deteriorates further. Only in severe, late ARF are patients unable to excrete CO_2.

POSITIVE END EXPIRATORY PRESSURE VALVES

There are two different types of PEEP valves: threshold and flow resistors (Figs 8-6 and 8-7). A water column over a diaphragm is an example of a threshold-resistor PEEP device. Despite expiratory flow changes PEEP remains constant. Flow resistors alter the radius of the exhalation orifice and hence flow, causing PEEP to vary, depending on expiratory flow rate. If expiratory flow suddenly increases, flow resistor valves may deliver a higher PEEP than intended (Fig 8-8).

CHEST TUBES

We do not advocate prophylactic chest tube placement during PEEP therapy even if subcutaneous or mediastinal emphysema is present. A loculated pneumothorax can occur if the visceral pleura has adhered to the chest wall. When that area is not contiguous with the chest tube, drainage does not

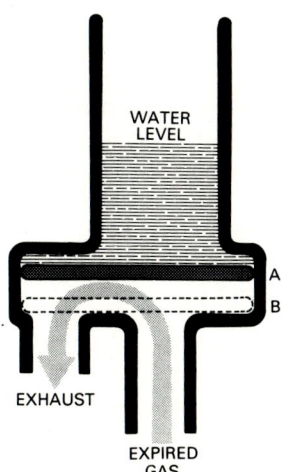

Fig 8-6. Threshold resistor: water column over a diaphragm. During exhalation, gas does not flow until the diaphragm moves from B to A. Pressure to move the diaphragm is just slightly greater than the water column (PEEP) pressure.

FLOW RESISTOR — PEEP

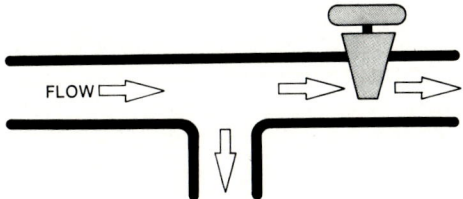

Fig 8-7. Flow resistor, PEEP. Expiratory/Pressure is inversely related to the size of the orifice.

occur. A new pneumothorax can develop, with both cardiovascular and pulmonary impairment. Additionally, fibrin or blood clots can impede chest tube function at any time.

CONTINUOUS POSITIVE AIRWAY PRESSURE MASK

A CPAP mask can sometimes simplify chest trauma management [24]. The anesthesialike mask is of soft, clear neoprene construction and fits snugly. Pressure is applied evenly over the face, making patient acceptance high. A continuous gas flow through a unidirectional valve, coupled with a PEEP device, maintains the desired end expiratory

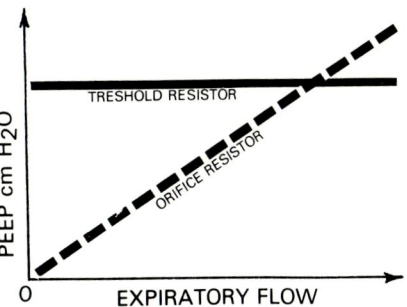

Fig 8-8. A flow resistor varies PEEP in proportion to expiratory flow rates. A threshold resistor maintains a constant PEEP regardless of flow rate.

pressure. FIO_2 can be maintained between 0.21 and 100%.

If respiratory failure causes only mild desaturation, intubation and mechanical ventilation may not be necessary. The positive expiratory pressure provided by the mask may be sufficient for effective restoration of oxygenation. If blood gas function deteriorates after extubation, reintubation can sometimes be avoided as well. When more than 10 to 15 cm H_2O is required, intubation and mechanical ventilation are advised to reexpand collapsed terminal airways. Gastric dilatation is not uncommon during CPAP mask therapy. The mask is designed to accommodate a nasogastric tube without loss of the facial seal.

UNILATERAL LUNG INJURY

Direct, blunt chest trauma is often unilateral. The standard treatment regimen previously described may then be inappropriate. A large unilateral contusion markedly reduces compliance only in the affected lung. When PEEP and mechanical ventilation are added to the entire airway, the raised airway pressure is directed through the path of least resistance to the more compliant lung. The high pressures redirect blood flow from the healthy to the diseased lung. Ventilation is primarily to the uninvolved lung and blood flow to the diseased side, a major ventilation-perfusion imbalance.

There are two possible solutions. The lateral position places the healthy lung down and promotes ventilation to that side. Perfusion is also distributed to the dependent lung. A special bed can help accomplish this function [30]. V/Q relationships are optimized and blood gas exchange improved. These efforts have no direct effect on the original disease process but improve blood gas exchange.

When those efforts are unsuccessful, independent lung ventilation can be employed. Ventilators are available that deliver synchronized, precise, independent tidal volumes and PEEP to each lung [13]. A double-lumen endotracheal tube isolates each lung. Precise PEEP and tidal volume can then be directed independently to each lung. Only the diseased, poorly compliant lung receives the high pressure necessary for ventilation and oxygenation.

BRONCHOPLEURAL FISTULA

A bronchopleural-cutaneous fistula presents difficult technical problems. A large air leak usually develops secondary to pulmonary rupture. Clinical signs include decreased exhaled tidal volume and increased $PaCO_2$. Large air losses through the underwater drain are evident. Desired PEEP levels may be difficult to maintain. Increased mechanical rate and tidal volume do not usually reduce $PaCO_2$ and may impair cardiac output.

The pathophysiology appears to be straightforward. Each mechanical breath moves gas through the path of least resistance, and it exits through the fistula. Gas does not remain in the lung long enough for any exchange. Theoretically, if gas can be trapped in the lungs for part of inspiration, some interaction with blood should occur. This can be accomplished by placing an exhalation valve between the chest tubes and the underwater seal [16]. The ventilator inspiratory limb pressurizes the simple mushroom valve. During inspiration the valve is charged shut, effectively occluding the chest tube. Gas is forced to remain in the lung and chest during the entire inspiratory cycle. The valve opens at beginning exhalation, and gas exits from the lungs and thorax. Inspiratory and expiratory chest roentgenography reveals a small pneumothorax during the inspiratory cycle. In most instances the diseased lungs have already formed chest wall adhesions, preventing total collapse. $PaCO_2$ returns to normal, while mechanical rate and tidal volume remain at baseline levels. Cardiovascular function is not impaired. Valves are placed on as many chest tubes as are leaking.

Continuous gas loss prevents PEEP maintenance. Conversion from a static device to a continuous flow Venturi PEEP device will solve the problem.

Other authors have advocated placing PEEP valves, set at the desired PEEP level, between the chest tubes and the underwater seal [10].

At least one clinical report indicates that high-frequency positive pressure ventilation has been successfully used to treat bronchopleural fistula [6].

SUMMARY

The management of the chest trauma patient is individualized according to the specific system or organ dysfunction. In some cases, oxygenation alone is affected, while in others, alveolar ventilation is abnormal. Modalities such as PEEP and IMV combined with a new generation of mechanical ventilators have provided a wide degree of flexibility in treatment. Goals include optimization and support of all functions, with minimal interference with unaffected systems. Early aggressive therapy then ensures a rapid return to a functional life-style.

REFERENCES

1. Allison SP: Metabolic aspects of intensive care. Br J Anaesth 49:689, 1977
2. Ashbaugh DG, Bigelow DB, Petty TL, et al: Acute respiratory distress in adults. Lancet 2:319, 1967
3. Ashbaugh DG, Petty TL: Positive end expiratory pressure. J Thorac Cardiovasc Surg 65:165, 1973
4. Banner MJ, Gallagher TJ, DeHaven CB: PEEP-CPAP. Curr Rev Respir Ther 1:11, 1978
5. Bork JL: Monitoring the patient in shock. Surg Clin North Am 55:713, 1975
6. Carlon GC, Howland WS, Klain M, et al: High frequency positive ventilatory support in patients with broncho-pleural fistula. Crit Care Med 7:89, 1979
7. Cullen P, Modell JH, Kirby RR, et al: Treatment of flail chest—use of intermittent mandatory ventilation and positive end expiratory pressure. Arch Surg 11:1099, 1975
8. Dane TEB, King EG: A prospective study of complications after tracheostomy for assisted ventilation. Chest 67:398, 1975
9. Dean RS, Shinozaki T, Morgan JG: An evaluation of the cuff characteristic and incidence of laryngeal complications using a new nasotracheal tube in prolonged intubation. J Trauma 17:311, 1977

10. Downs JB, Chapman RL: Treatment of bronchopleural fistula during continuous positive pressure ventilation. Chest 69:363, 1976

11. Downs JB, Klein EF, Jr., Desautels D, et al: Intermittent mandatory ventilation: A new approach to weaning patients from mechanical ventilators. Chest 64:331, 1973

12. Froese AB, Bryan AC: Effects of anesthesia and paralysis on diaphragmatic mechanics in man: Anesthesiology 41:242, 1974

13. Gallagher TJ, Banner MJ, Smith, RA: A simplified method of independent lung ventilation. Crit Care Med (in press)

14. Gallagher TJ, Civetta JM: Role of micropore blood filters in respiratory failure. Abs Sci Papr IARS, 1980

15. Gallagher TJ, Civetta JM, Kirby RR: Terminology update: Optimal PEEP. Crit Care Med 6: 323, 1978

16. Gallagher TJ, Smith RA, Kirby RR, et al: Intermittent chest tube occlusion to limit bronchopleural cutaneous fistula. Crit Care Med 4:328, 1976

17. Graybar GS: Letter to the editor. Chest 75:106, 1979

18. Grillo HC, Cooper JD, Geffin B, et al: A low pressure cuff for tracheostomy tubes to minimize tracheal injury: A comparative trial. J Thorac Cardiovasc Surg 62:898, 1971

19. Guyton AC: Interstitial fluid pressure: II. Pressure volume curves of interstitial space. Circ Res 26:452, 1965

20. Horovitz JH, Carrico CJ, Shires GT: Pulmonary response to major injury. Arch Surg 108:349, 1974

21. Kelman GA, Nunn JF, Prys-Roberts C, et al: The influence of cardiac output on arterial oxygenation. A theoretical study. Br J Anaesth 39: 450, 1967

22. Kirby RR: Mechanical ventilation in acute ventilatory failure: Facts, fiction and fallacies: Curr Probl Anesth Crit Care Med 1:9, 1977

23. Kirby RR, Downs JB, Civetta JM, et al: High level positive end expiratory pressure (PEEP) in acute respiratory insufficiency. Chest 67:156, 1975

24. Kirby RR, Smith RA, Gooding JM, et al: PEEP therapy by face mask. Abs Sci Papr Am Soc Anesthesiol 195, 1977

25. Klain M, Smith RB: High frequency percutaneous transtracheal jet ventilation. Crit Care Med 5:280, 1977

26. Kumar A, Falke KJ, Geffin B, et al: Continuous positive pressure ventilation in acute respiratory failure. N Engl J Med 283:1430, 1970

27. Laver ML: Dr. Starling and the "ventilator kidney." Anesthesiology 50:383, 1979

28. Pontoppidan H, Geffin B, Lowenstein E: Acute respiratory failure in the adult. N Engl J Med 287:690, 743, 799, 1972

29. Reynolds EOR, Taghizadeh A: Improved prognosis of infants mechanically ventilated for hyaline membrane disease. Arch Dis Child 49:505, 1974

30. Schimmel L, Civetta JM, Kirby RR: A new method to influence perfusion in critically ill patients. Crit Care Med 5:277, 1977

31. Staub NC: Pulmonary edema. Chest 74:559, 1979

32. Suter PM, Fairley HB, Isenberg MD: Optimum end-expiratory airway pressure in patients with acute pulmonary failure. N Engl J Med 292: 284, 1975

33. Taylor PA, Towley RM: The broncho-fiberscope as an aid to endotracheal intubation. Br J Anaesth 44:611, 1972

34. Teplitz C: The core pathobiology and integrated medical science of adult acute respiratory insufficiency. Surg Clin North Am 56:1091, 1976

35. Terry PB, Traystam RJ, Newball HH, et al: Collateral ventilation in man. N Engl J Med 298:10, 1978

36. Tonkin JP, Harrison GA: The effect on the larynx of prolonged endotracheal intubation. Med J Aust 11:581, 1966

37. Trinkle JK, Richardson JD, Franz JL, et al: Management of flail chest without mechanical ventilation. Ann Thorac Surg 19:355, 1975

38. Vriem CE, Snashall PD, Demling RH, et al: Lung lymph and free interstitial fluid protein. Am J Physiol 230:165, 1976

39. Weinstein M, Rice C, Peters R, et al: Hemodynamic and respiratory response to varying gradients between end expiratory and end inspiratory pressure in patients breathing on continuous positive airway pressure. J Trauma 18:231, 1978

40. Wenver DW, Ledgerwood AM, Lucas CE, et al: Pulmonary effects of allumin resuscitation for severe hypervolemic shock. Arch Surg 113:387, 1978

9. VASCULAR INJURIES OF THE THORAX RESULTING FROM BLUNT TRAUMA

Lewis H. Bosher, Jr.

Rupture or fracture of the intrathoracic great vessels is a common consequence of blunt trauma to the thorax. From postmortem studies Greendyke [52] found an incidence of rupture of the aorta in 16 percent of victims of automobile accidents. Statistics from Sweden are even more astounding; Voigt [129] noted aortic rupture in more than one-third of victims of vehicular accidents. In many instances early recognition of these injuries in hospitalized trauma patients makes it surgically possible to save these people.

In this age of mechanization and rapid transport, thoracic compression and impact injuries are occurring with increasing frequency. Although many such accidents are associated with deceleration, the role played by such forces in the mechanism of aortic rupture remains uncertain. Damage to the intrathoracic great vessels usually leads to sudden lethal hemorrhage, or the associated injuries cause immediate or early death. Initial survival in approximately 15 to 20 percent of such victims allows some chance for salvage by prompt surgical intervention [102]. Vehicular collisions, vehicular-pedestrian accidents, airplane disasters, cave-ins, falls from heights or parachute jumps, elevator drops, compression waves from explosions, and animal kicks or other direct blows and compression forces are the modes of violence most frequently cited as proved causative mechanisms. The majority of intrathoracic vascular disruptions result from vehicular crashes, however, and the incidence of aortic fracture increases with the magnitude of violence; minor collisions are rarely causative. Greendyke [52] cited two instances in which the driver and both passengers sustained aortic ruptures, and in one of these accidents the rupture in each of the three victims was located at the aortic isthmus.*

According to Parmley and colleagues [102], who analyzed the results of 275 postmortem examinations, the most common sites of aortic rupture in order of frequency were: isthmus (46 percent), ascending aorta (23 percent), descending thoracic aorta (13 percent), and aortic arch (8 percent). A smaller incidence was noted in the abdominal aorta (5 percent) or at multiple sites (6 percent). In the statistics from the Cologne Institute of Forensic Medicine [56] the ascending aorta was involved in 12.5 percent. Greendyke [52] found multiple tears in 19 percent. He also recorded 20 percent of aortic injuries at the diaphragmatic level and 7 percent in the ascending aorta; in only one case was the ascending aorta alone ruptured. This contrasts with Strassmann's autopsy series [122] in which a single rupture in the ascending aorta was found in 8 of 72 cases. Multiple aortic injuries and rupture at sites other than the isthmus occur far more frequently in postmortem series than in surgical series. In patients surviving long enough to undergo surgery, the incidence of isthmic ruptures is much higher than Parmley's experience [102] of 46 percent. The distribution of thoracic aorta injuries according to Voigt [129] is presented in Table 9-1.

The predilection for rupture of the aorta in the vicinity of the ligamentum arteriosum and of the ascending aorta just above the aortic valve has incited much interest and speculation regarding pathogenesis. Since 70 percent of patients sustaining fracture of the ascending aorta also have severe cardiac injury, only infrequently does such a patient survive long enough to reach a medical installation [102]. Associated rupture of the pericardium hastens death in many cases by allowing exsanguination, although tamponade has been reported. Cardiac injuries were observed by Parmley and colleagues [102] in only 23 percent of patients with rupture at the isthmus. It is not surpris-

---

* By rigid definition the term *isthmus* includes that portion of the aorta from the origin of the left subclavian artery to and including the origin of the ligamentum arteriosum. In this chapter, in order to facilitate the description, the meaning of isthmus is broadened to include that section of the aorta down to the first set of intercostal arteries. This is the sense in which the word is commonly used in the literature on rupture of the aorta.

Table 9-1. Ruptures of Thoracic
Aorta in Auto Passengers[a]

Place of Rupture	No. of Cases
Isthmus, isolated	49
Isthmus, ascending	5
Isthmus, descending	12
Isthmus, ascending and descending	4
Isolated, descending	19
Descending and ascending	3
Descending, arch	1
Isolated, ascending	6
Isolated arch	1
Total cases	100

[a] Derived from Voigt [129].

ing that with few exceptions the surgical successes have been reported in patients with isthmic rupture.

BIOMECHANICS AND PATHOGENESIS OF RUPTURED THORACIC AORTA

The biomechanics of ruptured thoracic aorta and its branches has been discussed by many authors [2, 18, 55, 67, 75, 82, 90, 93, 94, 101, 108, 109, 114, 116, 117, 119, 120, 122, 125, 134]. The variety of violent forces as causes and the finding of rupture at multiple aortic sites in some victims suggest that more than one mechanism is operative in the production of this lesion. In a small number of cases fracture dislocation of vertebral bodies is responsible for aortic injury, either by direct trauma or by a shearing mechanism, as recorded in 29 cases in Parmley's series [102]. Displaced rib or clavicular fragments also may directly lacerate the aorta or its branches.

Several theories have been proposed to account for the usual transverse tear at the so-called classic location, i.e., in the vicinity of the ligamentum arteriosum. Most cases of rupture in surgical series have occurred in relatively young individuals in whom intrinsic aortic disease is noncontributory and therefore atherosclerotic disease has not been a predisposing factor. When accurately documented, the rupture or resulting aneurysm is usually reported at or just beyond the ligamentum arteriosum, but in a few cases it occurs proximal to the ligamentum arteriosum. In the complete circumferential fracture the ligamentum remains unin-

jured and attached to the proximal segment, except in rare instances [20, 129]. Infrequently the tear extends proximally to or beyond the subclavian artery. Although Zehnder [134] in his combination compression-deceleration theory located incomplete tears on the convexity of the aorta in the isthmic region, a perusal of operative descriptions and other analyses indicates that the position on the circumference is not constant and, indeed, tears are frequently found on the concavity of the aorta or adjacent to it. Neither Parmley and colleagues [102] nor Greendyke [52] found a predilection for any particular position on the circumference in incomplete tears.

The relative mobility or fixation of aortic segments adjacent to the isthmus assumes importance in relation to the deceleration theory of aortic isthmic rupture. This theory, which was well enunciated by Rice and Wittstruck [108], perhaps originated with Hass [55] and Rindfleisch [109]. The theory postulates that rupture occurs from shear stress at a point of relative fixation, i.e., the ligamentum arteriosum, between two adjacent segments of aorta decelerating at different rates. It is unlikely that the descending aorta is displaced forward significantly during rapid horizontal deceleration since tears in the intercostal arteries and parietal pleura have not been reported in the absence of direct injury from rib fragments [129]. Indeed, the descending aorta seems relatively fixed by the intercostal arteries and pleura. The transverse arch is suspended by its branches and is considered more mobile than the descending aorta [90]. In all large series one finds examples of aortic rupture in which deceleration can be ruled out as a causative or contributing factor. Stapp [119, 120] concluded from animal and human experimentation that deceleration forces encountered in automobile collisions were generally insufficient alone to produce aortic rupture.

Zehnder [134] postulated that rupture of the aorta occurs when shear (radial) stress exceeds the tear strength of the aortic wall. He emphasized the shear stress forces induced by differential horizontal deceleration of aortic segments, but he maintained, as Stapp had contended, that these forces alone were insufficient in most instances to cause rupture. His conclusions were drawn from the results of tension—tear experiments on segments of aortic wall—and on calculations of aortic bursting tolerance. The aortic wall is capable of withstanding over 2000 mm Hg internal bursting forces [101, 133]. The Zehnder's deductions have been criticized on the grounds that he did not consider the rate of application of forces involved [18, 52]. Crucial to an accurate evaluation of deceleration forces is a correct estimation of the braking distance. The force of deceleration is inversely and linearly related to the braking distance or braking time of a moving object as it is decelerated from maximum to zero. This computation introduces considerations of vehicular collapsibility as well as thoracic compressibility. To supply the additional shear stress forces required for rupture, Zehnder [134] postulated a flexion bending of the aortic arch resulting from anteroposterior compression of the thorax.

Voigt [129] carefully analyzed the compression forces and the mechanism of aortic injury by making a study of damaged vehicles involved and injuries revealed at postmortem examinations in a large series of cases of ruptured aorta. On the basis of these studies and in contrast to Zehnder's concept of flexion injury, he proposed a theory of *deflexion* of the aortic arch when thoracic compression is delivered at the midpoint of the sternum or below in a sagittal plane, usually in a craniodorsal direction. This force results most often from the thrust of the steering wheel or the dashboard. In his convincing monograph Voigt traced the course of the displaced heart into the left hemithorax and upward into the arch of the aorta, and he emphasized the further deformity, which constitutes a straightening out or deflexion of the arch (Fig 9-1). In the absence of torsion, such a mechanism should initiate disruption along the concavity of the aorta. The absence of evidence of external thoracic injury does not exclude a severe sagittal compression of the thorax, even when rib fractures cannot be identified.

Voigt [129] also performed experiments on human cadavers by applying thoracic compression after the heart and aorta had been opacified with contrast media; he was then able to determine roentgenographically the resulting cardiovascular deformity. These results substantiated the postmortem observations. Especially crucial for acceptance of his theory was the experimental finding of rupture just distal to the ligamentum arteriosum, the classic location.

It is probable that the relative fixation of the aorta at the ligamentum arteriosum contributes to the mechanism of rupture in this region. Zehnder

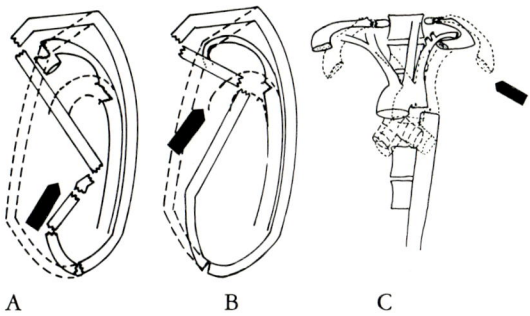

A   B   C

Fig 9-1. Proposed biomechanism of rupture of ascending aorta and isthmus from compression force applied to lower sternum (A), midsternum (B), or left lateral thorax (C). In A and B note deflexion of aortic arch. As shown in C the cranially directed force may cause fractures of the first ribs. (From G. E. Voight, Die Biomechanik stumpfer Brustverletzungen besonders von Thorax, Aorta und Herz, 1968. Used by permission of Springer-Verlag, New York.)

[133] pointed out that elasticity and tear strength are inherent properties of the aortic wall that determine its resistance to rupture. Loss of elasticity, as with aging, or dissipation of the elastic component with volume distention, renders the aorta more susceptible to rupture. The tear strength of the aorta diminishes progressively from the ascending aorta caudally [82, 101, 133]. Furthermore, experimentally, the aorta tears more readily when distracted in the longitudinal direction, no doubt a contributing factor in the production of the usual transverse fracture. The aorta is more susceptible to bending stress and fracture when it is distended and tense, as for example, at the end of cardiac systole and when abdominal compression or acute flexion of the lower extremities interferes with runoff from the thoracic aorta [133]. Similarly, in sudden, horizontal deceleration with the thorax and trunk collapsed forward, the axis shifts toward vertical deceleration and blood is displaced from the abdominal pool into the thoracic aorta.

In contrast to horizontal deceleration the force of vertical deceleration together with the weight of the attached heart appears more likely to rupture the aorta through the mechanism of shear stress alone. We have been unable to substantiate from the literature the oft-quoted statement that pure vertical deceleration, as exemplified by the uncontrolled dropping of an elevator or free falls, usually results in rupture of the *ascending* aorta. Zehnder [133] emphasized the common mechanism of aortic arch flexion by which vertical deceleration produces rupture of the isthmus.

A convincing example of the importance of decelerative forces is seen in those rare cases of isthmic rupture resulting from a direct fall on the back from a standing position [134]. Here the braking distance is very short because of the incompressibility of the spine and posterior thorax, and the inertial mass of the heart and ascending aorta is applied at the most effective angle to cause hyperflexion of the arch. In the car-pedestrian accident a centrifugal force is added. After a careful consideration of the theories of both Zehnder and Voigt, we have concluded that the theories, as applied to isthmic rupture, are not mutually exclusive and that either aortic arch *flexion* or *deflexion* together with deceleration forces may act under varying etiological circumstances.

Rupture of the ascending aorta usually results from a direct force applied at or just below the midpoint of the sternum [129]. The heart is displaced well into the left hemithorax, and torsion as well as flexion contribute to the rupture of the ascending aorta along its posterolateral convexity (Fig 9-1A). The injury is usually close to the aortic valve. The experiments of Moffat, Roberts, and Berkas [93], Roberts, Moffat, and Berkas [111], and Jackson, Berkas, and Roberts [67] lend support to the importance of direct force.

Ruptures of the branches of the aortic arch occur by a somewhat different mechanism. Voigt [129] contended that if the sagittal force of compression is applied superiorly, the resulting caudal displacement of the heart and ascending aorta produces a distraction at the origin of the great vessels that are tethered distally by attachments in the upper thorax and neck. The innominate artery is maximally affected. Impact by the inwardly displaced sternum may contribute to the avulsion. Simultaneous hyperextension of the cervical spine and rotation of the head stretches out the carotid arteries and distracts them even farther. Fracture of the upper sternum, right costochondral cartilages and ribs, and rupture of the right main stem bronchus may occur as associated injuries. Indeed, sternal fractures should tend to focus attention on the ascending aorta, arch, and branch vessels rather than the isthmic aorta where only a 10 percent associated incidence of sternal fracture has been reported.

Entrapment of the transverse aortic arch between the posteriorly displaced sternum and the vertebral column produces a direct aortic injury, usually on the posterior wall, that may occur as an isolated lesion or in conjunction with avulsion of the arch branches. Intrathoracic ruptures have occurred in all of the aortic branches and in the right subclavian artery, as will be discussed in more detail in the section dealing with surgical treatment.

Stenosis may occur as a secondary complication in a branch vessel as a result of exuberant scar tissue formation in the distal angle between the reflected adventitia and the inverted inner wall. The distal obstruction no doubt may contribute to the evolution of the associated aneurysm, which in turn increases the pressure against the distal shelf. A somewhat similar pathogenesis subsequent to incomplete rupture may be responsible for purely stenotic lesions occurring at unusual locations in the great vessels, as suggested by Freed and Bosher [46]. In a young adult without rib fracture we have observed contusion of the intrathoracic left subclavian artery, which led to thrombosis even in the absence of intimal rupture [81]. Thus direct impact from the deformed or subluxated rib cage may occasionally serve as the major or sole causative factor in vascular injury.

With a few exceptions, those patients who survive the initial aortic injury exhibit rupture at the isthmus or in the aortic branches. The tear extends transversely through the intima and media, and the developing aneurysm is often initially confined by the adventitia, which is said to provide a great portion of the strength of the aortic wall [17, 63]. Even circumferential transection of all the layers of the wall is not synonymous with early demise. Of 9 patients with this condition who survived initially, Parmley and colleagues [102] reported that 8 lived longer than 5 days. Complete circumferential transection of the inner layers with retraction has been encountered in at least 25 percent of patients who underwent operation, but this estimate is probably much too low in relation to current early recognition of aortic rupture [110]; the true figure probably approximates 50 percent. Separation of the transected segments up to 7 cm has been observed [44] or even farther after the development of a chronic aneurysm [3]. In many other instances only a narrow tongue of full-thickness wall remains intact. Tears involving only the intima usually remain unrecognized, and multiple intimal tears have been described in several postmortem studies [5, 12, 85, 116, 129]. Limited dissection of the adventitia away from the inner layers is commonly seen on either end of the rupture and occasionally this separation may extend over a much wider area. Parmley and colleagues [102] noted a few instances in which a true dissection occurred for a variable distance from the site of rupture before breaking through the adventitia externally. More extensive dissections have also been reported.

The role of trauma in the production of dissecting aneurysms is often disputed. In Table 9-2 are listed some cases of extensive dissection in which preexisting disease of the aortic wall was apparently absent and in which the trauma cited seemed of a magnitude sufficiently great or was applied critically enough to predispose to traumatic rupture of the aorta. In many instances the dissection

and a remote rupture contributed materially to the patient's death. In at least two operative cases a retrograde dissection around the arch led to uncontrollable hemorrhage [44]. Other cases are difficult to evaluate or are not available for review [114].

Within several weeks of the rupture a significant fibrous tissue reaction adds to the strength of the adventitia and surrounding layers. The traumatic aneurysm thus tends to stabilize and soon the danger of free rupture is temporarily lessened. Within a few years calcification is added in many aneurysms, but even this barrier does not guarantee protection against future expansion with consequent rupture (Fig 9-2).

The term *complete transection* has been loosely used in the literature and the integrity of the adventitia often not clearly defined. It is probable that seepage of blood through the adventitia and surrounding layers occurs quite frequently as a re-

Table 9-2. Extensive Dissecting Aneurysms Secondary to Traumatic Rupture of Aorta

Author	Postinjury Interval to Death	Rupture Site	Direction of Dissection	Extent of Dissection	Operation Performed
Zehnder [133]	5 days	Isthmus	Distal	Abdominal aorta	No
Stoney et al. [121]	6 days	Isthmus	Proximal	Ascending aorta	Yes
Nelson and Ashley [100]	1 day	Ascending aorta	Distal	Carotid artery	No
Leonard	15 days	Descending aorta	Proximal	Descending aorta	No
Spencer et al. [118]	4 days	Isthmus	Proximal	Carotid artery	Yes
Rice and Wittstruck [108]	18 days	Isthmus	Distal	Abdominal aorta	No
Mazzitello (Case 2) [87]	3 mo.	Ascending aorta	Distal	Innominate artery	No
Aufrance et al. [5]	1 day	Isthmus	Distal and proximal	Abdominal and ascending aorta	Yes
O'Sullivan (Case 9)	4 yr.	Isthmus	Distal	Bifurcation of aorta	No
Marshall (Case 2) [85]	2 days	Isthmus	Distal and proximal	Abdominal aorta and arch	No
Simpson (Case 1) [116]		Aortic arch	Distal and proximal	Diaphragm and ascending aorta	No
Pierce (Case 2)	10 days	Ascending aorta		Unknown	No
Marshall (Case 1) [85]	1 day	Isthmus	Distal	Descending aorta	No
Heberer [56]	8 yr.	Isthmus		Unknown	Yes
Fleming and Green [44]		Unknown	Proximal	Aortic arch	Yes

For other possible cases see T. Shennan, Dissecting aneurysms (Medical Research Council (Gt. Brit.). Special Report Series No. 193. Cases 173, 178, 185, 135, 29, 133.

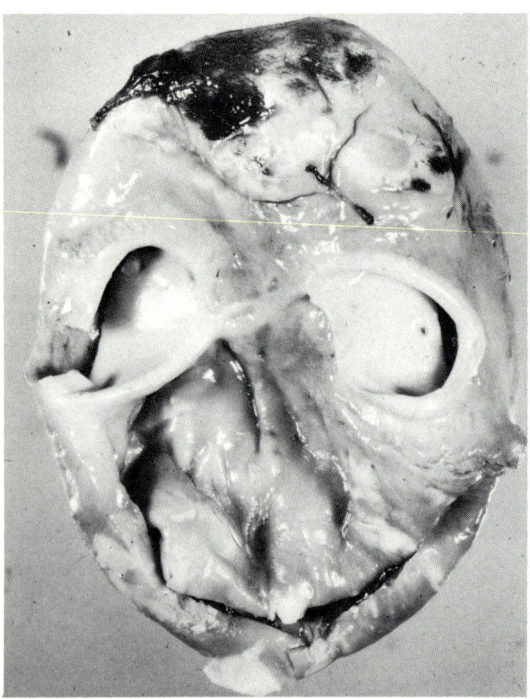

Fig 9-2. Specimen from same patient as in Fig 9-5. The aneurysm has been opened. The transection of the aorta is nearly complete, although there is a narrow isthmus of communicating intima. Much of the aneurysmal wall is composed of densely fibrosed adventitia with outer portions of the media. In some areas elastic tissue is completely absent. The rupture occurred at the level of the second intercostal artery and is therefore slightly below the "classic" level.

sult of stretching prior to frank rupture. One may liken this to the sanguineous pericardial fluid sometimes seen before final rupture of a dissecting aneurysm. Beyond the adventitia the hematoma is confined by the perivascular sheath that extends distally along the aorta and cephalad in communication with the perivascular carotid artery sheath. In discussing traumatic rupture, few surgeons and pathologists have identified this structure as distinct from the mediastinal pleura, but this sheath may possess surprising strength and is undoubtedly of great importance in prolonging the interval prior to free rupture and exsanguination.

In an exhibit and an unpublished work Mac-Kenzie and associates [84] have described studies on cadavers in which blood was injected beneath the perivascular sheath at different sites. With less than 50 cc injected beneath the sheath at the isthmus but proximal to the ligamentum, blood flowed upward and presented in the neck within the carotid artery sheath long before widening of the mediastinum was roentgenographically apparent. When it was injected at the base of the innominate artery, the presentation was first in the right carotid artery sheath. When blood was injected at the ascending aorta in the pericardium, a pericardial fusion barrier was not traversed. If blood was injected distal to the ligamentum arteriosum, a similar fusion barrier at the ligamentum was encountered. The jugular vein also has its own perivascular sheath, which is in communication with the superior vena cava. A second perivascular sheath, the well-known carotid sheath, extends from the aortic arch and commonly surrounds the carotid arteries and jugular veins. Mac-Kenzie and associates [84] examined 41 victims of fatal accidents; 15 showed blood in the carotid artery sheath. All had rupture of the aortic arch or its major branches. No false positives were found, but the authors do not deny the possibility of false negatives.

If these findings can be substantiated and found to apply also to clinical cases, their importance lies in the possibility of early, even inadvertent detection of aortic rupture before mediastinal widening is roentgenographically apparent and when aortography is not available to the physician. However, the pericardial fusion barrier at the ligamentum, the classic rupture below the ligamentum, and proximal extension of blood in the periaortic space can only be reconciled if the fusion barrier is incomplete or torn.

The occasional extension of the hematoma into the viscerovascular compartment in the pretracheal space may lead to the unforeseen catastrophic complication of exsanguinating hemorrhage during the performance of a preoperative tracheostomy [34]. Endotracheal intubation is a safer alternative prior to surgical repair in the event of serious airway obstruction.

The long-term prognosis for the patient with a traumatic aneurysm has been reviewed most adequately by Bennett and Cherry [9]. They collected information on 105 chronic traumatic aortic aneurysms of more than 3 months' duration. Of the 105, 41 percent were stable without symptoms or enlargement, 21 percent showed roentgenographic enlargement, and 50 percent produced symptoms, of which pain was the most frequent.

In 17 percent, complications first developed after 10 years. In a recent review Fleming and Green [44] analyzed 33 patients in whom aortic injury had progressed to a chronic aneurysm. In 39 percent late enlargement or symptoms, or both, occurred prior to subsequent surgery. Failure to detect the aortic rupture resulted either from minimal evidence of thoracic trauma or because other injuries such as major fractures or cerebral concussion diverted attention from the aortic rupture.

On the basis of these and other observations, conservative treatment of traumatic aneurysm in the good-risk patient does not seem justified. However, the prognosis for patients with chronic traumatic aortic aneurysms does appear to be distinctly more favorable than is ascribed for those with luetic and arteriosclerotic aneurysms.

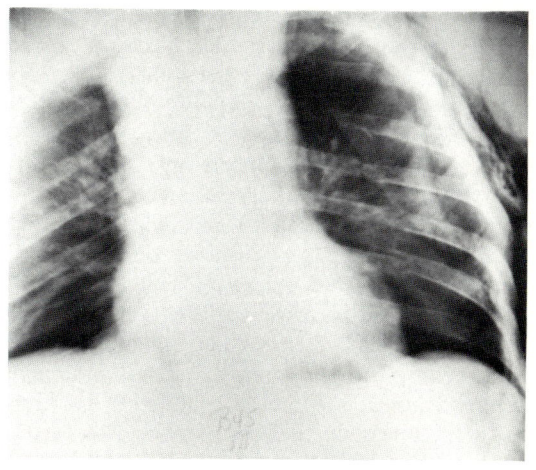

Fig 9-3. Ruptured aortic isthmus in a 34-year-old male. Other injuries included multiple left rib fractures with pneumothorax. Pulse volume was disproportionately weak in lower extremities; blood pressure was 130/80; and there was severe metabolic acidosis. Patient underwent resection of the transected aorta segments and insertion of a Dacron graft 24 hours post-injury. There was an associated tear in the left side of the pericardium. The oxygenator was required during left atrial-femoral artery bypass because of severe hypoxemia. He developed complete renal shutdown on the fifth postoperative day and died the ninety-third postoperative day of complications from a ruptured bile duct that was not recognized until late.

CLINICAL MANIFESTATIONS AND DIAGNOSIS

Because of the potential of the ruptured aorta for sudden lethal hemorrhage, prompt recognition of the vascular lesion has become the great responsibility of those surgeons initiating treatment of the trauma patient. Serious injuries involving long bones, pelvis, spleen, liver, diaphragm, other intra-abdominal organs, and the brain tend to divert attention from the mediastinal problem. In an opposite situation, we lost one patient despite a successful aortic repair, because recognition of a tear in a major bile duct was delayed (Fig 9-3). Of 48 cases of aortic rupture studied postmortem and reported from Stockholm, 35 percent were associated with liver rupture, 12 percent with splenic rupture, and 23 percent with involvement of both organs [59]. Backstrom [6] and Jensen [69] also found liver rupture to be two to three times as common as splenic rupture when either was associated with aortic rupture. This contrasts with the frequency of isolated organ rupture due to blunt trauma in which splenic injury occurs several times more frequently than liver injury.

Skeletal injuries of the thorax are often present, particularly rib fractures, but the absence of skeletal thoracic injuries by no means excludes the possibility of a ruptured aorta. In one series, one-third of the patients showed no significant external trauma to the thorax [102]. Forces of great magnitude (which often accompany rupture of the aorta) may be inferred in the presence of fractures of the first and second ribs.

In some instances clinical manifestations of ruptured aorta may be conspicuously absent, or the thoracic complaints may seem entirely explicable on the basis of obvious skeletal and pulmonary injuries. Shock, if present, is often determined by associated injuries. A high incidence (50 percent) of major abdominal injury has been encountered in patients with acute aortic rupture in some series [44]. A large amount of blood can be lost into the mediastinum before hemothorax develops. Whenever possible, blood pressure in upper and lower extremities should be compared since a measurable aortic obstruction may be present. An ultrasonic Doppler instrument greatly facilitates this measurement. Anterior chest or interscapular pain not related to respiration should arouse suspicion, particularly if persistent or recurrent. Dyspnea is often not related primarily to the vascular lesion, but expanding hematomas or aneurysms, when critically located, can compress the trachea or left main stem bronchus. If the hematoma is large and compresses the esophagus, dysphagia may be experienced. Necrosis of the esophagus with resulting intraesophageal hemorrhage has been reported, but this is rare and is more likely to follow surgical intervention [43, 115]. Four instances of hoarseness due to primary recurrent nerve injury following acute rupture [88, 110] have been documented.

Certain specific clinical manifestations may lead one to the correct diagnosis of isthmic rupture. Careful auscultation often discloses a systolic murmur over the left anterior chest, interscapular region, or epigastrium, a finding that is indicative of turbulence at the site of rupture; it has been heard in at least 25 percent of cases [44, 110]. The actual incidence is probably far higher and will increase in proportion to the care with which auscultation in the parascapular and infraclavicular areas is done. Murmurs are much less frequently heard over chronic traumatic aneurysms. The hematoma may extend proximally to compress the left subclavian artery, in which case a diminished pulse will be felt at the corresponding wrist. Hypertension in the upper extremities and diminished or absent pulses in the lower extremities are being reported with increasing frequency [73]. This manifestation of serious aortic obstruction may be concealed by reduced blood volume. Acquired coarctation of this type may produce advanced aortic obstruction to the point of acute left ventricular failure with pulmonary edema [47].

From operative descriptions one can usually attribute the mechanism of aortic obstruction to an infolding or inversion of the distal aortic segment. The pressure in the expanding "false" aneurysm and hematoma adds to the compression of the distal wall where it has dissected away from the adventitia. Partial thrombotic occlusion is often found in the surrounding aneurysmal sac. The pulse in the distal thoracic aorta, when examined at surgery, is weak or absent.

Aortic obstruction may not only cause hypertension, but interference with aortic flow at the site of acute rupture may be severe enough to cause spinal cord ischemia and resulting paraplegia. Fourteen such cases observed prior to surgical intervention have been reported in the English literature [8, 33, 49, 60–62, 66, 76, 96, 105, 117, 118]. The aortic transection was complete in less than half of the total. Absence of lower extremity pulses was noted in the majority, and upper extremity hypertension was recorded in several. Oli-

guria or anuria was often noted. Paraplegia was sometimes present on admission or was observed during the first day, but in 2 cases it was delayed until the fifth and fifteenth days, respectively [66, 76]. Two patients walked into the hospital. Operation was performed in 12 with survival in 5. In 2 patients operated upon promptly, one within 65 minutes of the accident [33] and the other after several hours [61], the paraplegia cleared completely; there was significant partial recovery in a third patient [8].

In three instances, however, paraplegia was attributed to a different mechanism. In 2 cases Beall and co-workers [8] reported adequate pulses in the lower extremities; they considered compression of intercostal arteries by a mediastinal hematoma to be important. This probably implied extension of the hematoma beneath the tense perivascular sheath. In the third patient, reported by Hughes [66], paraplegia developed on the fifth postinjury day; at postmortem examination the second, third, fourth, and fifth intercostal arteries were compressed by mural hematoma in the tunica media and adventitia, presumably a true traumatic dissecting aneurysm.

Chronic traumatic aneurysms in the region of the isthmus tend to expand ventrally and produce pressure on the left main stem bronchus, the esophagus, and the recurrent laryngeal nerve. They may rupture into the lung, bronchus, or esophagus.

Clinical manifestations of traumatic rupture of the ascending aorta are not usually seen because even temporary survival is infrequent. Cardiac tamponade is uncommon because pericardial laceration usually accompanies the injury. Superior vena cava obstruction due to acute intrapericardial expansion of a ruptured ascending aorta has been reported. Aortic valve incompetence may result from fracture of the ascending aorta [19, 87, 89]. We have corrected one traumatic aorta–right ventricular fistula occurring in association with an intimal tear of the aortic root. Successful repair of acute, traumatic rupture of the proximal ascending aorta has not been reported.

Clinical manifestations associated with rupture of the aortic arch vessels are variable and obviously depend on the vessel involved and the location of the injury. A differential in systolic blood pressure and pulse amplitude between right and left arms has been noted in at least 50 percent of cases of such arch ruptures. A bruit over the base of the neck is common. Venous engorgement, cyanosis, and even dysphagia are occasional manifestations of avulsion of the innominate artery and rupture of the transverse arch. The trachea may be displaced to the right and posteriorly.

A critically located rupture of the posterior wall of the transverse aortic arch, confined by fascial planes, may produce extreme dyspnea with obstruction of the trachea and left main stem bronchus, as well as engorgement of the upper veins. We have noted these manifestations in 2 patients undergoing exploratory operation prior to the availability of extracorporeal circulation. Paralysis of the left vocal cord was present in 1.

Roentgenographic Diagnosis

Patients with injuries to the long bones, pelvis, or spleen should also have a standard chest roentgenogram. A widened superior mediastinum, obscuration of the aorta and aortic knob, displacement of the lower trachea to the right and the left main stem bronchus inferiorly, esophageal displacement to the right, left hemothorax or sanguineous pleural effusion: all these features constitute the classic roentgenographic changes produced by aortic isthmic rupture. Any or all of these findings may not be present initially but will be revealed in a subsequent roentgenogram.

In 1966 MacKenzie and associates [84] reported that widening of the mediastinum could not be detected roentgenographically until 400 cc of blood had been injected beneath the perivascular aortic sheath. A widened superior mediastinum may be present without concomitant aortic rupture, however, and bleeding into the loose areolar tissue can occur from a fractured sternum or ribs and torn internal mammary and intercostal arteries as well as small veins. Under these circumstances even 100 cc of blood may produce widening. Paravertebral hematoma from fractured vertebrae also produces a widened mediastinum with obliteration of the aortic knob. Attar and co-workers [4] found aortic rupture in only 25 to 30 percent of trauma patients showing roentgenographic widening of the superior mediastinum. And again, an approximately equal number of patients with aortic rupture have a normal chest roentgenogram on admission.

On the other hand, a wide mediastinum has too often been unwisely disregarded because of expected distortion in the anteroposterior projection and close patient-to-film distance. Displacement of the lower trachea to the right can be observed in a high percentage of cases, and Flaherty and associates [42] claimed that this sign is more important than widening of the mediastinum in early detection. An overpenetrated supine film is required. Sanborn and colleagues [113] emphasized widening of the parasternal lines, apparent on overpenetrated film, as an important diagnostic sign. Downward displacement of the left main stem bronchus also occurs frequently but is less reliable than tracheal deviation, since the former may also be found in mediastinal hematoma unrelated to aortic rupture [74]. In the lateral view the aortic window becomes obliterated and the left main stem bronchus shows displacement forward. Blurring of the apical area due to subpleural extension from the mediastinum constitutes a late and infrequent finding. Within several weeks the generalized widening of the mediastinum develops into a well-defined mass in the region of the aortic knob as mediastinal hemorrhage resorbs. Widening of the upper mediastinum is also characteristic of rupture of the aortic branch vessels. Furthermore, left hemothorax and obscuration of the aortic knob are not specific for rupture at the isthmus.

When aortic rupture is suspected, aortography should be performed unless continuing intrathoracic or intra-abdominal hemorrhage dictates the need for immediate operation. Aortography is an indispensable tool without which the diagnosis is not always certain, and without which localization of one or more tears in the aorta and its major branches cannot be precisely determined. The radiologist may express a preference for performing the procedure via the femoral artery or the right axillary artery, but in each instance the entire thoracic aorta and its branch vessels up to the base of the neck should be visualized. The axillary approach may seem slightly less hazardous than the retrograde femoral route, but it is usually more time-consuming and more difficult and one may still have to transgress the region of an innominate artery tear. When the femoral route is elected, a J-shaped guide wire allows traversal of the site of rupture with safety. Furthermore, the transfemoral route permits investigation of the visceral organs. The antegrade venous method often fails to provide adequate definition, particularly of tears in the branch vessels. Instances of missed diagnosis when this technique has been used have been cited.

Aortographic studies are decisively diagnostic and reveal irregularity and dilatation at the site of the rupture, often with a translucent defect corresponding to the torn and inverted inner wall. Rarely is extravasation beyond the adventitial envelope seen. The angiographic picture is more striking in those patients with complete circumferential disruption and distraction, in which case proximal and distal ends of the transected aorta can be visualized (Fig 9-4). Thomford et al [128] emphasized the slow clearing of the radiopaque medium from the false aneurysm when obstruction is present at the distal segment. False positive diagnoses have been made in the presence of atherosclerotic plaques with ulceration, and the recess at the ligamentum arteriosum may lead to misinterpretation [4].

Because many trauma patients with ruptured aorta fail to show a widened mediastinum in the early period after admission, De Meules and associates [32] urged liberalization of the indications for aortography to include the following: multiple rib fractures, fractured sternum, first rib fracture, posteriorly displaced fractured clavicle, and pulse deficits in the upper extremities.

Surgical Treatment

The surgical importance of the ruptured aorta can be viewed in appropriate perspective by examining the survival statistics gathered by Parmley and colleagues [102]. Of 275 people with aortic rupture in all locations, 237 were dead on arrival at a hospital. Of the remaining 38, 12 died during the first hospital day, 11 from the second through the seventh day, 5 during the second week, and 1 each on the fifteenth and twenty-second days, respectively. Thus 82 percent of the 38 initial survivors died within 3 weeks after the accident. Eight patients (3 percent) survived beyond 2 months and all developed chronic aneurysms. Thus although the majority of patients initially surviving aortic rupture succumb from hemorrhage within the first few days or weeks, rupture is not always fatal and may lead to a stable or progressively enlarging traumatic aneurysm. Only 4 of 60 patients with rupture of the ascending aorta survived the initial injury and only 2 lived longer than 1 day after sustaining the trauma.

The survival statistics gathered by Parmley and colleagues [102] and others [56, 122] leave little doubt that repair of acute aortic rupture should be considered a relative surgical emergency. Delay in thoracotomy after a definitive diagnosis is made can be condoned only under special circumstances, for example, to allow for the treatment of active intra-abdominal hemorrhage or partial recovery from other injuries that would temporarily render aortic repair unsafe such as serious cerebral injury or severe myocardial damage. The definitive operative treatment of major orthopedic problems can usually be postponed. The relatively quiescent period between the initial injury and rupture to the final lethal exsanguinating or compressive hemorrhage should not lull the surgeon into a philosophy of conservatism. However, the report of Rittenhouse and associates [110] in 1969 revealed that in only 13 of 110 reported cases of repair of traumatic rupture or aneurysm was this aortic repair done during the first 24 hours postinjury, and only 19 during the first 48 hours. This record is now undoubtedly much improved.

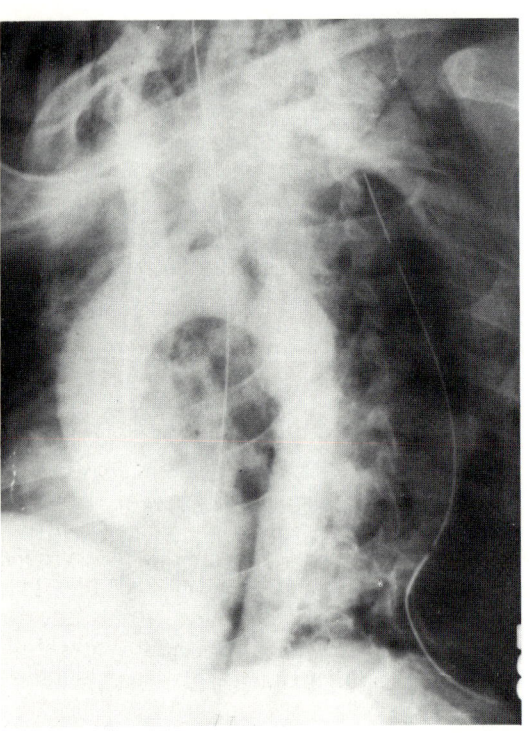

Fig 9-4. Aortogram in oblique projection. "Complete" transection of aorta just below ligamentum arteriosum with wide separation of segments and dilatation of "false" aneurysm in a 34-year-old male. At surgery dissection of the adventitia back to the origin of the left subclavian artery was noted.

As in the case of dissecting aneurysm, judicious use of Arfonad,* propranolol, and methyldopa to control blood pressure and protect against rupture during the interval between diagnosis and actual operation may occasionally be indicated, providing renal function is adequate and distal aortic flow is unimpaired. These pharmacological aids should be used only when associated severe injuries preclude early definitive aortic surgery, however. Geiger [50] mentioned 13 patients whose operative repair was delayed into the chronic stage of aortic healing and Dart and Braitman [29] 3 such patients, all "protected" by drug therapy.

ASCENDING AORTA. Of 10 recorded patients with acute rupture of the ascending aorta who survived longer than 1 hour after admission to the hospital, in none was the correct diagnosis made [12, 18, 86, 100, 102, 121, 123, 132]. Rupture followed external cardiac massage in one instance [100]. Operation was undertaken in only one, but with an erroneous diagnosis of isthmic rupture [18]. A recent case in which the ascending aorta was involved, reported by Appelbaum and colleagues [3], is considered by us as primarily a rupture of the transverse aorta. For acute rupture of the ascending aorta, the use of complete cardiopulmonary bypass followed by a direct repair or graft replacement is the only rational surgical approach.

The older literature on chronic traumatic aneurysms of the ascending aorta has been reviewed by Holmes and Netterville [64]. We have found 10 additional cases in more recent reports, 2 of which were associated with aortic insufficiency [16, 26, 37, 44, 76, 87, 89, 123]. A variety of compression injuries and direct blows caused the aneurysms. In one instance a dislocated clavicle contused the aorta [76]. A transverse tear just above the aortic valve, associated with limited dissection, may allow prolapse of the aortic commissure and incompetence of the valve, as reported by Mazzitello [87] and Heller [58] in 2 patients who died of chronic congestive heart failure. Mc-Clenathan and Brettschneider [89] listed a patient with traumatic aneurysm of the ascending aorta associated with aortic insufficiency who was observed to be in good condition 23 years after injury. Five chronic traumatic aneurysms have

* Roche Laboratories, Division of Hoffman-LaRoche, Inc., Nutley, N.J.

been resected, 4 of them successfully [16, 26, 37, 44, 76]. In one patient an aortic valve was replaced [16]. Death is thus not inevitable following rupture of the ascending aorta even though serious multiple injuries, major cardiac damage, and laceration of the pericardium limit the possibility for survival.

ISTHMUS AND DESCENDING THORACIC AORTA. Although Klassen (as reported by Passaro and Pace [103]) is usually credited with the first repair of an acute rupture of the thoracic aorta in 1959, accomplished within the first day after injury, Forsee and Blake [45] in 1958 published an account of a rupture resected and grafted about 3 days postinjury.

Current concepts eliminate any consideration of general body hypothermia to 30°C as an appropriate modality in the operative treatment of acute ruptured aorta because it is cumbersome and time-consuming in the adult. General body hypothermia has been used successfully in the resection of many chronic traumatic aneurysms but is not currently favored (Fig 9-5).

Repair of acute rupture of the isthmus or descending thoracic aorta has been performed successfully without any form of circulatory support or hypothermic protection. Until recently, however, this seemed advisable only under urgent circumstances, such as in the case of hemorrhage or ischemic paraplegia. When the upper thoracic aorta is occluded in excess of 20 minutes the consequences of spinal cord and visceral ischemia cannot be disregarded [1, 38, 39, 104]. The dangers are enhanced in the presence of shock and reduced blood flow. However, success has been reported without spinal cord complications even after simple cross-clamping up to 50 minutes [24, 27, 32, 131]. Crawford and colleagues [27] have recently contended that in the absence of hypotension, dissecting aneurysm, or extensive aortic resection, the period of safe aortic occlusion may be extended to 45 minutes or more. The results of Appelbaum and associates [3] support these recommendations. Seven patients with acute aortic rupture, who were treated without shunt or bypass survived without complications. They now prefer simple aortic cross-clamping for isthmic ruptures, if the repair can be completed in less than 30 minutes. Body temperature was not stated, but induced hypothermia was not employed.

A detailed discussion of paraplegia resulting from division of intercostal arteries in extensive

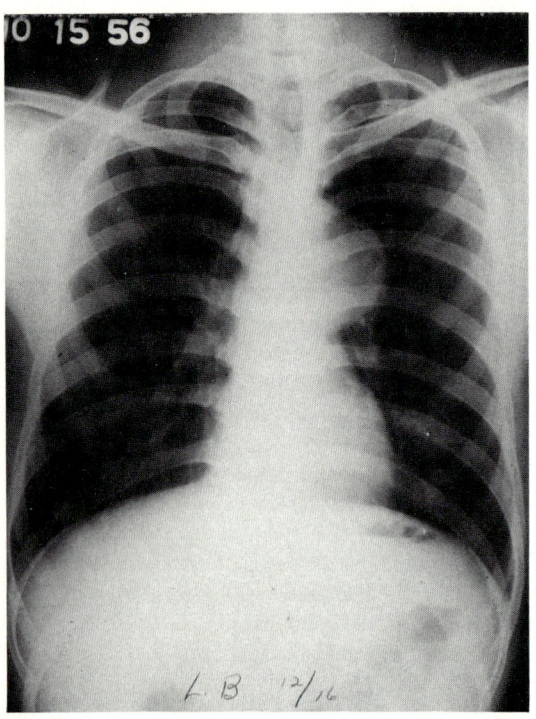

Fig 9-5. Traumatic aneurysm in an asymptomatic 21-year-old male. Patient suffered compound leg fracture one year previously, but recalled only slight chest pain. There were no rib fractures. The aneurysm was resected successfully under 32°C hypothermia and replaced with homograft. Aortic occlusion time was fifty minutes. There were no spinal cord complications.

importance of maintaining a normal or elevated proximal blood pressure in order to achieve adequate distal collateral circulation to the spinal cord during simple cross-clamping. The problem of acute left ventricular failure during simple aortic cross-clamping cannot be casually dismissed and constitutes a particular threat in the presence of myocardial contusion, aortic insufficiency, hypertension, or inadvertent volume overload. Methods of circulatory support are presently undergoing reappraisal, with a shift away from those techniques requiring heparinization. Simple aortic cross-clamping has already been discussed.

For rupture of the thoracic aortic isthmus, left atrial to femoral bypass or femoral vein to femoral artery bypass with an oxygenator have proved equally satisfactory in most instances. We have encountered less difficulty in cannulation of the left atrium than in cannulation of the inferior vena cava through the left iliofemoral route when the patient is placed in the right lateral decubitus position. Flow rates are generally suboptimal when the catheter cannot be passed into the inferior vena cava. Although the right femoral vein is less accessible, particularly in the male, it offers a more favorable route to the inferior vena cava. We have preferred to avoid obstruction of the deep veins of the leg in the patient with acute trauma, even under the protection of heparinization, and for this and other reasons have favored left atrial cannulation when feasible. However, under conditions of active intrathoracic bleeding, cannulation of the femoral or iliac vein should prove more expeditious.

In order to avoid release of the mediastinal hematoma prior to aortic occlusion, the pericardium should be entered anterior to the phrenic nerve and control of the aorta established proximal to the left subclavian artery, a maneuver that also reduces the likelihood of injury to the left recurrent nerve. When the left atrial appendage is used for cannulation, the catheter tip should be anchored just beyond the base of the appendage. If the catheter is advanced too far, mitral insufficiency or occlusion of the catheter in the valve or against the atrial wall may cause unsatisfactory venous drainage and disappointment with this method. A special atrial drainage catheter is available* that insures accurate placement and allows a continu-

resections of the descending aorta is not appropriate here, but the reader may wish to refer to the papers of Adams and Geertruyden [1] and Eiseman and colleagues [38, 39]. Unexplained cases of postoperative paraplegia continue to be reported sporadically even when bypass support or shunt has been utilized [3]. A recent lucid article by Pasternak, Boyd, and Ellis [104] emphasizes the variability in continuity of the anterior spinal artery as a determining factor in the development of ischemic spinal cord damage after division of intercostal and lumbar arteries. Ischemic injury of the cord has been most commonly reported in resections of the lower thoracic aorta below T8, in the region from which the arteria radicularis magna originates. Thus rupture and aneurysms of the aortic isthmus and upper thoracic aorta do not involve a highly vulnerable segment.

Pasternak, Boyd, and Ellis [104] emphasize the

---

* U.S. Catheter and Instrument Corp., Box 566, Billerica, Mass. 01821.

ous measurement of the left atrial pressure, a measurement that should preferably be monitored even when femoral vein to femoral artery bypass is employed. Left heart overload is thereby avoided, and the potential danger of aspiration of air into the left atrium from excessive negative pressure or sudden volume depletion is eliminated. The arterial system, which is divided into cephalic and caudal segments by aortic occlusion, appears peculiarly sensitive to small changes in blood volume, and the contused heart tolerates poorly the added resistance of aortic occlusion or an increased volume load. If preexisting aortic valve or myocardial disease is present, exquisite control of left heart bypass is required. Hug and Taber [65] have demonstrated the devastating pulmonary effects that occur during partial left heart bypass when left atrial hypertension occurs and is allowed to persist.

These factors are particularly pertinent when the aortic occlusion is extended proximal to the left subclavian artery, as is usually necessary. When simple aortic cross-clamping is employed, deliberate control of left ventricular afterload by pharmacological manipulation should prove safer and more physiological than induced hypovolemia. A bypass flow of approximately 30 to 35 cc per kilogram of body weight maintains adequate distal pressures, and appropriate volume control can be exercised by attention to the left atrial and right brachial blood pressures. A heat exchanger in the circuit should be provided for the maintenance of normothermia since ventricular fibrillation resulting from a combination of moderate hypothermia, myocardial contusion, and myocardial overload will immeasurably complicate the procedure.

Hypoxemia may result from one or more factors: preexisting lung disease, fat emboli, pulmonary contusion, pulmonary dysfunction caused by shock, chest wall damage, or possibly from the effects of the high pulmonary venous pressure wave that accompanies sudden thoracic compression. When hypoxemia is already present, it is extremely important not to impose further pulmonary damage by a poorly conducted bypass. An oxygenator in a partial bypass circuit provides only limited, indirect protection against cephalic hypoxemia through raising the level of oxygenation in the mixed venous blood (in the case of left atrial bypass) or by reducing the total blood flow through the lungs (in the case of femorofem-

oral bypass). We have preferred to exercise the option of left lung collapse by means of a Carlens tube in order to facilitate the operative procedure and to minimize trauma to the left lung. One may occlude the left main pulmonary artery rather readily and thus reduce the magnitude of the resulting right-to-left pulmonary shunt.

In the presence of severe pulmonary contusion or intracerebral or intra-abdominal injury, one would certainly favor those techniques with which heparinization is avoided. Kahn and co-workers [70] have demonstrated the feasibility of utilizing direct aorta-to-aorta bypass in nonheparinized patients by means of a short polyvinyl chloride tube and cannulas with a 9 mm inside diameter. The method can be further improved by utilizing tubes coated with antithrombogenic material, such as those popularized by Murray, Brawley, and Gott [98]. These are now commercially available. Such a mode of bypass is probably not ideal or even possible in every instance. Operating time and total amount of blood transfused are significantly reduced. If unexpected blood loss is encountered, conversion to a heparinized system may be necessary to salvage large volumes of blood or for autotransfusion to be employed. English [41], Molloy [95], Powley [107], Gunning [53], and Ketharanathan and co-workers [72] have successfully used a direct ventriculoaortic bypass without heparinization in traumatic rupture of the aorta and in other conditions.

Murray and Young [99] have recently shown a preference for ventriculofemoral to that of aorta-aorta shunts because of potential difficulties in cannulating the ascending aorta or aortic arch in some patients. They have used the technique successfully in 3 patients. Diastolic return to the left ventricle through the shunt has apparently not constituted a physiological drawback. Despite the convenience of this approach, there are clearly patients for whom this technique would seem inappropriate.

An added argument in favor of ventricle or aorta to femoral shunting relates to the potential benefit of pulsatile flow on renal function. Many patients with acute aortic rupture will already have suffered renal damage from low flow and low pressure states. Urine excretion with high flow, nonpulsatile partial perfusion during aortic occlusion, using 2500 to 3000 ml/min, has often been disappointing in our experience.

The importance of occluding the aorta proximal to the left subclavian artery by dissection from within the pericardium has already been mentioned. This prevents sudden release of a hematoma. The distal clamp should be placed beyond the level of mediastinal hematoma. The clamp is subsequently advanced toward the site of rupture after the hematoma is evacuated and the rupture exposed within the false aneurysm.

Although a single transverse tear is most commonly found, occasionally two or more transverse lacerations separated by 1 to 4 cm have been noted [35, 80, 103]. In one patient there were three transverse lacerations involving 50, 75, and 100 percent of the circumference. An L- or T-shaped longitudinal tear may extend proximal to the ligamentum arteriosum as far as the left subclavian artery [22, 77, 97] or even to the left common carotid artery [12, 61]. Herenden and King [61] found it necessary in 1 case to occlude just distal to the innominate artery as did also Dart and Braitman [29]. These variations from the single standard transverse lesion emphasize the desirability of initial placement of the proximal clamp between the left subclavian and the left common carotid artery.

Although several surgeons have advocated and practiced direct end-to-end approximation of the ruptured aorta, friability and other pathological alterations in the traumatized tissues have induced most operators to interpose a vascular prosthesis. The ends of the transected aorta are frequently fragmented and must be trimmed. Since to gain a strong anastomosis the adventitia should be included in the suture line, preferably beyond the limits of the mural dissection, a graft is often preferable. However, Appelbaum and associates [3] found primary repair possible in 7 of 17 patients with acute rupture. Primary repair may be more easily accomplished with a partial tear. In some instances a patch repair may be appropriate. After the first day or two following injury, hemorrhagic infiltration, edema, and inflammation weld the tissues together and thus enhance the difficulties of surgical dissection and mobilization.

Esophageal injuries during aorta repair have been reported and can best be avoided by localizing this structure with a Levine tube and by leaving the posteromedial wall of the aorta or aneurysm in situ. Blood supply to the esophagus may already have been compromised by the expanding diffuse hematoma or aneurysm. Esophageal rupture and massive hematemesis have been

reported from an expanding hematoma or chronic aneurysm as well as following operative intervention. The diaphragm should always be explored at thoracotomy since associated rupture of this organ has been reported in approximately 10 percent of cases (Fig 9-6).

In a recent article Heberer [56] published a report of 72 patients collected up to 1970 with traumatic rupture of the aortic isthmus who were operated upon less than 2 months after injury. Fifty-four patients survived; 18 of the total number were treated by direct suture. Most of the chronic aneurysms are either fusiform or saccular with a wide mouth and expanding anteriorly (Fig 9-7); tangential resection is thus not appropriate, although it was employed in some of the early attempts at operative treatment. Several recurrences have been reported after tangential resection [25, 83, 103, 128]. Heberer [56] summarized 204 patients from the literature in whom the traumatic isthmic aortic aneurysms were resected more than 2 months after injury; 186 were repaired with a prosthesis or homograft (20 deaths), 18 by direct suture (1 death), and 5 by endoaneurysmal implantation of a prosthesis (no deaths). Although primary repair in chronic traumatic aneurysm has been accomplished, an interposed prosthesis should minimize surgical dissection and potential hazards.

INNOMINATE ARTERY. The operative treatment of rupture of the transverse arch and branch vessels introduces special considerations. We have reviewed the salient features of 19 operative cases

Fig 9-6. Isthmic aortic rupture in an adult male. Plain chest film illustrates prominence of aortic knob, displacement of trachea and esophagus to right, and rupture of left diaphragm. (Courtesy of Dr. James W. Brooks.)

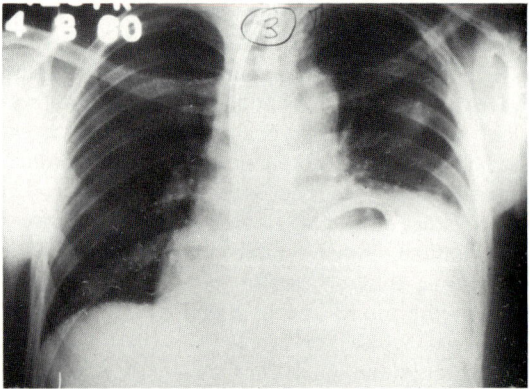

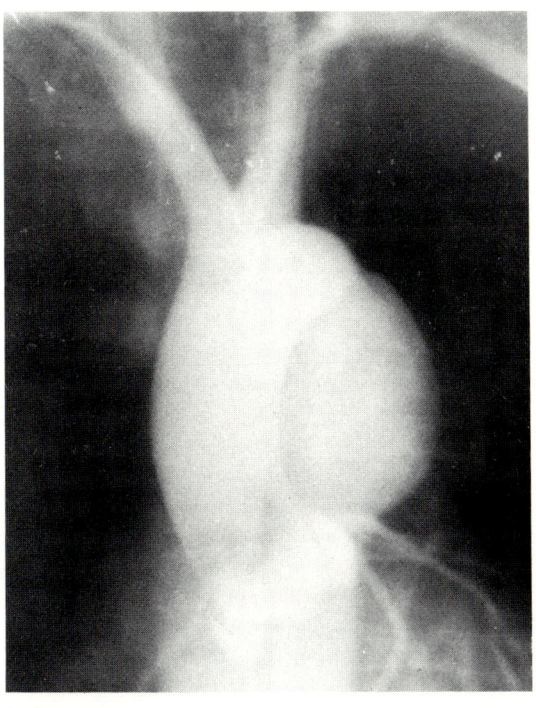

A

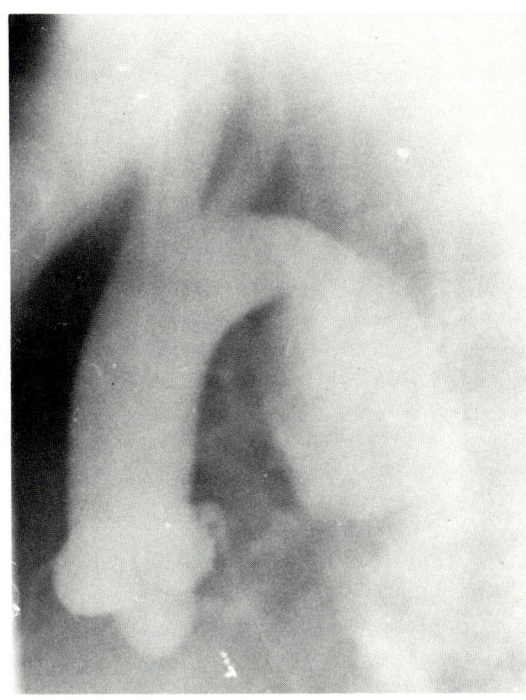

B

Fig 9-7. PA and lateral aortogram. Asymptomatic traumatic aneurysm in a 26-year-old male, resulting from injury four years previously. Other injuries included left pneumothorax and fractures of the left ribs. Distracted ends of transected aorta were 2 to 3 inches apart. Aneurysm was successfully resected under partial bypass support.

of rupture of the innominate artery known to us or recorded in the recent English literature (Table 9-3) [10, 11, 13, 19, 23, 28, 30, 40, 57, 68, 76, 79, 81, 98, 106, 130]. In addition, Piwnica and co-workers [106] referred to 4 other cases in the French literature. Bowen [14] reported a patient who did not undergo operation in whom the innominate artery ruptured into the trachea 1 month after injury. Innominate artery rupture is less frequently encountered but should carry a lower operative mortality than isthmic rupture. Of the 19 patients reported, 4 died.

Characteristically, the rupture is circumferentially complete and represents an avulsion of the origin of the innominate artery confined by adventitia. However, Clarke [23] found a localized tear of the anterior wall, which he repaired directly. More distally located ruptures were encountered by Heggtveit, Campbell, and Hooper [57] and Carlsson and Silander [19] in 3 cases, all of which were more suitably treated by resection of the innominate bifurcation at a later stage. Distal ruptures treated in the acute stage should be amenable to reanastomosis by mobilizing the bifurcation of the innominate artery. In 2 patients lacerations extended to the origin of the left common carotid artery and in 1 case the arch itself was extensively involved [13, 76, 106].

A midsternotomy incision extended into the neck serves admirably for exposure of the innominate artery and base of the left common carotid artery (Figs 9-8, 9-9). A ligneous infiltration into the anterior mediastinum is a common finding following mediastinal hemorrhage. When the dissection is difficult or hazardous, complete circulatory arrest under moderate or deep hypothermia during extracorporeal circulation facilitates the operation and offers protection against sudden, catastrophic hemorrhage. Prior to aortotomy the head of the table should be lowered to avoid the trapping of air in his arch vessels. If he is cooled to 15 to 18°C esophageal temperature,

Table 9-3. Innominate Artery Fracture or Avulsion

Author and Year	Interval from Injury to Operation	Location	Bypass Support			Repair			Result
			ECC	Hypothermia	Carotid Perfusion	Shunt to Carotid Artery	Graft to Ascending Aorta	Direct Reconstruction	
Acute or Subacute (less than 30 days)									
Binet, 1962 [10]	7 days	Origin	+	Deep; arrest	0	0	+	NA	S
Jahnke, 1964 [68]	7 days	Origin	0	0	0	0	NA	+	S
Jahnke, 1964 [68]	16 days	Origin	+	30°	0	0	NA	+(g)	S
Bosher, 1967 [13]	4 days	Origin	+	Deep; arrest	+	NA	+	NA	S
Danielson, 1968 [28]	few hr.	Origin	+	0	+	NA	+	NA	S
Davies, 1970 [30]	?	?	0	+	0	0	NA	+	D
Wexler, 1970	?	Origin(?)	0	?	NA	+	+(?)	?	S
Eller, 1970 [40]	1 day	Origin	?	NA	NA	?	NA	+(g)	D
Eller, 1970 [40]	?	Origin	?	NA	NA	?	NA	+	S
Eller, 1970 [40]	?	Origin	?	NA	NA	?	+	NA	S
Lower, 1971 [81]	2 days	Origin	+	34°	+	0	+	NA	S
Murray, 1971 [98]	5 hr.	Origin	0	0	0	+	+	NA	D(late)
Langlois, 1971 [76]	?	Origin	+	Deep; arrest	0	NA	+	NA	S
Chronic (more than 30 days)									
Carlsson, 1963 [19]	?	Distal	0	30°	0	0	NA	+	S
Clarke, 1964 [23]	7 mo.	Origin	+	0	+	NA	NA	+	D
Heggtveit, 1964 [57]	4 mo.	Distal	0	0	0	0	NA	+(g)	S
Heggtveit, 1964 [57]	11 mo.	Distal	0	0	0	0	NA	+(g)	S
Lim, 1968 [79]	17 yr.	Origin Distal	0	30°	NA	+	+	NA	S
Piwnica, 1971 [106]	3 mo.	Origin	+	30°	+	NA	+	NA	S

g = graft; ? = information not available; NA = not applicable; S = survived; D = died; ECC = extracorporeal circulation; 0 = ECC not used; + = ECC used.

and with the use of the adjunctive measure of 5% carbon dioxide in the gas mixture to facilitate cerebral cooling, interruption of the circulation for 30 minutes is safe. In the gas mixture 100% oxygen is used during the final 5 minutes of prearrest perfusion. Circulatory arrest allows time for isolation of the rupture, most commonly the origin of the innominate artery, and closure of the aortic wall by patch or direct suture (Fig 9-10). Extracorporeal circulation is reinstituted and carotid circulation is then maintained by separate catheter perfusion. Continuity is restored by an appropriately sized tube graft from the ascending aorta to the distal innominate artery or to both the subclavian and the carotid arteries. This method of reconstruction is simpler and safer than reanastomosis of the innominate artery or suture of a tube graft to the point of avulsion, at

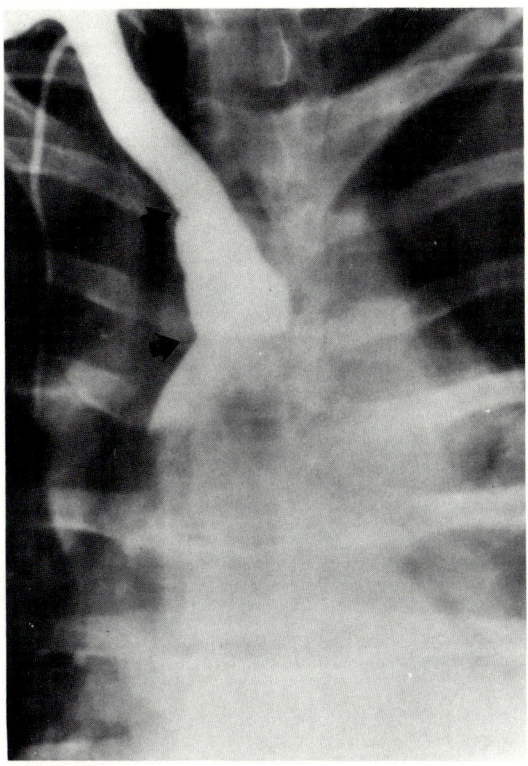

Fig 9-8. A 20-year-old female sustained crushing injury to the chest in an auto accident. There was minimal hemopneumothorax on the right. A widened mediastinum was noted on chest roentgenogram and a systolic bruit was heard in the epigastrium. Aortogram revealed an avulsion of the innominate artery. Extent of distraction and "false" aneurysm indicated by arrows. (From Bosher and Freed [13]. Courtesy of C. V. Mosby Co.)

which point the aortic wall is both friable and fragmented.

Total cardiopulmonary bypass has been employed in about half of the cases of innominate artery avulsion and provides additional safety since the tear may extend along the wall of the aorta. In specific cases circulatory support can be modified; for example cardiopulmonary bypass is obviously not needed when the innominate artery is injured at a more distal point. In some instances repair of the avulsion site can be accomplished safely after application of an exclusion clamp to the aortic wall, as was done in many of the cases reviewed. If the distal innominate artery pressure is less than 50 mm Hg, it is wise to employ a shunt or perfusion to protect the brain. Murray,

Brawley, and Gott [98] have emphasized the special adaptability of the heparin-coated bypass shunt in surgery of the innominate artery.

TRANSVERSE ARCH. Few cases of operative repair of acute rupture or resection of chronic traumatic aneurysms of the transverse arch have been reported. Piwnica and co-workers [106] encountered an avulsion of the innominate artery with a transverse tear into the aorta that required reanastomosis of the entire circumference of the aorta. The innominate and left common carotid arteries were perfused distally through separate catheters; this is undoubtedly the technique to be preferred when a prolonged period of isolation of the transverse arch is required. A similar technique was employed by Bosher and Freed [13] in closing a tear that extended to the base of the left carotid artery. In 1958 DeBakey and colleagues [31] referred to three traumatic aneurysms of the aortic arch, two resected successfully, but did not specify the exact location of the lesions. Most impressive is the successful case reported by Appelbaum, Karp, and Kirklin [3] in which extensive injury involved the entire aortic arch. During the period of 44 minutes the patient was under profound hypothermia, the arch was replaced by a Dacron tube to which a strip of aortic wall containing the origins of the head vessels was anastomosed.

The usefulness of deep hypothermia and complete circulatory arrest in the treatment of a chronic traumatic aneurysm of the posterior aspect of the transverse aorta was again demonstrated by Dumanian and associates [36]. The complex aneurysm was approached through a midline sternotomy and readily managed by patch closure of its mouth from within the lumen of the aorta.

A similar type of traumatic aneurysm of 34 years' standing, involving the transverse arch and presenting superiorly between the innominate and left common carotid arteries, was corrected by Mittal, May, and Samson [92]. He used a midline sternotomy and extended it into the left second intercostal space. The transverse arch was isolated by occluding the ascending and descending aorta and perfusing the innominate and carotid arteries separately. The aneurysm was excised and the defect closed directly.

LEFT SUBCLAVIAN ARTERY. Symbas and co-workers [124] repaired a fracture of the aortic arch at the origin of the left subclavian artery associated with transection of the latter vessel. We

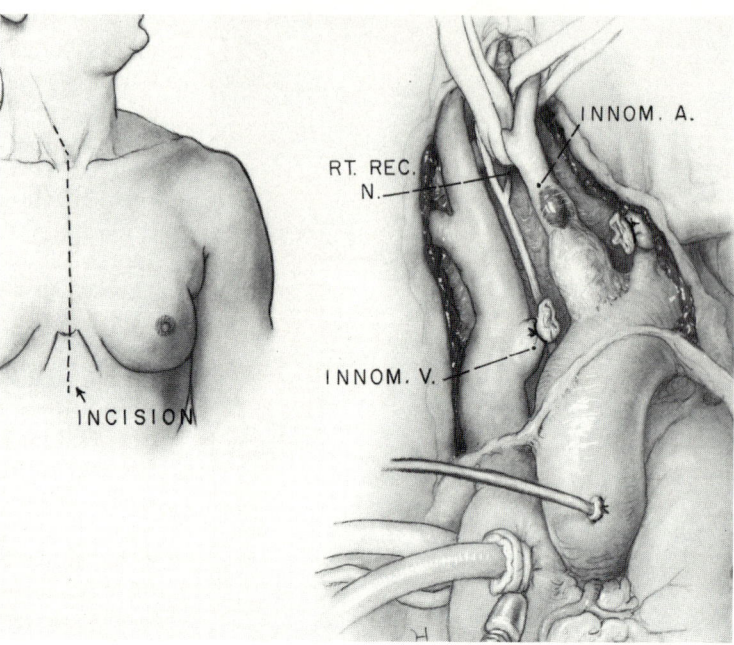

Fig 9-9. Same patient as in Fig 9-8. Surgery performed four days following injury. The incision was extended into the neck. Division of the sternal head of the sternomastoid muscle and strap muscles provided excellent exposure. Transection of the left innominate vein was essential. (From Bosher and Freed [13]. Courtesy of C. V. Mosby Co.)

believe that this represents the acute stage of a type of chronic aneurysm that has been reported in a less extensive form by several other authors. Symbas surmised that direct impact from the flail sternum caused the injury, but the mechanism is probably more complex and either distraction of the subclavian artery or kinking of this vessel at its origin are probably also involved. This segment of aorta was resected by Symbas, a graft interposed, and continuity with the subclavian artery reestablished by means of a second graft.

A traumatic avulsion of the left subclavian artery in a patient suffering first rib and clavicular injuries was also reported by Clarke and Allen [21]. The vessel was avulsed at its origin, but a short sleeve of adventitia prevented exsanguination. The aortic wall was repaired tangentially. De Meules, Cramer, and Perry [32] mentioned rupture of the proximal left subclavian artery in 2 patients, but it is not clear that these were clinical cases. Nelson and Ashley [100] found a complete tear of the intima of the left subclavian artery 2 cm from its origin in a patient in whom isthmic aortic rupture had been suspected.

Temple [126] in 1950 reported the first transpleural approach to an aneurysm of the left subclavian artery undertaken 2 years after the patient suffered blunt trauma to the chest. In 1953 Bahnson [7] reported the definitive repair of a chronic

traumatic aneurysm at the origin of the left subclavian artery with involvement of the adjacent aortic wall. The defect was directly sutured from within the opened aneurysm after the aorta was cross-clamped above and below the subclavian artery. Holmes and Netterville [64] wrapped a similar type of aneurysm with reactive polyethylene. Two chronic aneurysms, probably resulting from avulsion injuries of the left subclavian artery, were treated by Thomas [127]. The aorta was repaired tangentially in both, and, in 1 case, the left subclavian artery was restored by end-to-side anastomosis to the left common carotid.

LEFT COMMON CAROTID ARTERY. Judging from the paucity of operative reports, injury to the intrathoracic left common carotid artery is infrequently recognized clinically, although it may be seen not uncommonly at postmortem examination. Three cases have been reported, and in 2 instances associated avulsion of the innominate artery was also present [13, 30, 32]. Michaud and colleagues

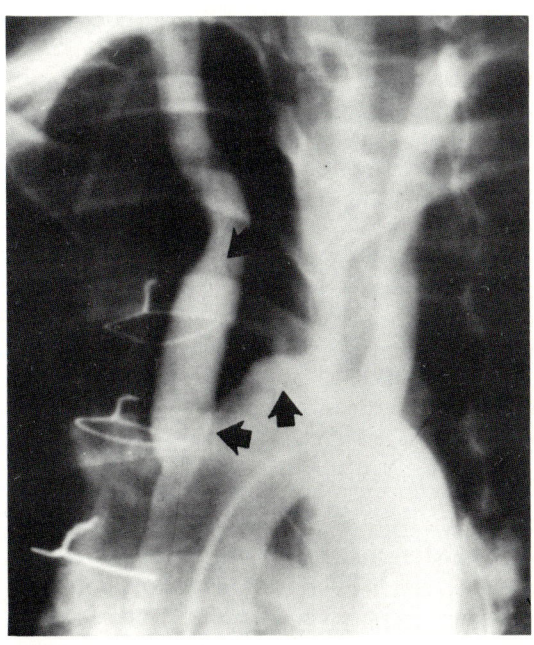

Fig 9-10. Same patient as in Figure 9-8. Aortogram done six weeks post-repair demonstrates reconstruction of the innominate artery with a prosthesis to the ascending aorta, closure of avulsion site with patch, and retarded flow into left common carotid artery. A previously unrecognized fracture of this carotid artery has developed a stenotic lesion. (From Bosher and Freed [13]. Courtesy of C. V. Mosby Co.)

[91] reported a rupture of the aorta between the left subclavian and left common carotid arteries but provided no additional information.

It is important to emphasize the posttraumatic pathological changes that may occur in the branch vessels of the aorta, first described by Heggtveit, Campbell, and Hooper [57]. Scarring and thickening occur rapidly at the angle formed by the reflected adventitia and the media. Loss of elasticity and stricturing at the distal segment produce a significant stenosis, one which must be resected along with the aneurysm if a satisfactory reconstruction is to be obtained [13] (see Fig 9-10).

MULTIPLE RUPTURES AND ANEURYSMS. In the summary of Parmley and colleagues [102] all patients with multiple tears of the aorta died immediately or lived less than 30 minutes. However, the outlook is not so gloomy, particularly when branch vessels are involved. Several patients have undergone surgery for isthmic aortic rupture only to die from a previously unrecognized rupture at

a remote site. Callaghan described a patient who died from a second rupture near the diaphragm (referred to by Beall and associates [8]), and Lipchik and Robinson [80] have recorded an instance of death from a second rupture in the abdominal aorta. Lim and co-workers [79] resected an expanding 6-cm innominate artery aneurysm, but the patient later refused surgery for an associated asymptomatic isthmic aneurysm. Garamella and colleagues [48] noted a healed laceration of the ascending aorta at postmortem examination in a patient who died after resection of an isthmic aneurysm that had ruptured into the esophagus. In 3 patients who died without operation, Blazek [12] found a rupture at the isthmus and ascending aorta, Lewis [78] found one at the isthmus and in the abdominal aorta, and Matloff and Morton [86] found one in the right subclavian artery and ascending aorta.

Hardin [54] successfully resected two chronic aneurysms in the descending thoracic aorta. Bosher and Freed [13] have repaired a rupture of the innominate and left common carotid arteries in two stages, and Brawley and associates [15] have repaired rupture of the innominate and left subclavian arteries in a single stage. Davies and Roylance [30], reporting on a remarkable series of patients with multiple ruptures, reported rupture of combinations of (1) the aortic isthmus and innominate artery, (2) innominate artery and left common carotid artery, and (3) aortic isthmus and right subclavian artery. Two of these patients were treated with operation and 1 recovered. Because of the wide variety and combination of vascular lesions that have been seen, it is obvious that emphasis should be placed on a thorough arteriographic study of the entire aorta and its major branches whenever possible. Analysis of the forces and mechanisms of injury involved should lead to a higher index of suspicion and more aggressive methods of detection. The opportunity for complete operative treatment and salvage of these patients is by no means remote.

RUPTURES IN CONGENITALLY ANOMALOUS VESSELS. Ruptures in congenitally anomalous vessels have been reported in 3 patients, including an anomalous left vertebral artery that was avulsed from the aortic arch [96]. In this instance the hematoma extended toward the right and displaced the superior vena cava.

An expanding aneurysm due to rupture of an aberrant right subclavian artery behind the esophagus and trachea caused death from mediastinal tamponade [112]. Symptoms of tracheal and esophageal compression, distention of the cervical veins, and a blood pressure differential between the arms dominated the clinical picture. The injury was localized to the anomalous vessel as it crossed in front of the third thoracic vertebra. The aorta remained intact.

Langlois, Binet, and Jegou [76] encountered rupture of a right aortic arch with a retroesophageal left subclavian artery. The exact location of the injury was not stated. Successful repair was accomplished using total bypass and proximal and distal arterial cannulations.

BRONCHIAL RUPTURE COMPLICATING VASCULAR RUPTURE. The rare combination of rupture of a main stem bronchus and aorta, or aortic branch vessel, has been reported in 6 patients (Table 9-4). The ability of a patient to survive such massive thoracic trauma is remarkable. The right main stem bronchus has been reported as having been ruptured twice in combination with innominate artery avulsion [57], once with right subclavian artery rupture [51], and, in a contralateral injury, with the aortic isthmus [105]. Transections of the left main stem bronchus have been associated with a rupture of the isthmus [20] and a traumatic aneurysm of the transverse arch [71]. Two patients died of hemorrhage from the vascular injury during operation; in the others both lesions were successfully corrected. Chalant and associates [20] reported an interesting case of detachment of the left main stem bronchus just below the tracheal bifurcation as a result of a crush injury in a 4-year-old child. No abnormality of the aorta was noted during exploration, but 3 weeks later signs of an aortic rupture developed and were verified by angiography. Thoracotomy revealed a complete rupture of the isthmic aorta, which was repaired successfully.

It is comforting to know that in most instances the two ruptures will occur in the same hemithorax. The gravity of each lesion makes immediate surgery mandatory, with repair of the respiratory tract being the most urgent unless active hemorrhage is present. Under the circumstances of pleural contamination, a major effort should be made to accomplish an end-to-end vascular anastomosis and avoid the use of a prosthesis.

Postoperative Complications

If there is preoperative pulmonary parenchymal injury and chest wall damage, postoperative pulmonary complications are likely to be serious. Continued postoperative tracheal intubation or tracheostomy with assisted ventilation is often required, and end-expiratory positive pressure is helpful. Acute tubular necrosis is not uncommon following the combination of shock, multiple trauma, transfusions, and partial bypass. Postoperative paraplegia is now rare unless it existed prior to surgery, but it does continue to be a threat whenever prolonged cross-clamping of the aorta without bypass support is required [110], or when crucial intercostal arteries are sacrificed. Injury to the left recurrent laryngeal nerve and esophageal necrosis have previously been alluded to, together with preventive measures. Cardiac ar-

Table 9-4. Bronchial Rupture Complicating Vascular Rupture

Author	Interval to Bronchial Repair	Interval to Vascular Repair	Bronchus Injured	Vessel Injured	Outcome
Pate [105]	1 day	1 day	Right	Isthmus	Died
Chalant [20]	1 day	3 wk.	Left	Isthmus	Survived
Katz [71][a]	2 mo.	2 mo.	Left	Transverse arch	Died
Giragos [51]	7 wk.	7 wk.	Right	Right subclavian artery	Survived
Heggtveit [57]	1 day	4 mo.	Right	Innominate	Survived
Heggtveit [57]	1 day	11 mo.	Right	Innominate	Survived

[a] This patient also had a blocked right subclavian artery.

Note: One additional case with aortic rupture and perforation of the right main stem bronchus and esophagus was apparently successfully treated, although complete information is lacking. (L. Johansson, Surgery of Aortic Aneurysms. Analysis of 36 operation cases. Acta Chir Scand 128:630, 1964.)

rhythmias may be expected in proportion to the extent of cardiac contusion and circulatory disturbance as well as preexisting cardiac disease.

REFERENCES

1. Adams HD, van Geertruyden HH: Neurologic complications of aortic surgery. Ann Surg 144:574, 1956
2. Aldman B: Biodynamic studies on impact protection. Acta Physiol Scand (Suppl.):192, 1962
3. Appelbaum A, Karp RB, Kirklin JW: Surgical treatment for closed thoracic aortic injuries. J Thorac Cardiovasc Surg 71:458, 1976
4. Attar S, Ayella RJ, McLaughlin JS: The widened mediastinum in trauma. Ann Thorac Surg 13:435, 1972
5. Aufrance OE, Jones WN, Stewart WG Jr: Delayed aortic rupture accompanying major musculoskeletal trauma. JAMA 191:666, 1965
6. Backstrom CG: Traffic injuries in South Sweden with special reference to medico-legal autopsies of car occupants and value of safety belts. Acta Chir Scand (Suppl.):308, 1963
7. Bahnson HT: Definitive treatment of saccular aneurysms of the aorta with excision of sac and aortic suture. Surg Gynecol Obstet 96:383, 1953
8. Beall AC Jr, et al: Aortic laceration due to rapid deceleration (surgical management). Arch Surg 98:595, 1969
9. Bennett DE, Cherry JK: The natural history of traumatic aneurysms of the aorta. Surgery 61:516, 1967
10. Binet J-P, et al: A case of recent traumatic avulsion of the innominate artery at its origin from the aortic arch. J Thorac Cardiovasc Surg 43:670, 1962
11. Binet J-P, et al: Two instances of traumatic rupture of the aortic arch. Mem Acad Chir (Paris) 93:44, 1967
12. Blazek JV: Acute traumatic rupture of the thoracic aorta demonstrated by retrograde aortography. Radiology 85:253, 1965
13. Bosher, LH Jr, Freed TA: The surgical treatment of traumatic rupture or avulsion of the innominate artery, with report of a case involving both the innominate and left common carotid arteries. J Thorac Cardiovasc Surg 54:732, 1967
14. Bowen DA: Traumatic aneurysm of the innominate artery. Med Sci Law 7:132, 1967
15. Brawley RK, et al: The management of wounds of the innominate, subclavian, and axillary blood vessels. Surg Gynecol Obstet 131:1130, 1970
16. Bross W: Injuries of the thoracic aorta. J Cardiovasc Surg (Torino) 12:95, 1971
17. Butcher HR Jr: The elastic properties of human aortic intima, media, and adventitia: The initial effect of thromboendarterectomy. Ann Surg 151:480, 1960
18. Cammack K, et al: Deceleration injuries of the thoracic aorta. Arch Surg 79:90, 1959
19. Carlsson E, Silander T: Rupture of the subclavian and the innominate artery due to nonpenetrating trauma of the chest. Acta Chir Scand 125:294, 1963
20. Chalant Ch-H, et al: Surgical treatment of post-traumatic aneurysms of the thoracic aorta. J Cardiovasc Surg (Torino) 12:108, 1971
21. Clarke CP, Allen GL: Traumatic avulsion of the left subclavian artery. Ann Thorac Surg 3:154, 1967
22. Clarke CP, et al: Traumatic rupture of the thoracic aorta: Diagnosis and treatment. Br J Surg 54:353, 1967
23. Clarke DB: Traumatic aneurysm of the innominate artery at its origin from the aortic arch. Br J Surg 51:668, 1964
24. Clegg J, Charlesworth D: Traumatic rupture of the thoracic aorta. J Cardiovasc Surg (Torino) 13:206, 1972
25. Cooley DA, DeBakey ME: Resection of the thoracic aorta with replacement by homograft for aneurysms and constrictive lesions. J Thorac Cardiovasc Surg 29:66, 1955
26. Cooley DA, DeBakey ME: Resection of entire ascending aorta in fusiform aneurysm using cardiac bypass. JAMA 162:1158, 1956
27. Crawford ES, et al: Reappraisal of adjuncts to avoid ischemia in the treatment of thoracic aortic aneurysms. Surgery 67:182, 1970
28. Danielson GK, Wood R, Holloway JB Jr: Traumatic avulsion of the innominate artery from the aorta. Successful immediate repair utilizing cardiopulmonary bypass. Ann Thorac Surg 5:451, 1968
29. Dart CH, Braitman HE: Traumatic rupture of thoracic aorta. Arch Surg 111:697, 1976
30. Davies ER, Roylance J: Aortography in the investigation of traumatic mediastinal haematoma. Clin Radiol 21:297, 1970
31. DeBakey ME, et al: Aneurysms of the thoracic aorta. Analysis of 179 patients treated by resection. J Thorac Cardiovasc Surg 36:393, 1958
32. DeMeules JE, Cramer G, Perry JP Jr: Rupture of aorta and great vessels due to blunt thoracic trauma. J Thorac Cardiovasc Surg 61:438, 1971

33. DeMuth WE Jr, Roe H, Hobbie W: Immediate repair of traumatic rupture of thoracic aorta. Arch Surg 91:602, 1965

34. DeMuth WE Jr: Exsanguination during tracheostomy. A complication of mediastinal arterial injury. Ann Surg 163:643, 1966

35. Dobell ARC, MacNaughton EA, Crutchlow EF: Successful early treatment of subadventitial rupture of the thoracic aorta. N Engl J Med 270:410, 1964

36. Dumanian AV, et al: Profound hypothermia and circulatory arrest in the surgical treatment of traumatic aneurysm of the thoracic aorta. J Thorac Cardiovasc Surg 59:541, 1970

37. Edwards JE: Pathologic aspects of cardiac valvular insufficiencies. Arch Surg 77:634, 1958

38. Eiseman B, Rainer, WG: Clinical management of post-traumatic rupture of the thoracic aorta. J Thorac Cardiovasc Surg 35:347, 1958

39. Eiseman B, Summers WB: Factors affecting spinal cord ischemia during aortic occlusion. Surgery 38:1063, 1955

40. Eller JL, Ziter FMH Jr: Avulsion of the innominate artery from the aortic arch. An evaluation of roentgenographic findings. Radiology 94:75, 1970

41. English TAH: Direct left ventriculofemoral bypass during resection of coarctation of the aorta with anomalous subclavian arteries. Thorax 20:36, 1965

42. Flaherty TT, et al: Nonpenetrating injuries to the thoracic aorta. Radiology 92:541, 1969

43. Fleischaker RJ, Mazur JH, Baisch BF: Surgical treatment of acute traumatic rupture of the thoracic aorta. J Thorac Cardiovasc Surg 47:289, 1964

44. Fleming AW, Green DC: Traumatic aneurysms of the thoracic aorta. Ann Thorac Surg 18:91, 1974

45. Forsee JH, Blake HA: The recognition and management of closed chest trauma. Surg Clin North Am 38:1545, 1958

46. Freed TA, Bosher LH Jr: Arteriographic demonstration of laceration of great vessels secondary to blunt chest trauma. Radiology 90:88, 1968

47. Fry RD, et al: Severe coarctation of the aorta with pulmonary edema. Chest 70:76, 1976

48. Garamella JJ, et al: Traumatic aneurysms of the thoracic aorta. (Report of four cases, including one of spontaneous rupture into the esophagus.) N Engl J Med 266:1341, 1962

49. Gazzaniga AB, et al: Rupture of the thoracic aorta following blunt trauma. Arch Surg 110:1119, 1975

50. Geiger JP: Discussion, ref 44.

51. Giragos H, Faber LP, Weinberg M Jr: Concomitant intrathoracic aneurysm and bronchial rupture due to trauma. Successful repair. Ann Thorac Surg 5:47, 1968

52. Greendyke RM: Traumatic rupture of aorta (special reference to automobile accidents). JAMA 195:527, 1966

53. Gunning AJ: A disposable one-piece left ventriculo-aortic bypass cannula. Thorax 27:371, 1972

54. Hardin CA: Resection and Orlon graft of multiple aortic aneurysms due to trauma. J Thorac Cardiovasc Surg 32:251, 1956

55. Hass GM: Types of internal injuries of personnel involved in aircraft accidents. J Aviation Med 15:77, 1944

56. Heberer G: Ruptures and aneurysms of the thoracic aorta after blunt chest trauma. J Cardiovasc Surg (Torino) 12:115, 1971

57. Heggtveit HA, Campbell JS, Hooper GD: Innominate arterial aneurysms occurring after blunt trauma. Am J Clin Pathol 42:69, 1964

58. Heller A: Uber eine traumatische Insuffizienz der Aortenklappen. Arch Klin Med 79:306, 1903

59. Hellstrom G: Lesions associated with closed liver injury. A clinical study of 192 fatal cases. Acta Chir Scand 131:460, 1966

60. Henning BH, Agmar AR: Traumatic rupture of thoracic aorta. Report of a case. Milit Surg 103:260, 1948

61. Herenden L, King H: Transient anuria and paraplegia following traumatic rupture of the thoracic aorta. J Thorac Cardiovasc Surg 56:599, 1968

62. Heroy WW: Discussion, p. 96. In TF Nealon Jr, JY Templeton III, VD Cuddy, Instrumental perforation of the esophagus. J Thorac Cardiovasc Surg 41:75, 1961

63. Hiertonn T: Homologous transplantation of arterial segments preserved in a blood vessel bank. Preliminary report on an experimental investigation in dogs. Acta Orthop Scand 22:5, 1952

64. Holmes TW Jr, Netterville RE: Complications of first rib fracture, including one case each of tracheo-esophageal fistula and aortic arch aneurysm. Survey of literature: incidence and complications. J Thorac Cardiovasc Surg 32:74, 1956

65. Hug HR, Taber RE: Bypass flow requirements during thoracic aneurysmectomy with particular attention to the prevention of left heart failure. J Thorac Cardiovasc Surg 57:203, 1969

66. Hughes JT: Spinal-cord infarction due to aortic trauma. Br Med J 2:356, 1964

67. Jackson FR, Berkas EM, Roberts VL: Trau-

matic aortic rupture after blunt trauma. Dis Chest 53:577, 1968

68. Jahnke EJ, Fisher GW, Jones RC: Acute traumatic rupture of the thoracic aorta. J Thorac Cardiovasc Surg 48:63, 1964

69. Jensen OM: Traumatisk aortaruptur. En analyse af 68 fatale tilfaelde. Nord Med 71: 337, 1964

70. Kahn DR, Vathayanon S, Sloan H: Resection of descending thoracic aneurysms without left heart bypass. Arch Surg 97:336, 1968

71. Katz RI, Briggs JN: Traumatic ruptured bronchus and injury of major thoracic vessels. Ann Thorac Surg 3:235, 1967

72. Ketharanathan V, McConchie IH, Westlake GW: Left ventricle-femoral artery shunt in the management of acute traumatic rupture of the descending thoracic aorta. J Thorac Cardiovasc Surg 64:291, 1972

73. Kirsh MM, et al: Repair of acute traumatic rupture of the aorta without extracorporeal circulation. Ann Thorac Surg 10:227, 1970

74. Kirsh MM, et al: Roentgenographic evaluation of traumatic rupture of the aorta. Surg Gynecol Obstet 131:900, 1970

75. Klotz O, Simpson W: Spontaneous rupture of the aorta. Am J Med Sci 184:455, 1932

76. Langlois J, Binet J-P, Jegou D: Traumatic rupture of the thoracic aorta and of its branches. J Cardiovasc Surg (Torino) 12:83, 1971

77. Lemmon WM, et al: Traumatic aortic rupture. Penn Med 69:29, 1966

78. Lewis H: Some unusual features in a case of traumatic rupture of the thoracic aorta. J Trauma 5:665, 1965

79. Lim RC Jr, et al: Multiple traumatic thoracic aneurysms after nonpenetrating chest injury. Ann Thorac Surg 6:377, 1968

80. Lipchik EO, Robinson KE: Acute traumatic rupture of the thoracic aorta. Am J Roentgenol 104:408, 1968

81. Lower RR: Unpublished case, 1971.

82. Lundevall J: The mechanism of traumatic rupture of the aorta. Acta Pathol Microbiol Scand 62:34, 1964

83. MacIntyre RS: Traumatic aneurysm of the thoracic aorta. Am J Roentgenol 83:1011, 1960

84. MacKenzie JR, Hackett M, Munro DD: Diagnosis of ruptured great vessels of the thorax: A simple and reliable method. Presented at the 26th annual session of the American Association for the Surgery of Trauma, Santa Barbara, Calif., Oct. 6–8, 1966

85. Marshall TK: Traumatic dissecting aneurysms. J Clin Pathol 11:36, 1958

86. Matloff DB, Morton JH: Acute trauma to the subclavian arteries. Am J Surg 115:675, 1968

87. Mazzitello WF: Traumatic involvement of the thoracic aorta. Arch Intern Med 100:894, 1957

88. McBurney RP, Vaughan RH: Rupture of the thoracic aorta due to nonpenetrating trauma. Ann Surg 153:670, 1961

89. McClenathan JE, Brettschneider L: Traumatic thoracic aortic aneurysms. J Thorac Cardiovasc Surg 50:74, 1965

90. McKnight JT, Meyer JA, Neville JF Jr: Nonpenetrating traumatic rupture of the thoracic aorta. Ann Surg 160:1069, 1964

91. Michaud P, et al: Traumatic aneurysms of the aorta. Analysis of 11 observations. J Cardiovasc Surg (Torino) 12:121, 1971

92. Mittal A, May IA, Samson PC: Traumatic aneurysm of the aortic arch—Report of an unusual location. Ann Thorac Surg 13:494, 1972

93. Moffat RC, Roberts VL, Berkas EM: Blunt trauma to the thorax—development of pseudoaneurysms in the dog. J Trauma 6:666, 1966

94. Moffat RC, et al: Pathogenesis of experimental traumatic thoracic aneurysm. Vasc Surg 1: 11, 1967

95. Molloy PJ: Repair of the ruptured thoracic aorta using left ventriculo-aortic support. Thorax 25:213, 1970

96. Molnar W, Pace WG: Traumatic rupture of the thoracic aorta. Radiol Clin North Am 4: 403, 1966

97. Mulder DG, Grollman JH Jr: Traumatic disruption of the thoracic aorta. Am J Surg 118: 311, 1969

98. Murray GF, Brawley RK, Gott VL: Reconstruction of the innominate artery by means of a temporary heparin-coated shunt bypass. J Thorac Cardiovasc Surg 62:34, 1971

99. Murray GF, Young WG: Thoracic aneurysmectomy utilizing direct left ventriculofemoral shunt (TDMAC-heparin) bypass. Ann Thorac Surg 21:26, 1976

100. Nelson DA, Ashley PF: Rupture of the aorta during closed-chest cardiac massage. JAMA 193:681, 1965

101. Oppenheim F: Gibt es eine Spontanruptur der gesunden Aorta und wie kommt sie zustande? Munch Med Wochenschr 65:1234, 1918

102. Parmley LF, et al: Nonpenetrating traumatic injury of the aorta. Circulation 17:1086, 1958

103. Passaro E Jr, Pace WG: Traumatic rupture of the aorta. Surgery 46:787, 1959

104. Pasternak BM, Boyd DP, Ellis HE Jr: Spinal cord injury after procedures on the aorta. Surg Gynecol Obstet 135:29, 1972

105. Pate JW, Butterick OD, Richardson RL:

Traumatic rupture of the thoracic aorta. JAMA 203:1022, 1968

106. Piwnica AH, et al: Traumatic rupture of the aortic arch with disinsertion of the innominate artery. Report of a case with successful treatment. J Thorac Cardiovasc Surg 61:246, 1971

107. Powley PH: Traumatic rupture of the aorta: Repair using ventriculo-aortic bypass. Proc R Soc Med 64:1085, 1971

108. Rice WG, Wittstruck KP: Acute hypertension and delayed traumatic rupture of the aorta. JAMA 147:915, 1951

109. Rindfleisch E: Zur Entstehung und Heilung des Aneurysma dissecans aortae. Virchows Arch [Pathol Anat] 131:374, 1893

110. Rittenhouse EA, et al: Traumatic rupture of the thoracic aorta: A review of the literature and a report of five cases with attention to special problems in early surgical management. Ann Surg 170:87, 1969

111. Roberts VL, Moffat RC, Berkas EM: Blunt trauma to the thorax-mechanism of vascular injuries. In Proceedings of the 9th Stapp Car Crash Conference (Sec. 1, Chapter I), Oct. 20–21, 1965

112. Ryan JA: An unusual case of traumatic mediastinal aneurysm in a closed chest injury. Br J Surg 50:210, 1962

113. Sanborn JC, Heitzman ER, Markarian B: Traumatic rupture of the thoracic aorta, roentgen-pathological correlations. Radiology 95:293, 1970

114. Shennan T: Traumatic (false) aneurysm of the aorta. J Pathol Bacteriol 32:795, 1929

115. Shumacker HB, King H: Surgical management of rapidly expanding intrathoracic pulsating hematomas. Surg Gynecol Obstet 109:155, 1959

116. Simpson K: Traction rupture of the great vessels of the chest following injury to the head. Guys Hosp Rep 90:196, 1940

117. Slaney G, Ashton F, Abrams LD: Traumatic rupture of the aorta. Br J Surg 53:361, 1966

118. Spencer FC, et al: A report of fifteen patients with traumatic rupture of the thoracic aorta. J Thorac Cardiovasc Surg 41:1, 1961

119. Stapp JP: Human tolerance to deceleration, summary of 166 runs. J Aviation Med 22:42, 1951

120. Stapp JP: Human tolerance to deceleration. Am J. Surg 93:734, 1957

121. Stoney RJ, Roe BG, Redington JV: Rupture of thoracic aorta due to closed-chest trauma. Arch Surg 89:840, 1964

122. Strassmann G: Traumatic rupture of the aorta. Am Heart J 33:508, 1947

123. Stryker WA: Traumatic saccular aneurysm of thoracic aorta. Am J Clin Pathol 18:152, 1948

124. Symbas PN, Pourhamidi A, Levin JM: Traumatic rupture of the aortic arch between left common carotid and left subclavian arteries and avulsion of the left subclavian artery. Ann Surg 170:152, 1969

125. Tannenbaum I, Ferguson JA: Rapid deceleration and rupture of the aorta. Arch Pathol 45:503, 1948

126. Temple LJ: Aneurysm of the first part of the left subclavian artery. Review of the literature and a case history. J Thorac Cardiovasc Surg 19:412, 1950

127. Thomas TV: Intrathoracic aneurysms of the innominate and subclavian arteries. J Thorac Cardiovasc Surg 63:461, 1972

128. Thomford NR, Pace WG, Meckstroth CV: Traumatic rupture of the thoracic aorta. Am Surg 35:244, 1969

129. Voigt GE: Die biomechanik stumpfer brustverletzungen besonders von thorax, aorta und herz. Stuttgart, Springer-Verlag, 1968

130. Wexler L, Silverman J: Traumatic rupture of the innominate artery—a seat-belt injury. N Engl J Med 282:1186, 1970

131. Wilson RF, et al: Acute mediastinal widening following blunt chest trauma. Arch Surg 104:551, 1972

132. Wyman AC: Roentgenologic diagnosis of traumatic rupture of the thoracic aorta. Arch Surg 66:656, 1953

133. Zehnder MA: Zerreissfestigkeit und Elastizitat der Aorta. Beitrag zur traumatischen Aortenruptur. Schweiz Med Wochenschr 85:203, 1955

134. Zehnder MA: Unfallmechanismus und Unfallmechanik der Aortenruptur im gesschlossenen Thoraxtrauma. Thoraxchirurgie 8:47, 1960–61

ADDITIONAL READING

Alley RD, et al: Traumatic aortic aneurysms. Four cases of graftless excision and anastomosis. Ann Thorac Surg 2:514, 1966

Anastasia LF: Traumatic disruption of the thoracic aorta treated with external shunt. Am J Surg 120:810, 1970

Aronstam EM, et al: Recent surgical and phamacologic experience with acute dissecting and traumatic aneurysms. J Thorac Cardiovasc Surg 59:231, 1970

Athey P, et al: Transections of the thoracic aorta—special reference to routine chest roentgenograms. South Med J 63:971, 1970

Blank RH, Blackburn JP, Connar RG: Traumatic rupture of the thoracic aorta following blunt chest injury. Ann Thorac Surg 2:827, 1966

Bloodwell RD, Hallman GL, Cooley DA: Partial cardiopulmonary bypass for pericardiectomy and resection of descending thoracic aortic aneurysms. Ann Thorac Surg 6:46, 1968

Bryant LR, et al: Thoracic aneurysms with aortico-bronchial fistula. Ann Surg 168:79, 1968

Connolly JE, Kountz SL, Boyd RJ: Left heart bypass, experimental and clinical observations on its regulation with particular reference to maintenance of maximal renal blood flow. J Thorac Cardiovasc Surg 44:577, 1962

Cox WD, et al: Resection of descending thoracic aorta using peripheral cardiopulmonary bypass. Dis Chest 55:54, 1969

Dillon MC, Young WG, Sealy WC: Aneurysms of the descending thoracic aorta. Ann Thorac Surg 3:430, 1967

Ellis F: Surgical repair of a traumatic rupture of the thoracic aorta. Br J Surg 46:495, 1959

Fahlsing WC, Magoon CC, Sproul G: Subclavian artery aneurysm due to closed chest trauma. Calif Med 101:126, 1964

Fidler HK: Traumatic rupture of the thoracic aorta. Can Med Assoc J 60:590, 1949

Gerbode F, et al: Traumatic thoracic aneurysms: Treatment by resection and grafting with the use of an extracorporeal bypass. Surgery 42:975, 1957

Goggin MJ, Thompson FD, Jackson JW: Deceleration trauma to the heart and great vessels after road-traffic accidents. Br Med J 2:767, 1970

Goyette EM, et al: Traumatic aortic aneurysms. Circulation 10:824, 1954

Groves LK: Traumatic aneurysm of the thoracic aorta. N Engl J Med 27:220, 1964

Gwathmey O, Byrd CW: Clinical experience with acute traumatic rupture of the thoracic aorta in a general hospital. Ann Surg 159:846, 1964

Hamby RI, Gulotta SJ, Gruber F: Traumatic aortic aneurysm complicated by obstruction of the left pulmonary artery. Vasc Surg 1:179, 1967

Hughes RK: Thoracic trauma. Ann Thorac Surg 1:778, 1965

Jay JB, French SW III: Traumatic rupture of the thoracic aorta. Review of literature and case report. Arch Surg 68:657, 1954

Juanteguy JM, Wilder RJ: Treatment of dissecting aneurysm of the descending thoracic aorta. Am Surg 36:493, 1970

Kahn AM, Joseph WL, Hughes RK: Traumatic aneurysms of the thoracic aorta. Ann Thorac Surg 4:175, 1967

Keen G, Bradbrook RA, McGinn F: Traumatic rupture of the thoracic aorta. Thorax 24:25, 1969

Koroxenidis GT, et al: Traumatic rupture of the thoracic aorta simulating coarctation. Am J Cardiol 16:605, 1965

Kosak M: Traumatic rupture of the thoracic aorta caused by deceleration. J Cardiovasc Surg (Torino) 12:131, 1971

Laforet EG: Acute hypertension as a diagnostic clue in traumatic rupture of the thoracic aorta. Am J Surg 110:948, 1965

Lawrence MS, Ehrenhaft JL: Trauma to the thoracic aorta. J Iowa Med Soc 55:637, 1965

Leonard DW: Dissecting aneurysm of the thoracic aorta due to trauma. Am J Surg 69:344, 1945

Malm JR, Deterling RA Jr: Traumatic aneurysm of the thoracic aorta simulating coarctation. A case report. J Thorac Cardiovasc Surg 40:271, 1960

Marsh CL, Moore RC: Deceleration trauma. Am J Surg 93:623, 1957

Meyer JA, Neville JF Jr, Hansen WG: Traumatic rupture of the aorta in a child. JAMA 208:527, 1969

Nagel CB, Williams GR: Method of repair in the surgical treatment of aneurysms of the descending thoracic aorta. Am J Surg 112:709, 1966

Ochsner JL, Crawford ES, DeBakey ME: Injuries of the vena cava caused by external trauma. Surgery 49:397, 1961

Pearce CW, Weichert RF, delReal RE: Aneurysms of aortic arch. Simplified technique for excision and prosthetic replacement. J Thorac Cardiovasc Surg 58:886, 1969

Peterson HJ, Linder E: Closed avulsion of the thoracic aorta. Acta Chir Scand 130:611, 1965

Pierce RE: Traumatic dissecting aneurysms of the thoracic aorta. US Armed Forces Med J 5:1589, 1954

Pupello DF, Mark JBD, Iben AB: Surgical treatment of traumatic rupture of the thoracic aorta and diaphragm. Calif Med 112:27, 1970

Quast DC, et al: Surgical correction of injuries of the vena cava. An analysis of 61 cases. J Trauma 5:3, 1965

Reid RDW: Ruptured subclavian artery sutured. Proc Mine Med Off Assoc 47:71, 1967

Rey-Baltar E, Perez-Agote I: Traumatic rupture of the thoracic aorta. Arch Surg 91:344, 1965

Richardson RL, et al: Traumatic rupture of the thoracic aorta: A follow-up report. Am Surg 35:624, 1969

Rindfleisch E: Uber klammerartige Verbindungen zwischen Aorta und Pulmonalarterie (Vincula aortae). Virchows Arch [Pathol Anat] 96:302, 1884

Rutherford PS: Traumatic rupture of aorta. Br Med J 2:1337, 1951

Sandor F: Incidence and significance of traumatic mediastinal haematoma. Thorax 22:43, 1967

Schmitz W, et al: Die Akute Traumatische Ruptur

der Descendierenden Thorakalen Aorta. (In press)

Schonholtz GJ, Jahnke EJ Jr: Occult injury of the thoracic aorta associated with orthopaedic trauma. J Bone Joint Surg [Am] 46a:1421, 1964

Steinberg I: Chronic traumatic aneurysm of the thoracic aorta. (Report of five cases, with a plea for conservative treatment.) N Engl J Med 257:913, 1957

Steinberg I: Traumatic aneurysm of the thoracic aorta. A further report. Am J Roentgenol 91:1295, 1964

Storey CF, Nardi GL, Sewell WH: Traumatic aneurysms of the thoracic aorta. Report of two cases, one successfully treated by resection and graft replacement with the aid of a shunt. Ann Surg 144:69, 1956

Tarlov E, Greenfield LJ: Post-traumatic aortic arch aneurysm with arteriovenous fistula to the innominate vein. J Thorac Cardiovasc Surg 55:134, 1968

Thomas TV: Management of cardiac and intrathoracic great vessel injuries. Surg Gynecol Obstet 125:997, 1967

Valiathan MS, et al: Resection of aneurysms of the descending thoracic aorta using a GBH-coated shunt bypass. J Surg Res 8:197, 1968

Wagner JC, Miller JDR: Value of angiography in acute conditions affecting the thoracic aorta. Can Med Assoc J 103:57, 1970

Wilder RJ, Fishbein RH: Complete transection of the aorta. JAMA 188:176, 1964

Wright JS, Johnston JB: Lesions of the thoracic aorta and the place of emergency bypass. Aust NZ J Surg 36:301, 1967

Zehnder MA: Delayed post-traumatic rupture of the aorta in a young healthy individual after closed injury. Mechanical-etiological considerations. Angiology 7:252, 1958

Zehnder MA: Symptomatologie und Verlauf der Aortenruptur bei geschlossener Thorax-verletzung an Hand von 12 Fallen. Thoraxchirurgie 8:1, 1960–61

10. PENETRATING INJURIES OF
THE INTRATHORACIC GREAT VESSELS

Kenneth E. Thomas
Lewis H. Bosher, Jr.

From military and civilian experience with penetrating injuries of the thorax there has developed a considerable reservoir of information regarding the diagnosis and management of cardiac and pulmonary injuries but comparatively few reports concerning the problems of intrathoracic great vessel injury. Because of the highly lethal nature of penetrating injuries to these vessels, there is only a comparatively small experience with their management in any one center.

The incidence of injury to the intrathoracic great vessels varied from 0.3 percent to 1.5 percent in seven series from civilian practice comprising more than 3200 cases of penetrating thoracic trauma [4, 5, 25, 28, 48, 56, 119, 122]. Within the same series cardiac injury varied from 1.7 percent to 11 percent, averaging 7 percent. Injuries to the intrathoracic vessels were rarely seen in the Tokyo Army Hospital during the Korean conflict among a large number of patients with thoracic injuries [135]. In 1958 Parmley and co-workers [102] analyzed a postmortem series of penetrating wounds of the heart and aorta. Of 66 persons with missile or stab wounds of the aorta, 80.4 percent were dead on arrival at a medical facility; 19.6 percent survived longer than 30 minutes and 16 percent of these survived more than 6 hours. Major venous injuries have proved equally lethal. Of 27 persons with superior vena caval penetrating injuries reported from the Baylor Hospitals, only 2 were alive on admission [99].

The recent conflict in Vietnam has reemphasized the destructive nature of high-velocity missile wounds as compared to the more common stab wounds seen in civilian experience [103]. Nevertheless, because of prompt evacuation from the scene of injury in Vietnam Billy, Amato, and Rich [14] found that 20, or 19 percent of 105 men with penetrating wounds of the thoracic aorta reached a medical installation alive.

Among the initially surviving patients there is a further high mortality, resulting primarily from a delay in recognition of life-threatening injury and institution of operative treatment. Whereas most penetrating injuries of the great vessels are characterized by massive hemorrhage leading to rapid exsanguination, in surviving patients hemorrhage may be hidden and contained by the perivascular sheaths, pleura, and pericardium. The containment of hemorrhage by these structures is usually only temporary and delayed bleeding or exsanguination is a constant threat. If the hemorrhage is confined to the pericardium, cardiac tamponade follows and death ensues unless the tamponade is relieved. Bleeding may cease as a result of thrombotic occlusion in the lacerated wall, a favorable event that occurs most often in the vena cava and pulmonary vessels where the pressure is low. Hemorrhage may recur as the intravascular pressure rises or a poorly formed clot contracts or is partially lysed. False aneurysm is more commonly the result of blunt trauma but occasionally results from penetrating injuries. The formation of an acute arteriovenous fistula lessens the danger of intrathoracic bleeding by decompressing a false aneurysm into the adjacent vein. A systolic or continuous bruit may offer the first clue to the vascular injury. Rarely do the initial clinical manifestations result from peripheral embolization of the missile.

DIAGNOSIS

The diagnosis of great vessel injury in a patient in shock and with persistent massive hemorrhage is relatively easy for the physician to make, but the diagnosis may be obscure if bleeding has temporarily subsided, hemorrhage is moderate, and vital signs appear stable.

In a consideration of stab wounds, the type and length of weapon as well as the sex of the assailant are factors that may influence the direction and depth of the wound track. Females more often stab overhand with weapons such as household knives and ice picks, whereas males frequently stab upward with knives such as switchblades [64]. In the case of gunshot wounds knowledge of the type of gun and its position as

129

to distance and angle in relation to the victim provides useful information [116]. With low-velocity missiles the injury is generally limited to the permanent wound track, whereas with high-velocity missiles (minimum muzzle velocity of 2000 feet/sec within 200 yards) the damage extends a considerable distance beyond the permanent track. The temporary wound cavity produced by high-velocity missiles may be thirty times as great as the permanent track. High-velocity gunshot wounds are also sometimes seen in civilian practice. DeMuth [34] cited 19 civilian cases of high-velocity missile wounds of the chest; there were only 6 survivors after surgical treatment.

By appraising the location and direction of the wound track one can often predict the possibility and location of vascular injuries. Midline wounds should alert one to possible involvement of the heart and mediastinum, parasternal wounds to the internal mammary vessels, wounds above the second rib to thoracic outlet vessels, and those below the fourth intercostal space to combined thoracoabdominal injuries. Possible injury to mediastinal structures should always be considered when the wound is located at the base of the neck. More than one vessel may be involved. Circuitous bullet tracks may be conditioned by the interposition of bone and other dense tissue, especially when the bullet velocity is nearly spent.

Unstable vital signs, hemothorax, cardiac tamponade, hematoma at the base of the neck, distended neck veins, a bruit, and inequality of pulses are all clinical manifestations that suggest a great vessel injury. Important roentgenographic findings are fluid accumulation, enlarged pericardial shadow, widening of the mediastinum, and the specific location of the missile. The wound of entrance and of exit, if present, should be identified with metallic markers to facilitate estimation of the missile tract from the roentgenogram. A vascular injury is suspected whenever it appears that the mediastinum has been traversed by missile or wounding instrument. Injuries of the esophagus and major bronchi are often found in association with great vessel injury.

The manifestations of a centrally located arteriovenous fistula are typically unique and specific. The presence of a continuous bruit with systolic accentuation, in some instances associated with a thrill, usually leads to the recognition of the arteriovenous fistula. Of such cases 25 percent were recognized within 24 hours of injury and 50 percent within 2 weeks. Some cases, however, remained undetected for more than 5 years. Other prominent findings include a wide pulse pressure with peripheral manifestations, pulsating cervical and retinal veins, hilar dance, and cardiomegaly. Venous blood near the fistula is arterialized. Unlike peripheral arteriovenous fistulas, in which congestive heart failure is unusual unless the fistula is of long duration or of great size, the central arteriovenous fistula from penetrating great vessel trauma resulted in congestive heart failure in over 70 percent of patients. This higher incidence of congestive heart failure can be attributed to the large volume flow through a proximally located fistula, which results from the higher energy level in the proximal aorta as well as the lower resistance in the receiving veins, as compared to more distally located vessels.

Until recently, arteriography has seldom been used for the detection of acute penetrating intrathoracic vascular injury. Its value in locating and analyzing chronic traumatic arteriovenous fistulas and false aneurysms has been well established, but in many acute cases the urgency of the situation does not permit surgery to be delayed in favor of arteriography. Furthermore, false negative results have been reported [61, 122]. Recent experience in Vietnam, however, has demonstrated the value of arteriography in selected cases [26]. In a well-documented report Brawley and colleagues [17] supported the routine use of arteriography in patients with potential wounds of the great vessels in whom there was no indication for immediate exploration. Similar views have been expressed by Symbas [126]. Brawley also stressed the value of arteriography in the detection of *multiple* vascular injuries. Details regarding aortography are included in the section on blunt vascular injuries. Cleveland, Kemp, and Lower [27] demonstrated by aortography an acute aorto-right ventricular fistula associated with aortic insufficiency that had resulted from a gunshot wound. Successful repair of the injury was undertaken a few hours after the patient's admission. With emergency aortography Treiman and associates [132] demonstrated an acute fistula between the aorta and left innominate vein secondary to a stab wound. In a patient with multiple gunshot wounds of the thorax who had stable vital signs and a wide mediastinum, Thomas and Brooks [131] used aortography to demonstrate the exact site of aortic injury, a procedure that greatly contributed to a successful operative outcome.

MANAGEMENT

Although conservative treatment of penetrating injuries to the heart may prove satisfactory in some cases, the only rational treatment for known penetrating injuries of the intrathoracic great vessels is operation. However, since a true diagnosis of such injury may be uncertain or even unlikely, a decision in favor of surgery may hinge on the early hospital course of the patient and close observation of his vital signs. Uncertainty should usually dictate exploration. In some cases the definitive thoracotomy will follow emergency resuscitation [5].

If the patient arrives in the emergency room in extremis from a penetrating intrathoracic injury, emergency thoracotomy should be performed for immediate resuscitation of the patient and control of hemorrhage or cardiac tamponade. If a great vessel injury remains a distinct possibility in a patient in stable condition, he should be observed and evaluated in the operating room until arteriography can be performed. Initial management includes insertion of a central venous line, large intravenous cannulas, appropriate chest roentgenograms, electrocardiogram, and possibly an arterial pressure line. If injury to the major superior venous channels is suspected, the intravenous cannulas should be inserted into the venous system of the lower extremities. If the patient remains in stable condition without signs or proof of great vessel injury, he may be removed to the recovery room for further observation. If the patient's condition deteriorates, hemorrhage persists or recurs, cardiac tamponade intervenes, or there is a strong suspicion of vascular injury, thoracotomy should be performed. Most of the uncertainties regarding great vessel injury can be eliminated by definitive, well-performed arteriography, and this should be carried out whenever it is not contraindicated by the urgency of the situation.

In the treatment of massive or continuing intrapleural hemorrhage the surgeon may consider the use of autotransfusion as a lifesaving technique. Although autotransfusion has been used successfully for more than a century, this modality for resuscitation has often been forgotten or disregarded because of the widespread availability of blood transfusions [139]. When these facilities are limited or when hemorrhage is massive, autotransfusion offers an effective and relatively safe way to replace blood. It was first used in thoracic trauma in 1917 by Elmendorf [46]. Recent reports also describe its successful use in the treatment of chest trauma [75, 127].

Symbas [127] advocated the collection of intrapleural blood in a bottle containing 400 ml of normal saline without an anticoagulant and reinfusion to the patient through a standard blood filter. His experimental and clinical data revealed normal half-life survival of autotransfused erythrocytes. Although there was a marked decrease in platelets and fibrinogens within the autotransfused blood, there was no decrease in these factors within the circulation of the experimental animals or patients.

Klebanoff [75] described a disposable system for autotransfusion that incorporates a modified Bentley cardiotomy reservoir, which can be readily used to recover blood from a tube thoracostomy as well as from the pleural cavity during thoracotomy. The reservoir is loaded with 300 ml of Ringer's solution for each 500 cc of blood removed.

A variety of thoracotomy incisions have been utilized to approach the intravascular structures of the thorax. The median sternotomy incision provides excellent exposure of the vascular structures of the anterior and middle mediastinum. It has the distinct advantage that it may be carried out rapidly and with minimum disturbance to the hemodynamic state of the patient. Injuries of the ascending aorta, pulmonary artery, and great veins are readily managed through this approach. The incision may be extended into the right and left cervical region and the heads of the sternomastoid muscle and the strap muscles divided for improved access to the innominate artery, the right subclavian artery, and the carotid arteries. Division of the anterior scalene muscle uncovers the middle portion of the subclavian artery and allows limited exposure of the distal subclavian artery; resection of the clavicle may aid this exposure. Many hilar vascular injuries also can be satisfactorily repaired by this route, but if additional exposure is needed, this can be obtained by an interspace counterincision.

The descending aorta and distal arch at the origin of the left subclavian artery are best exposed through a standard posterolateral thoracotomy. However, for acute injuries of the subclavian artery this approach is suitable only when it is known that the injury is limited to the proximal portion of the vessel. The proximal left subclavian artery can also be exposed satisfactorily through an anterolateral thoracotomy incision in the third intercostal space with the patient in the supine position. With the patient in this position it is not necessary to reposition the arm to gain distal control above the clavicle. Brawley and coworkers [17] have shown that when the injury is found in the distal intrathoracic subclavian artery, the whole artery can be mobilized through the anterolateral approach with its distal portion being delivered into the supraclavicular wound for repair. Although the so-called trapdoor incision (median sternotomy incision to the third or fourth interspace with extension in the interspace, supraclavicular extension with resection of the clavicle) is often recommended, good exposure is not always obtained with facility and closure can be troublesome. However, this approach can be developed from an initial emergency anterolateral incision as additional exposure becomes necessary.

When urgent thoracotomy is required to cope with massive hemothorax, unless the descending aorta is suspected of being injured, an anterolateral thoracotomy in the third and fourth interspace provides the most expeditious and usually the most useful operative approach. Temporary tamponade of the bleeding site can be established until additional exposure is obtained. This maneuver is especially useful when the subclavian artery is bleeding at the thoracic apex. With the left chest tilted anteriorly the incision can be carried well posteriorly if exposure of the descending aorta becomes necessary or converted to a midsternotomy incision for improved exposure of the mediastinum and proximal control of the great vessels. In other instances, it may be more useful to extend the anterolateral incision across the sternum into the opposite hemithorax. Temporary clamping of the descending thoracic aorta, by limiting the vascular bed, has occasionally proved useful in emergency resuscitation. Amato and colleagues [1] have described an emergency approach to the subclavian and innominate vessels that apparently has not been widely used but may offer certain advantages. He utilizes a parasternal

approach obtained by resecting the medial portion of the clavicle and sectioning the first and second cartilages on either the left or right side. Bricker and associates [20] described an emergency approach to the left common carotid artery through a similar incision.

Immediate, if temporary, control of hemorrhage is mandatory and is usually most easily accomplished by finger and sponge pressure. Subsequently, proximal and distal control can be obtained at appropriate sites. In some instances, the location of the injury will permit tangential application of a partially occluding clamp. If this technique cannot be used, the wound may be sutured below the finger with horizontal mattress sutures. In other instances, a small intravascular balloon catheter passed into the vessel through the wound offers a possible means of controlling hemorrhage, at least in low pressure areas such as the atrium and cava [106]. Wounds of the ascending aorta can often be controlled by a partially occluding clamp after temporary digital control. When neither clamp application nor digital pressure permits suture control, balloon tamponade may be tried, although we are not aware of its successful use in the ascending aorta or arch. Temporary occlusion of the intrapericardial inferior vena cava is a useful method of achieving precipitous and easily reversible hypotension. The resulting softening of the aorta facilitates tangential application of a vascular clamp. When caval occlusion is not feasible, electrical fibrillation of the heart accomplishes the same end; although it may not be so easily reversible [18], it can provide a unique but rare opportunity to control hemorrhage.

In some instances the anatomy of the vascular injury simply does not allow complete control and repair even with the use of these special maneuvers. The use of a heparinized Gott shunt between the ascending aorta above and the femoral artery below may obviate the need for cardiopulmonary bypass and systemic heparinization. Cardiopulmonary bypass may still be required, however, particularly in the management of wounds of the aortic arch. Its special features and the use of deep hypothermia and circulatory arrest for injuries of the aortic arch have been described in the section on blunt vascular injuries (Chapter 9).

Injuries to the descending thoracic aorta are usually more easily managed. The descending thoracic aorta can be cross-clamped for periods of 10 to 15 minutes without fear of spinal cord damage; and if blood loss is initially incompletely replaced, acute hypertension with left ventricular failure can be avoided. When the repair is completed and the operating table has been placed in the Trendelenburg position, the clamps are released slowly. Blood volume is rapidly restored and vasopressors administered as needed. During aortic occlusion, blood pressure should not be allowed to fall below normal and a mild degree of hypertension is even preferred in order to optimize collateral circulation to the spinal cord.

A bypass circuit must be employed if a longer period of cross-clamping is required, particularly when hypotension existed before the procedure or is continuing. A local shunt from the proximal aorta to the lower thoracic aorta, a shunt from the left atrium to femoral artery, or a femoral artery to femoral vein bypass with oxygenator are all potentially satisfactory. However, under emergency conditions and in the interest of avoiding heparinization, a local bypass circuit is far simpler and should prove entirely satisfactory in most instances [71, 128]. If damage to the aortic wall is not extensive, closure by direct suture after minimal debridement can be accomplished. Infrequently, because of a larger wound and more widespread mural damage, a prosthetic patch closure will be required. Almost never will a patient survive a penetrating injury severe enough to require resection of an aortic segment for reconstruction.

Prosthetic tube grafts are employed for repair of the innominate artery or intrathoracic subclavian artery, whereas saphenous vein grafts are considered preferable for reconstruction of the extrathoracic great vessels when direct repair is not possible. Intravascular shunts may be used for the innominate and carotid arteries whenever complete cross-clamping of the cerebral vessels is contemplated, but a local bypass shunt between the aortic arch and carotid artery is more suitable for the innominate artery [95]. Vena caval and pulmonary artery lesions can usually be isolated and repair carried out in a dry field with clamp control or balloon tamponade as indicated. Posterior wall injury of the great veins can often be more easily approached through the anterior wall of the vessel and repair accomplished from within the lumen. Reul and co-workers [111] have stressed the use of bypass shunts for use in repair

of inferior vena cava and superior vena cava wounds; they believed that these were especially invaluable when liver injury had occurred or during the preceding repair of arterial injuries.

Thoracic Aorta Results

Dschaneledz [39] has been credited with the first successful repair of thoracic aortic injury anywhere in 1922; in 1932, Blalock [15] reported the first successful repair in the United States. From civilian practice, there have been over 50 documented cases of repair of penetrating injuries of the thoracic aorta not associated with significant fistula formation [3, 6, 7, 10, 15, 19, 21, 29, 33, 37–39, 42, 43, 48, 50, 61, 66, 77, 81, 83, 86–88, 96, 100, 101, 105, 109, 112, 121, 123, 128, 131, 138, 140]. Of these cases 47 percent involved the ascending aorta, 15 percent the aortic arch, and 38 percent the descending thoracic aorta. All repairs were accomplished with direct suture without cardiopulmonary bypass support, although DeMeester and co-workers [33] did use a heparinized Gott shunt in a complicated aortic arch injury. In several instances, the closure was reinforced with a homograft or Dacron patch. Additional repairs to the heart or major intrathoracic organs were often required. Paraplegia developed in 1 patient as a result of two periods of cross-clamping of the descending thoracic aorta [40].

Arteriovenous Fistulas

The formation of an arteriovenous fistula is a relatively rare manifestation of penetrating thoracic trauma. Fifty-one major cases have been described: 18 with communication between the intrapericardial aorta and the right heart; 12 between the aorta and pulmonary artery; 10 between the aorta and the left innominate vein; 8 between the innominate artery and innominate vein; and 1 each between the innominate artery and superior vena cava, between the aorta and superior vena cava, and between the right pulmonary artery and right superior pulmonary vein.

Eighteen aortocardiac fistulas have been diagnosed antemortem and in 14 of these successful repairs were achieved with the support of extracorporeal circulation [8, 12, 27, 51, 60, 74, 91, 93, 94, 98, 113, 120, 124, 125, 137]. Aortic insufficiency was present in 5. The time interval between injury and repair varied between 6 hours and 10 years, but the majority were repaired within 2 months. Knives inflicted 77 percent of the injuries. Fourteen of the 18 patients developed congestive heart failure. However, catheterization studies revealed right heart pressures to be normal or only mildly elevated, with the highest systolic right ventricular pressure 45 mm Hg.

Aorticopulmonary fistulas have been successfully closed in 11 of 12 patients and cardiopulmonary bypass was employed in all but 1 [38, 52, 58, 69, 78, 79, 97, 113, 128, 129, 142]. Congestive heart failure was present in over half the patients, but cardiac catheterization data revealed normal or only mildly elevated right heart pressures. In most instances, repairs were carried out within 6 months of injury. In 5 cases, the fistula was closed from within the pulmonary artery and in 3, from within the aorta. The latter approach is required for a very proximal injury where direct visualization of the left coronary ostium is essential. Proper evacuation of the air from the ascending aorta is of the utmost importance.

Fistulas between the ascending aorta and the overlying left innominate vein have been repaired on 10 occasions [9, 16, 30, 53, 89, 107, 115, 128, 130, 132]. Meredith and Bradshaw [92] reported the only repair of a fistula between the aorta and superior vena cava. Over 60 percent of these 11 injuries were secondary to stab wounds, the others to various missiles. Congestive heart failure was present in more than two-thirds of the patients. Although 2 repairs were accomplished within several hours of the time of injury, the majority of the fistulas were not recognized and repaired for more than a year. In 2 patients significant pulmonary hypertension was present. Successful repair was reported in all 11 cases. The left innominate vein was sacrificed in 4 patients without sequelae in any of these, but it should be repaired if feasible. Local or total bypass procedures were required in only 3 of the 11 patients.

Repair of fistulas between the innominate artery and either the right or left innominate vein have been attempted on 8 occasions with 2 fatalities [11, 44, 47, 55, 82, 85, 143]. Fistulas between the innominate artery and right innominate vein were present in 4 patients, between the innominate artery and left innominate vein in 2, and between the innominate artery and both innominate veins in 2. Congestive heart failure was present in more than 70 percent of the patients, and in most patients the vein was sacrificed at the time of repair. A single case of a fistula between the innominate artery and superior vena cava has been reported [32]. In none was bypass employed.

In 1975, Arom and Lyons [2] reported the only known case of a traumatic pulmonary arteriovenous fistula occurring after a stab wound. The patient had a 7-year interval of being asymptomatic and then had a 3-year history of exertional dypsnea and clubbing. Cardiac catheterization revealed a 75% right-to-left shunt. At operation, there was a 1-cm fistula between the right pulmonary artery and right superior pulmonary vein; this was closed from within the right pulmonary artery. Unfortunately, the patient died of sepsis on the tenth postoperative day.

Miscellaneous traumatic arteriovenous fistulas involving the chest wall have been reported; 9 of the internal mammary vessels [22, 45, 54, 57, 62, 70, 73, 117, 134], two of the intercostal vessels [90, 110], and 1 of a chest wall-lung fistula [31]. Various types of chest wall trauma were involved, including thoracostomy for tube drainage and subclavian vein catheterization. None of the fistulas were hemodynamically significant, but some were confused with more serious defects because of the presence of a continuous murmur. They were treated by quadruple ligation and excision.

Missile Embolization

Missile embolization is a rare complication of a penetrating wound of the intrathoracic great vessels. Twenty-four such injuries involving the thoracic aorta have been reported with 13 survivors [14, 37, 38, 49, 72, 74, 76, 79, 80, 121, 133, 136]. Early repair of the aortic wound was undertaken in 6, 12 underwent embolectomy, and 5 survivors received no treatment for the entrance wound. The bullet embolized to the left iliofemoral system in 62 percent, to the right iliofemoral system in 24 percent, and was found at some other site in 14 percent. Less common missile embolizations have originated from the pulmonary artery, pulmonary vein, or vena cava [59, 72, 114]. Survival from missile wounds to the chest wall with either arterial or venous embolization is not rare, but the exact site of entrance in many of the survivors remains in doubt.

Thoracic Outlet

Penetrating wounds of the vessels of the thoracic outlet and base of the neck have proved considerably less lethal than those involving more centrally located vessels, but the injuries can nevertheless prove extremely treacherous. Sudden hemorrhage may obstruct the airway or decompress into the pleural space. One-half of the 14 patients with penetrating injuries at the base of the neck reported by Hunt and co-workers [65] were thought initially not to have vascular involvement. In 1915 Wakeley [55] reported successful ligation of the innominate artery 6 weeks after injury from shrapnel. Since that time, many successful repairs of the innominate, carotid, and subclavian vessels have been reported [23, 35, 36, 55, 67, 84, 118]. In 1970 Bricker and colleagues [20] reported 27 cases with 33 injuries to major vascular structures of the thoracic outlet. In this series, there were 8 deaths, a mortality rate of 29.6 percent.

Proximal control can often only be obtained by extension of the incision into the chest, and with the exception of injuries to the left subclavian artery, median sternotomy has proved the most useful of the various incisions. This is true also for injuries of the great veins at the base of the neck. Intrathoracic control is usually required for wounds of the second portion of the subclavian artery. Ligation rather than reconstruction should be considered only in the most desperate situations. Ligation of the innominate arteries carries a mortality of 9 percent from cerebral complications and ligation of the common carotid artery a mortality of 20 to 30 percent [23].

Caval Injuries

The high lethality of vena caval injuries has previously been noted [6, 108]. In 1933 Bigger and Wilkinson [13] reported the first successful repair of a superior vena caval injury that involved the intrapericardial portion of the vessel. Since that time, other successful repairs have been reported on the intrathoracic vena cava [87, 108, 111, 141]. In several of these cases, local thrombus formation was noted in the vascular wound and active bleeding had ceased. As stated before, the use of either balloon tamponade or intravascular bypass shunt in the repair of caval injuries has been advantageous.

REFERENCES

1. Amato JJ, et al: Emergency approach to the subclavian and innominate vessels. Ann Thorac Surg 8:537, 1969
2. Arom KV, Lyons GW: Traumatic pulmonary arteriovenous fistula. J Thorac Cardiovasc Surg 70:918, 1975
3. Baret AC, et al: Transfixion of the aorta accompanied by a Brown-Sequard syndrome. A case report. J Thorac Surg 35:359, 1958
4. Beall AC Jr, et al: Considerations in the management of penetrating thoracic trauma. J Trauma 8:408, 1968
5. Beall AC Jr, et al: Surgical management of penetrating thoracic trauma. Dis Chest 49: 568, 1966
6. Beall AC Jr, et al: Surgical management of penetrating cardiovascular trauma. South Med J 60: 698, 1967
7. Beall AC Jr: Penetrating wounds of the aorta. Am J Surg 99:770, 1960
8. Beall AC Jr, et al: Surgical management of traumatic intracardiac injuries. J Trauma 5: 133, 1965
9. Beall AC Jr, Roof WR, DeBakey ME: Successful surgical management of through and through stab wound of the aortic arch. Ann Surg 156:823, 1962
10. Beattie EJ, Greer D: Laceration of the aorta. A case report of successful repair forty-eight hours after injury. J Thorac Surg 23:293, 1952
11. Belcher JR: Innominate arteriovenous fistula. Report of a case. Br J Surg 44:627, 1956–57
12. Berger RL, et al: Traumatic aortic regurgitation, ventricular septal defect, and fistula of the sinus of Valsalva. N Engl J Med 281:887, 1969
13. Bigger IA, Wilkinson BW: Wound of the superior vena cava treated by suture. Arch Surg 27:392, 1933
14. Billy LJ, Amato JJ, Rich NM: Aortic injuries in Vietnam. Surgery 70:385, 1971
15. Blalock A: Successful suture of a wound of the ascending aorta. JAMA 103:1617, 1935
16. Borst HG, Schandig A, Rudolph W: Arteriovenous fistula of the aortic arch: Repair during deep hypothermia and circulatory arrest. J Thorac Cardiovasc Surg 48:443, 1964
17. Brawley RK, et al: Management of wounds of the innominate, subclavian, and axillary blood vessels. Surg Gynecol Obstet 131:1130, 1970
18. Brewer LA III, Carter R: Elective cardiac arrest for the management of massively bleeding heart wounds. JAMA 200:1023, 1967
19. Brewer LA III, Carter R: Wounds of the great vessels of the thorax: Diagnosis and surgical approach in 24 cases. Am J Surg 114:340, 1967
20. Bricker DL, et al: Vascular injuries of the thoracic outlet. J Trauma 10:1, 1970

21. Bross W: Injuries of the thoracic aorta. J Cardiovasc Surg 12:95, 1971

22. Brownlee WE, McGannon PT: Arteriovenous fistula between the internal mammary artery and vein following stab wound of the chest: A case report. J Thorac Cardiovasc Surg 38:271, 1959

23. Buckner F, Lyons C, Perkins R: Management of lacerations of great vessels of upper thorax and base of neck. Surg Gynecol Obstet 107:135, 1958

24. Burnett W, Baillie HD: Surgical repair of a traumatic laceration of the extrapericardial superior vena cava. Br J Surg 50:16, 1962

25. Cameron DA Jr, O'Rourke PV, Burt CW: The management of penetrating and perforating wounds of the chest in civilian practice. Am J Surg 79:361, 1950

26. Chambers A, Thomas KE: Personal communication, 1969

27. Cleveland RJ, Kemp VE, Lower RR: Acute aortic valve insufficiency as a result of a bullet wound. Report of a case of successful treatment. J Thorac Cardiovasc Surg 55:123, 1968

28. Conn JH, et al: Thoracic trauma; analysis of 1022 cases. J Trauma 3:22, 1963

29. Conn JH, et al: Challenging arterial injuries. J Trauma 11:167, 1971

30. Conrad JK, Cartwright RS, Mostyn EM: Arteriovenous fistula of the aortic arch. Report of a case with hemodynamic data. N Engl J Med 267:15, 1962

31. Cox PA, Keshishian JM, Blades BB: Traumatic arteriovenous fistula of the chest wall and lung secondary to insertion of an intercostal catheter. J Thorac Cardiovasc Surg 54:109, 1967

32. Creech O Jr, Gantt J, Wren H: Traumatic arteriovenous fistula at unusual sites. Ann Surg 161:908, 1965

33. DeMeester TR, Cameron JL, Gott VL: Repair of a through and through gunshot wound of the aortic arch using a heparinized shunt. Ann Thorac Surg 16:193, 1973

34. DeMuth WE Jr: High velocity bullet wounds of the thorax. Am J Surg 115:616, 1968

35. Dickinson EH, Hood RM, Spencer FC: Traumatic aneurysm of the innominate artery. US Armed Forces Med J 3:1871, 1952

36. Dickinson JF, Hornberger HR: The operative management of thoracic and thoracoabdominal wounds in the combat zone in Korea. J Thorac Cardiovasc Surg 41:318, 1961

37. Dillard BM, Staple TW: Bullet embolism from the aortic arch to the popliteal artery. Arch Surg 98:326, 1969

38. Diveley WL, Daniel RA Jr, Scott HW Jr: Surgical management of penetrating injuries of the ascending aorta and aortic arch. J Thorac Cardiovasc Surg 41:23, 1961

39. Dschaneledze II: Manuscript Petrograd 1922. Cited by Lilienthal H, Thoracic Surgery: The Surgical Treatment of Thoracic Disease. Philadelphia, Saunders, 1926

40. Eiseman B, Summers WB: Factors affecting spinal cord ischemia during aortic occlusion. Surgery 38:1063, 1955

41. Elkan W: Repair of through and through laceration of the superior vena cava with survival. Am J Surg 96:458, 1958

42. Elkin DC: The diagnosis and treatment of cardiac trauma. Ann Surg 114:619, 1941

43. Elkin DC: Wounds of the heart. Ann Surg 120:817, 1944

44. Elkin DC: Arteriovenous aneurysm; the approach to the innominate vessels. JAMA 129:26, 1945

45. Elkin DC, Warren JV: Arteriovenous fistulas. JAMA 134:1524, 1947

46. Elmendorf: Ueber Widerinfusion nach Punktion eines frischen Haematothorax. Munch Med Wochenschr 64:36, 1917

47. Franklin RB, Mankin JW: Arteriovenous aneurysms of the innominate vessels: Review of the literature and report of one case. Arch Intern Med 96:413, 1955

48. Fromm SH, Carrasquilla C, Lucas C: The management of gunshot wounds of the aorta. Arch Surg 101:388, 1970

49. Garzon AA, Omer N, Karlson KE: The management of penetrating wounds of the chest. Arch Surg 88:397, 1964

50. Garzon AA, Gliedman ML: Peripheral embolization of a bullet following perforation of the thoracic aorta. Ann Surg 160:901, 1964

51. Gerbode F: Surgical treatment of emergencies of the heart and vessels in the thorax. JAMA 154:898, 1954

52. Gillanders AD: Traumatic aorta-pulmonary fistula. Br Heart J 17:411, 1955

53. Giraud RM: Arteriovenous fistula of aortic arch complicating stab wound of the neck. S Afr Med J 39:474, 1965

54. Glenn F, Steinburg I: Arteriovenous fistula of the right internal mammary vessels following radical mastectomy: Visualization by angiocardiography. J Thorac Surg 23:719, 1957

55. Gordon-Taylor G: The surgery of the innominate artery, with special reference to aneurysm. Br J Surg 37:377, 1949–1950

56. Gray CR, et al: Penetrating injuries to the chest. Clinical results in the management of 769 patients. Am J Surg 100:709, 1960

57. Greenfield LG, Hatcher CR, Jr: Post-traumatic

internal mammary arteriovenous fistula: Diagnostic considerations and report of a case. Ann Surg 158:129, 1963

58. Halonen PI, Siltanen P, Laustela E: Traumatic aortopulmonary fistula. Ann Chir Gynaecol Fenn 52:541, 1963

59. Harken DE, Williams AC: Foreign bodies in and relation to the thoracic blood vessels and the heart. Am J Surg 72:80, 1946

60. Heller RF, et al: Traumatic ventricular septal defect with aorto-right ventricular fistula and aortic regurgitation: Surgical considerations. Chest 62:343, 1972

61. Hewitt RL, et al: Penetrating vascular injuries of the thoracic outlet. Surgery 76:715, 1974

62. Holland RH: Arteriovenous fistula of the left internal mammary vessels simulating a patent ductus arteriosus. J Thorac Cardiovasc Surg 39:767, 1960

63. Hudson TR: Wound of the superior vena cava with survival. J Thorac Surg 24:101, 1952

64. Hughes RK: Thoracic trauma. Ann Thorac Surg 1:778, 1965

65. Hunt TK, Blaisdell FW, Okimoto J: Vascular injuries of the base of the neck. Arch Surg 98:586, 1969

66. Hyman RA, Finby N: Varicose aneurysm of the thoracic aorta with aorto-azygos fistula. Am J Roentgenol Radium Ther Nucl Med 122:788, 1974

67. Imamoghi K, Read RC, Huebl HC: Cervicomediastinal vascular injury. Surgery 61:274, 1967

68. Intonti F, Beltram V: Successful surgical repair of intrathoracic rupture of the inferior vena cava. J Trauma 5:433, 1965

69. Jeresafy RM, Khan AH, Knight HF: Traumatic aorticopulmonary fistula. Cardiology 57:358, 1972

70. Jordan D: Personal communication, 1975

71. Kahn DR, Vathayanon S, Sloan H: Resection of descending thoracic aneurysms without left heart bypass. Arch Surg 97:336, 1968

72. Keeley JL: A bullet embolus to the femoral artery following a thoracic gunshot wound. J Thorac Surg 21:608, 1951

73. Ketharanathan V, Westlake GW: Traumatic arteriovenous fistula between internal thoracic artery and vein. Aust NZ J Surg 38:278, 1969

74. King HB, Shumacker HB Jr: Surgical repair of a traumatic aortico-right ventricular fistula. J Thorac Cardiovasc Surg 35:734, 1958

75. Klebanoff G: Early clinical experience with a disposable unit for the intraoperative salvage and reinfusion of blood loss (intraoperative autotransfusion). Am J Surg 120:718, 1970

76. Klein CP: Gunshot wounds of the aorta with peripheral arterial bullet embolism. Am J Roentgenol Radium Ther Nucl Med 119:547, 1973

77. Kleinert HE: Homograft patch repair of bullet wounds of the aorta. Experimental studies and report of a case. Arch Surg 76:811, 1958

78. LaFleche LR, et al: Communication aortico-pulmonaire traumatique. Union Med Can 92:999, 1963

79. Lam CR, McIntyre R: Air-pistol injury of pulmonary artery and aorta. Report of a case with peripheral embolization of the pellet and residual aortico-pulmonary fistula. J Thorac Cardiovasc Surg 59:729, 1970

80. LaRoque GP: Penetrating bullet-wound of the thoracic aorta followed by lodgement of the bullet in the femoral artery. Ann Surg 83:827, 1926

81. Lawrence MS, Ehrenhaft JL: Trauma to the thoracic aorta. J Iowa Med Soc 55:637, 1965

82. Lexer E: Operation unes arteriell-venosen anonyma-aneurysma. Schweiz Med Wochenschr 64:645, 1934

83. Lindberg EJ: Bullet wound of the thoracic aorta with survival. Md State Med J 8:285, 1959

84. Lindskog GE: Surgery of the innominate artery. N Engl J Med 235:71, 1946

85. MacLean LD, Mazzitello WF: Innominate arteriovenous fistula: A report of one case and review of the literature. J Thorac Cardiovasc Surg 39:770, 1960

86. Mattila SP: Penetrating chest injuries. Ann Chir Gynaecol Fenn 63:297, 1974

87. Maynard A, Brooks HA, Froch CJL: Penetrating wounds of the heart. Report on a new series. Arch Surg 90:680, 1965

88. McCann WJ: Successful repair of a stab wound of the ascending aorta. NY State J Med 58:3177, 1958

89. McCook WW: Arteriovenous fistula of the aortic arch. J Thorac Surg 23:299, 1952

90. McLaughlin JS, et al: Traumatic intercostal arteriovenous fistula: Case report. Ann Surg 161:218, 1963

91. McNalley MC, Sugg WL: Traumatic communication between the aorta, right atrium, and left atrium. A case report. J Thorac Cardiovasc Surg 54:150, 1967

92. Meredith JH, Bradshaw HH: Fistula between aorta and superior vena cava. Report of a traumatic case with surgical repair. J Thorac Surg 34:278, 1957

93. Morris GC Jr, et al: Traumatic aortico-ventricular fistula; report of two cases successfully repaired. Am Surg 24:883, 1958

94. Mulder DG: Stab wound of the heart. Ann Surg 160:287, 1964

95. Murray GF, Brawley RK, Gott VL: Reconstruction of the innominate artery by means of a

temporary heparin-coated shunt bypass. J Thorac Cardiovasc Surg 62:34, 1971

96. Nissen R: Effect of reduced blood flow in a case of combined cardioaortic injury. Exp Med Surg 18:124, 1960

97. Norman JC, et al: Post-traumatic fistula of the aorta, pulmonary artery and right ventricle. Ann Surg 161:357, 1965

98. Nowlan JA, et al: Traumatic aortic-right ventricular fistula. JAMA 181:159, 1962

99. Ochsner JL, Crawford ME, DeBakey ME: Injuries of the vena cava by external trauma. Surgery 49:397, 1961

100. Ochsner JL, Zuber W: Immediate repair of penetrating wounds of the thoracic aorta. JAMA 186:1170, 1963

101. Overbeck W, Gruenagle HH: Iron splinter injury of the intrapericardial aorta. Thoraxchirurgie 16:274, 1968

102. Parmley LF, Mattingly TW, Manion WC: Penetrating wounds of the heart and aorta. Circulation 17:953, 1958

103. Patterson LT, Schmitt HJ Jr, Armstrong RC: Intermediate care of war wounds of the chest. J Thorac Cardiovasc Surg 55:16, 1968

104. Paul M: Penetrating wounds of the superior vena cava. Br J Surg 46:178, 1958

105. Perkins R, Elchos T: Stab wound of the aortic arch. Ann Surg 147:83, 1958

106. Pierce CW, McCool E, Schmidt FE: Control of bleeding from cardiovascular wounds; balloon catheter tamponade. Ann Surg 163:257, 1966

107. Proctor WH Jr: Arteriovenous fistula of the aortic arch. JAMA 144:818, 1950

108. Quast DC, et al: Surgical correction of injuries of the vena cava; an analysis of sixty-one cases. J Trauma 5:3, 1965

109. Ramanathan T, Somesundarem K, Young NK: Successful repair of a penetrating wound of the thoracic aorta. Thorax 30:348, 1975

110. Reid MR, McGuire J: Arteriovenous aneurysms. Ann Surg 108:643, 1938

111. Reul GJ Jr, et al: Early operative management of injuries to great vessels. Surgery 74:862, 1973

112. Reul GJ Jr, Rubio PA, Beall AC Jr: The surgical management of acute injury to the thoracic aorta. J Thorac Cardiovasc Surg 67:272, 1974

113. Rogers MA, Chesler E, DuPlessis L: Surgical management of traumatic cardiac fistulae. Thorax 24:543, 1969

114. Samson PC: Battle wounds and injuries of the heart and pericardium. Ann Surg 127:1127, 1948

115. Sealy WC, Fawcett B: Arteriovenous fistula of ascending aorta and left innominate vein. A report of a case with successful surgical repair. Ann Surg 142:302, 1955

116. Shefts LM: Thoracoabdominal injuries. Am J Surg 105:490, 1963

117. Shirkey AL, et al: Arteriovenous fistula of the internal mammary vessels: Report of a case and review of the literature. J Thorac Cardiovasc Surg 48:49, 1964

118. Shumacker HB Jr, Carter KL: Arteriovenous fistulas and arterial aneurysms in military personnel. Surgery 20:9, 1946

119. Smyth NPD, Hughes RK, Cornwell EE: Penetrating thoracic wounds. Am Surg 27:770, 1961

120. Smyth NPD, et al: Traumatic aortic right ventricular fistula. Surg Gynecol Obstet 109:566, 1959

121. Stanford W, et al: Gunshot wounds of the thoracic aorta with peripheral embolization of the missile. Ann Surg 165:139, 1967

122. Steichen FM: Penetrating wounds of the chest and the abdomen. Curr Probl Surg August 1967

123. Stelzner F, Horatz K: Successful correction of gunshot wound of extrapericardial ascending aorta. Thoraxchirurgie 10:632, 1963

124. Summerall CP, Lee WH Jr, Boone JA: Intracardiac shunts after penetrating wounds of the heart. N Engl J Med 272:240, 1965

125. Swanepoel A, et al: Traumatic aortico-right atrial fistula: Report of a case corrected by operation. Am Heart J 61:120, 1961

126. Symbas PN: Traumatic injuries of the heart and great vessels. Springfield, Ill, Thomas, 1972

127. Symbas PN, et al: A study of autotransfusion from hemothorax. South Med J 62:671, 1969

128. Symbas PN, Sehdeva JS: Penetrating wounds of the thoracic aorta. Ann Surg 171:141, 1970

129. Symbas PN, et al: Traumatic aortico-pulmonary fistula complicated by postoperative low cardiac output treated with dopamine. Ann Surg 165:614, 1967

130. Tarlov E, Greenfield LJ: Post-traumatic aortic arch aneurysm with arteriovenous fistula to the innominate vein. J Thorac Cardiovasc Surg 55:134, 1968

131. Thomas KE, Brooks JW: Personal communication, 1971

132. Treiman RL, et al: Early surgical repair of acute post-traumatic arteriovenous fistulas. Arch Surg 102:559, 1971

133. Trimble C: Arterial bullet embolism following thoracic gunshot wounds. Ann Surg 168:911, 1968

134. Tumacder OC: Traumatic arteriovenous fistula between the internal mammary artery and innominate vein. Vasc Surg 8:224, 1974

135. Valle AR: War injuries of the heart and mediastinum. Arch Surg 59:398, 1955

136. Valle AR: Management of war wounds of the chest. J Thorac Surg 24:457, 1952

137. Villareal R, et al: Traumatic aortico-right ventricular fistula. A case with delayed appearance and successful repair. Ann Thorac Surg 5:36, 1968

138. Williams DJ: Embolization of a bullet to the right posterior tibial artery following a gunshot wound of the thorax. J Trauma 4:258, 1964

139. Wilson JD, Taswell HF: Autotransfusion: Historical review and preliminary report on a new method. Mayo Clin Proc 43:26, 1968

140. Wilson RF, Bassett JS: Penetrating wounds of the pericardium or its contents. JAMA 195:513, 1966

141. Yadusky RJ, Demos NJ, Timmes JJ: Successful management of laceration of superior vena cava. J Med Soc NJ 63:193, 1966

142. Zajtchuk R, et al: Traumatic aorta to pulmonary artery fistula. Thorax 26:219, 1971

143. Zhmur VA: The method of surgical treatment of innominate arteriovenous fistula. Vestn Khir 81:121, 1958

11. TRAUMA TO THE HEART

Donald L. Bricker
Arthur C. Beall, Jr.

The life-threatening potential of injury to the heart has been recognized since antiquity. It was not until relatively recently, however, that truly effective therapy for these injuries became available. With an increasingly aggressive approach to resuscitation and therapy and the development of effective cardiopulmonary bypass, the mortality rate of patients with severe cardiac injury being brought alive to hospitals has decreased progressively.

This fact is particularly meaningful considering the increasing numbers of patients presenting to hospital emergency rooms with trauma from all causes. Although automobile accidents account for the majority of these cases of heart injury nationwide, knife wounds and gunshot wounds are appearing with ever greater frequency in heavily populated urban areas, paralleling the violence of our times. Cardiac involvement may occur in as many as 76 percent of cases of serious bodily injury, and it has been estimated that as many as 150,000 individuals suffer heart injury in automobile accidents annually [63, 77]. Penetrating wounds of the chest and abdomen involve the heart in 2 to 4 percent of cases that reach the hospital [64, 74, 86]. The magnitude of the problem is shown by the fact that as many as 50 percent of patients with penetrating wounds of the heart may reach a medical facility alive [64].

ETIOLOGY

Trauma to the heart occurs basically from two types of injuries: penetrating and nonpenetrating. Most of the penetrating injuries seen in civilian hospitals today are the result of gunshot wounds or knife wounds. These two wounding agents vary in relative frequency according to geographic areas. It is unfortunate that gunshot wounds of the heart have become progressively more common, for they have been associated with a higher overall mortality rate than stab wounds in the larger reported series [5, 61, 79, 90]. Approximately 30 percent of patients suffering gunshot wounds to the heart will die even after reaching a hospital alive, in contrast to only 10 percent of those with stab wounds. This can be understood when one realizes that while stab wounds usually lacerate the right ventricle, which is more easily repaired, gunshot wounds are more likely to produce damage to the left ventricle and intracardiac structures, none of which are so amenable to repair [65, 74].

Whether the heart has been penetrated by either of these agents, or shell fragments, glass, wooden splinters, cardiac catheters, or any of the other myriad of wounding agents described, two common factors contribute to disturbance of myocardial function. These are disruption of myocardial continuity and cardiac tamponade. The magnitude and precise location of myocardial disruption determines the degree of alteration of effectiveness of the heart as a mechanical pump. Relatively minor injuries to the heart may result in great disturbance of cardiac function should cardiac tamponade develop. This occurs when bleeding from the heart is contained within a relatively intact pericardial sac. As the pericardial accumulation increases, ventricular diastolic filling is progressively diminished until cardiac output is inadequate. Relief must then be afforded or death results. This is how a symptomatic penetrating wound of the heart is most commonly first seen by the emergency room physician. Less commonly, isolated pericardial injuries may result in tamponade. Those persons with more extensive wounds of the myocardium with wider rents in the pericardium are usually first seen in shock from hemorrhage with massive hemothorax, or they fail to reach a medical facility alive. Thus, pericardial integrity is an important determinant of survival [18]. Occasionally, a penetrating agent will cause neither tamponade nor severe hemorrhage but may damage intracardiac structures. The patient may then be seen with myocardial failure secondary to valvular injuries, severed papillary muscles or chordae tendinae, septal defects, or aorta to right ventricular fistulas [7, 10, 11, 18, 22, 29, 48, 55, 65, 87]. These injuries may go unrecognized in the immediate postinjury period and only be diagnosed later as myocardial decompensation occurs.

Coronary artery laceration occurs in about 4 percent of penetrating cardiac wounds [71]. This injury may result in hemorrhage, tamponade, myocardial infarction, arteriocameral fistulas, or aneurysm formation, with all the problems attendant thereof, and it is therefore associated with a higher mortality than cardiac injuries without coronary artery involvement [1, 24, 51, 82].

Nonpenetrating injuries can also result in disruption of myocardial continuity. Kemmerer and colleagues [43] in a study of 585 people with thoracic injury who had died in traffic accidents found a 4 percent incidence of myocardial laceration. Parmley, Manion, and Mattingly [63] in a review of 546 postmortem examinations of patients with fatal cardiac injury, found 353 patients with rupture of one or more cardiac chambers. Although they found that ventricular rupture occurred almost twice as often as atrial rupture, Bright and Beck [20], in an earlier study, found almost equal incidences of chamber rupture in 152 cases. Nonetheless, ventricular rupture is usually immediately fatal, while the patients able to reach the hospital alive will have atrial tears in the majority of instances [62, 85].

Ventricular septal defects secondary to nonpenetrating trauma are slightly more common than chamber rupture in the surviving patient; these may result from septal rupture at the moment of trauma or from late muscular necrosis secondary to a traumatic infarction. These lesions may be repaired with an excellent likelihood of success [25, 73].

Valvular injury, while present in 5 percent of fatal cardiac injuries, is rare in the patient surviving blunt trauma [63]. The aortic valve appears to be functionally impaired most frequently [9, 42, 47, 49, 52, 67]. The mitral valve is the next most commonly injured, with damage to the subvalvular mechanism and ruptures of papillary muscles and chordae tendinae [3, 57]. Damage to the tricuspid valve appears least significant functionally [21, 41, 53].

Nonpenetrating injury to the coronary arteries also occurs, usually being seen as a tearing injury that produces tamponade [63]. Coronary occlusion and thrombosis, secondary to a severe compression injury, have been reported [70]. Rupture of the coronary arteries and fistulas have also been reported following blunt trauma [31, 36].

Difficulty arises in determining the exact cause of myocardial infarctions occurring in non-fatally injured patients in the age group most susceptible to atherosclerotic disease.

Nonpenetrating injuries much more commonly take the form of myocardial contusion with interstitial hemorrhage, edema, and destruction of muscular fibers with varying degrees of actual muscle necrosis. This injury probably occurs in at least 15 percent of all patients arriving at a hospital with blunt trauma to the chest. The resultant alteration in myocardial function is proportionate to the area and amount of myocardium damaged. Gross cardiac failure may result and arrhythmias are common [12, 52, 53]. If the degree of myocardial necrosis is extensive, a true infarction pattern may appear and the late formation of a ventricular aneurysm can result in myocardial decompensation. These aneurysms should be repaired when diagnosed, for the complication of rupture, cardiac failure, peripheral emboli, and arrhythmias seem to be particularly prominent in posttraumatic aneurysms [45].

Attempts have been made to classify the types of external force precipitating these nonpenetrating injuries, but this hardly seems necessary. While the injury may have resulted from a direct blow or a concussive or blast effect, the pathophysiology involved is essentially the same. That is, whether the heart has sustained compression from externally applied air, water, or solid substances, or from adjacent intrathoracic structures in either accelerative or decelerative types of motion, the myocardium in each case has absorbed externally applied force and energy that have tended to damage and disrupt it. Although the etiological mechanisms may differ, the pathological anatomy is the same, as are the therapeutic applications.

The pericardium also sustains damage in virtually every case of traumatic injury to the heart, whether it be from a penetrating or nonpenetrating source. The pericardial injury, per se, is usually of little consequence in terms of immediate management in the emergency situation, except in the unusual case of hemorrhage from pericardial vessels or the rare instance of herniation of the heart through a large pericardial rent wherein cardiac output may be seriously impaired [60]. Late sequelae of pericardial injuries are not uncommon, however, and both suppurative and nonsuppurative pericarditis and recurrent pericardial effusions are seen with some frequency [63, 81]. A postpericardiectomy syndrome similar to that seen after cardiac surgery may appear, and constrictive pericarditis has been reported [34, 40, 46, 81].

DIAGNOSIS

The diagnosis of injury to the heart is established in proportion to the frequency and diligence with which it is sought. Most patients with injury to the heart have other associated injuries that not uncommonly divert the attention of the physician away from this potentially fatal lesion. The victim of a penetrating wound may have more obvious sources of blood loss to account for a hypotensive state, and be agitated, apprehensive, combative, or intoxicated. Although a patient with a wound of entrance over the precordium who is hypotensive with an elevated central venous pressure and distant heart sounds may readily suggest the diagnosis of a penetrating heart wound with tamponade, the problem is not usually so well delineated. The wound of entrance, particularly in the case of gunshot wounds, may not be in proximity to the precordium. The patient may not be hypotensive and may initially have normal vital signs. If severe hypovolemia is present, the central venous pressure may not be elevated, even if tamponade is present [58]. The heart sounds may be clear and undiminished. Most authors describing a large series of penetrating wounds of the heart found a minority of patients with Beck's classic triad of symptoms that establish the diagnosis of cardiac tamponade [5, 61, 90]. A high index of suspicion, therefore, is required and should be exercised in the management of any patient with a wound about the precordium or a wound that conceivably could extend in that direction.

When time permits roentgenographic examination, suggestive clues are available from such findings as obvious increase in heart size, hemomediastinum, or pneumopericardium. The course of a bullet or shell fragment from the point of entrance to its resting place may suggest cardiac injury, although it is axiomatic that missiles do not traverse straight lines through the body. In such individuals, while airways are being established, obvious sources of hemorrhage are controlled, and hypovolemia is corrected, the physician must diligently search for signs of myocardial injury and the development of tamponade. Elevation of the central venous pressure in an anxious, apprehensive patient is the most consistently reliable indication of significant tamponade. The anxiety these patients manifest, often appearing disproportionate to the obvious degree of injury, has been a very valuable clinical sign of tamponade, in our experience. The diagnosis becomes clear when elevation of central venous pressure coexists with persistent hypotension. Placement of a central venous pressure catheter is therefore mandatory in the evaluation of these patients and should be placed immediately upon admission, preferably by the percutaneous, subclavian route.

It should be emphasized that varying degrees of cardiac tamponade occur with progressive diminution of cardiac output and corresponding compensatory increase in peripheral vascular resistance, which may maintain arterial pressure until a critical level of tamponade is reached, beyond which complete cardiovascular collapse occurs [54]. It has also been documented, both clinically and experimentally, that even in the face of severe tamponade, volume expansion alone may return cardiac output and arterial pressures to normal values, although the central venous pressure will demonstrate a significant rise [23, 27, 76]. Thus, apparent improvement of the patient's condition with fluid administration should not relieve the physician of the worry of progressive tamponade.

When central venous pressures and roentgenograms are equivocal in a hypotensive, anxious patient with a penetrating wound, pericardiocentesis should be performed without hesitation. A long 17- or 18-gauge needle is inserted by the paraxyphoid route into the pericardial sac, aspirating fluid gently as the needle is advanced (Fig 11-1). The precordial lead from an electrocardiograph may be attached to the needle and will indicate myocardial contact by a sudden change in the electrocardiographic pattern, a forewarning of impending chamber puncture. Contact of the needle with ventricular myocardium is signaled by a striking elevation of the S-T segment, while atrial contact is revealed by a deviation in the P-Q segment, atrial arrhythmias, or atrioventricular conduction abnormalities [13, 44]. This is more important than commonly supposed, for in every series of heart wounds there are those with tamponade caused by iatrogenic ventricular puncture. It is understandable that this may occur in the desperate situations these patients often present, with physicians making frantic efforts to re-

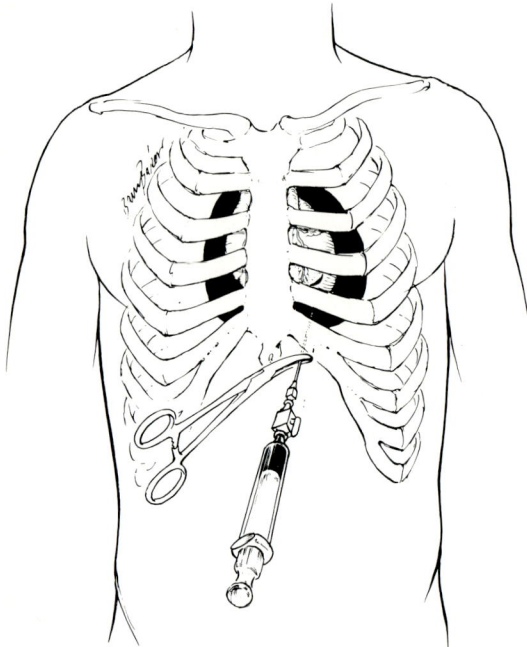

Fig 11-1. Pericardiocentesis by paraxyphoid route. A hemostat placed on the needle at skin level prevents inadvertent advancement of needle.

suscitate a hypotensive, combative, apparently dying patient.

Relief of symptoms with aspiration of blood from the pericardial sac confirms the diagnosis of cardiac tamponade. Aspiration of surprisingly small amounts can result in significant clinical improvement [26]. It is often stated that blood from the pericardial sac in cases of tamponade will be nonclotting, having been defibrinogenated by the beating heart, and that blood that clots has been aspirated from a cardiac chamber. This is not true, as clotting blood is frequently present in acute tamponade. A negative pericardiocentesis, unfortunately, does not rule out tamponade or significant hemopericardium [88].

Occasionally with large pericardial wounds tamponade never develops, and the diagnosis of cardiac injury is established at thoracotomy undertaken for control of hemorrhage in the face of massive hemothorax or continued bleeding from a large wound of entrance. As mentioned previously, this type of presentation is less common, as most of these patients die before reaching a physician.

In an undetermined percentage of patients, the

diagnosis of a penetrating cardiac injury will not be established immediately, or even during the initial hospitalization. Late pericardial effusion, tamponade, pericarditis, or a typical postpericardiotomy syndrome may occur up to several weeks after the original injury. In these cases, the diagnosis usually is readily established, in retrospect, by the history, the presenting symptoms, and roentgenographic and electrocardiographic findings. Less commonly, valvular injuries, septal defects, intracardiac fistulas, and aneurysms at sites of ventricular lacerations are late sequelae. Rarely being diagnosed initially, these lesions may appear years after the original injury and are diagnosed by cardiac catheterization and appropriate angiography findings following the onset of symptoms and suggestive auscultatory findings.

While the diagnosis of cardiac injury is occasionally obscure with penetrating wounds, it is even more so with nonpenetrating trauma. Although myocardial contusion probably occurs in at least 15 percent of patients with blunt injuries to the chest severe enough to warrant hospitalization, the physician's attention to these cases is very likely to be directed toward treatment of obvious fractures and other visceral injuries that appear more immediately threatening. The diagnosis of a cardiac injury is established electrocardiographically with the appearance of conduction disturbances, T-wave changes, and S-T segment alterations.

These changes are seen with nonpenetrating injuries from all causes and are not specific for the various types of nonpenetrating trauma [38, 88, 89]. A pattern of infarction may develop when actual myocardial necrosis is present. An electrocardiogram should be a routine part of the initial evaluation of all patients sustaining severe blunt trauma. Unfortunately, the electrocardiographic changes may be transient, and the rapid evolution and recovery of the abnormality may result in failure to diagnose the injury [35]. Serum enzyme levels are of less value in establishing this diagnosis because of other visceral injuries that may produce similar enzyme elevations. Radionuclide imaging of areas of injured myocardium offers promise of more accurate diagnosis, and noninvasive impedence techniques have been described that accurately document accompanying depression of cardiac output [30, 64]. Significant contusions continue to be underdiagnosed, and a higher degree of suspicion for them is warranted.

Late complications of nonpenetrating injury include aneurysm formation at a site of myocardial necrosis, septal rupture, and papillary muscle necrosis with valvular insufficiency. Acute valvular rupture or torn chordae tendineae may be unapparent until hypovolemia is corrected and the characteristic murmurs appear. Cardiac decompensation in the recovery period is too often the presenting sign and daily auscultation, as well as serial electrocardiograms and chest roentgenograms, should be considered an integral portion of the care of these individuals. Specific diagnosis is again established by cardiac catheterization and angiography.

TREATMENT

The initial treatment of penetrating wounds of the heart and nonpenetrating wounds resulting in cardiac tamponade probably should be pericardiocentesis. A controversy, which was more apparent than real, existed for years as to whether pericardiocentesis should be utilized for initial therapy in cases of penetrating wounds with tamponade [5, 32, 83]. There is no doubt that this form of therapy is often successful per se in many cases of penetrating wounds, but the current consensus is that cardiac wounds are best managed by early exploration with precise cardiac repair and evacuation of the pericardial accumulation [16, 61, 79, 83, 90]. This approach obviates the possibilities of recurrent tamponade, residual clotted hemopericardium, or missed injury and has resulted in an overall increase in survival. We have employed primary thoracotomy in a progressively increasing percentage of patients with penetrating heart wounds and currently utilize this approach exclusively, reserving pericardiocentesis for diagnostic and resuscitative maneuvers [6, 8, 16, 69]. When pericardiocentesis has been effective in relieving acute tamponade and a decision to proceed with thoracotomy has been made, it is wise to leave the needle in place while preparations for operation are completed and the pericardium is opened. The induction of anesthesia in such patients is extremely hazardous, and the surgeon should be gloved and gowned and the operating team in readiness before induction is carried out. However, while it may be preferable to delay induction of anesthesia and avoid administration of positive pressure ventilation until the patient has been surgically prepped and draped, anesthesia should not be delayed in the combative patient who is performing repeated Valsalva maneuvers and aggravating tamponade with each breath.

The incision usually employed for penetrating heart wounds is a left fourth or fifth intercostal space entry unless isolated right atrial injury is strongly suspected. However, the chest should always be prepared and draped in such a manner that the incision can be extended across the sternum into the right fourth intercostal space, if necessary (Fig 11-2). A median sternotomy incision has been recommended routinely by some and may provide superior access in cases of chamber rupture [4, 85]. Unfortunately, this incision does not provide adequate exposure of other posterior mediastinal structures that may also be damaged, particularly with penetrating injuries [84]. Pump oxygenator equipment should be available on a standby basis, if at all possible, as the emergency use of cardiopulmonary bypass occasionally allows repair of an otherwise hopelessly damaged heart. A portable pump for emergency room use has been utilized with limited success [84]. Unfortunately, its use will not always be feasible due

Fig 11-2. Position of patient and incision(s) usually employed for penetrating wounds of the heart. The right side of the chest should be draped into surgical field and required surgical instruments should be available for transecting sternum, if that procedure should become necessary.

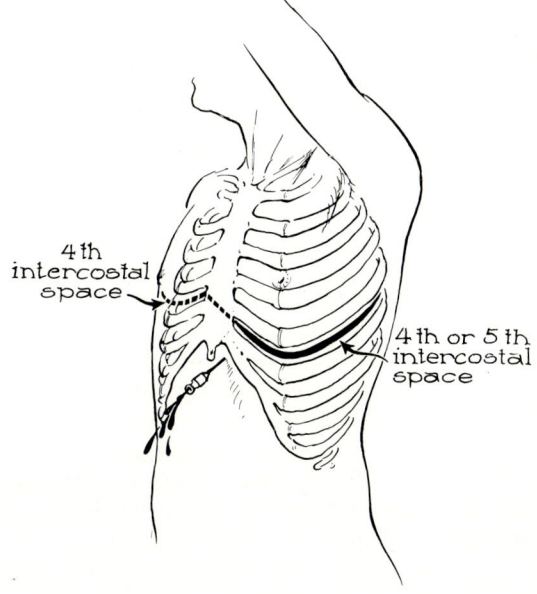

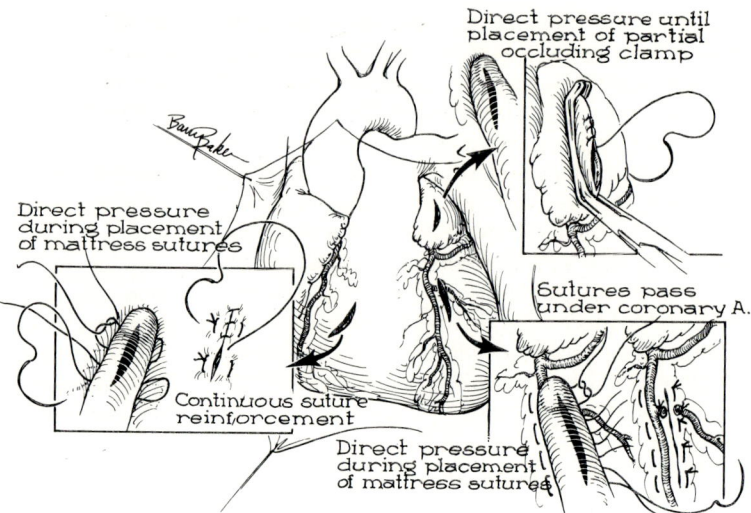

Direct pressure until
placement of partial
occluding clamp

Direct pressure
during placement
of mattress sutures

Sutures pass
under coronary A.

Continuous suture
reinforcement

Direct pressure
during placement
of mattress sutures

to the extreme urgency and the time many of these patients arrive at the hospital.

The precise method of repair of the cardiac injury itself has been well outlined (Fig 11-3) [5]. Digital compression usually suffices to control hemorrhage while precise approximation of the myocardium is carried out. While adequate margins of myocardium must be taken within the suture, very gross technique encompassing a large quantity of myocardium strangulated within a figure-eight or mattress suture should be avoided unless absolutely necessary. Particular care must be taken to avoid injury to the coronary arteries; horizontal mattress sutures passed beneath the artery will avoid this complication in wounds located in close proximity to a major coronary vessel. Occasionally, but rarely, a patient with loss of myocardial wall sufficient to obviate repair without cardiopulmonary bypass will reach the operating room alive, and manual tamponade (such as a digit in the defect) must be carried out until bypass can be instituted. This is often true in cases of rupture of one of the cardiac chambers with high velocity gunshots, although large atrial tears have been repaired successfully without bypass [15, 17, 28, 62].

In the case of very large wounds or tears of the myocardium, exsanguination may well occur before control and repair can be carried out. In these desperate situations, the surgeon may be wise to accept the inevitable onset of ventricular fibrillation and complete the repair rapidly before attempting volume replacement and resuscitation.

Fig 11-3. *Method of repair of cardiac injury. Small branches of coronary artery transected at time of injury should be ligated to prevent subsequent hemorrhage* (inset, lower right).

Manual techniques for elective cardiac arrest to allow repair of large defects without cardiopulmonary bypass have been described for use in such situations [19]. Obviously, if bleeding can be controlled with pressure, it is safer to institute cardiopulmonary bypass to allow performance of the repair in a precise, unhurried manner.

Injuries to the coronary arteries were managed in the past by ligation, accepting the myocardial infarction that usually followed [71]. These injuries carried a high degree of mortality because of associated arrhythmias and cardiogenic shock. Techniques currently utilized in reconstructive coronary artery surgery have been applied to save an increased number of these patients [50, 82].

Immediate repair of intracardiac injuries is seldom done, usually being managed later in the patient's course in a manner similar to that utilized for elective repair of acquired or congenital heart lesions [7, 80]. However, hemodynamically significant lesions may be repaired at the time the patient is first seen if they have been accurately diagnosed [50]. The paucity of case reports documenting successful early repairs would seem to indicate infrequent opportunities or necessity for such repairs [39, 80, 87]. There are valid reasons for delaying repair of intracardiac defects, if possible, until an elected time. Traumatic septal defects, for example, usually are seen low in the muscular portion of the septum in an area where the tissues hold sutures poorly [73]. This problem is aggravated if the muscular defect is bordered by friable, necrotic tissue as is often the case when immediate repair is attempted [75]. The routine use of an intracardiac patch to close these defects has been advocated as a solution to minimize the appearance of residual shunts [78]. Rarely, traumatic septal defects may close spontaneously [33, 78]. Ventricular aneurysm usually appears late in the course of evolution of either penetrating or nonpenetrating injuries, and these should be repaired in a manner similar to that used for postinfarction aneurysm secondary to coronary artery disease [2, 45].

Management of retained foreign bodies in the heart is a problem of surgical judgement. Unless migration of the foreign body is demonstrated or symptoms are produced, such as recurrent pericardial effusion or conduction difficulties, or unless the foreign body is serving as a nidus for continuing infection or thrombus formation with recurrent emboli, those artifacts embedded in the myocardium usually should be left alone [37, 66]. Emboli to cardiac chambers such as bullets that have entered large peripheral veins have successfully been removed. This has been done because of the size of the missiles, their contaminated nature, and the danger of damage to the subvalvular mechanism of the tricuspid valve, where they usually lodge [59].

The majority of nonpenetrating injuries probably go unrecognized and therefore untreated, and it is thus difficult to assess the efficiency of treatment in these cases. Bedrest, supplemental oxygen, and digitalis glycosides when myocardial failure becomes evident would appear to be indicated. The administration of anticoagulant therapy is of questionable efficacy. Arrhythmias are managed by conventional therapy as are pericarditis, postpericardiotomy syndromes, and late constrictive pericarditis.

The majority of patients with cardiac injury arriving alive at hospital emergency rooms will survive with expeditious resuscitation, diagnosis, and therapy. Almost all have injuries that are amenable to correction with current surgical techniques. A further reduction of mortality can be achieved only with more rapid transport of these particular patients to a medical facility and earlier diagnosis and treatment.

REFERENCES

1. Aaron BL, Doohen DH: Traumatic coronary artery-right atrial fistula caused by a penetrating metal fragment. J Trauma 13:81, 1973
2. Aronstam EM, et al: Traumatic left ventricular aneurysm. J Thorac Cardiovasc Surg 59:239, 1970
3. Bailey CP, Vera CA, Herose T: Mitral regurgitation from rupture of chordae tendinaea due to "steering wheel" compression. Geriatrics 24:90, 1969
4. Beall AC Jr, et al: Considerations in the management of penetrating thoracic trauma. J Trauma 8:408, 1968
5. Beall AC Jr, et al: Surgical management of penetrating cardiac injuries. Am J Surg 112:686, 1966
6. Beall AC Jr, Gasior RM, Bricker DL: Gunshot wounds of the heart: Changing patterns of surgical management. Ann Thorac Surg 11:523, 1969
7. Beall AC Jr, et al: Surgical management of traumatic intracardiac lesions. J Trauma 5:133, 1965
8. Beall AC Jr, et al: Penetrating wounds of the heart. Changing patterns of surgical management. J Trauma 12:468, 1972
9. Beall AC Jr, Shirkey AL: Successful surgical correction of traumatic aortic valve regurgitation. JAMA 187:507, 1964
10. Berger RL, et al: Traumatic aortic regurgitation, ventricular septal defect and fistula of the sinus of Valsalva. N Engl J Med 281:887, 1969
11. Berkowitz R, et al: Traumatic aorto-right atrial fistula and intraventricular septal defect: A case report. J Trauma 13:735, 1973
12. Bharte S, et al: Atrial arrhythmias related to sino-atrial node. Chest 61:331, 1972
13. Bishop LH Jr, Estes HJ, McIntosh HD: The electrocardiogram as a safeguard in pericardiocentesis. JAMA 162:264, 1956
14. Bland EF, Beebe GW: U.S. Navy Medical Newsletter. 48:3, 1966
15. Bogedain W, et al: Traumatic rupture of myocardium. Successful surgical repair. JAMA 197:154, 1966
16. Bolonowski PJP, Saminathan AP, Neville WE: Aggressive surgical management of penetrating cardiac injuries. J Thorac Cardiovasc Surg 66:52, 1973
17. Borja AR, Lansing AM: Traumatic rupture of the heart: A case successfully treated. Ann Surg 171:438, 1970

18. Boyd RF, Streider JW, Scarpato RA: Immediate surgery for traumatic heart disease. J Thorac Cardiovasc Surg 50:305, 1965

19. Brewer LA III, Carter R: A rational treatment of small and large wounds of the heart. Surg Gynecol Obstet 126:977, 1968

20. Bright EF, Beck CS: Non-penetrating wounds of the heart: A clinical and experimental study. Am Heart J 10:293, 1935

21. Cahill NS, et al: Isolated traumatic tricuspid regurgitation, prolonged survival without operative intervention. Chest 61:689, 1972

22. Carter RL, Albert HM, Glass BA: Traumatic ventricular septal defect. Ann Thorac Surg 4:256, 1967

23. Carey JS, et al: Cardiovascular responses to acute hemopericardium, compression by balloon tamponade, and acute coronary artery occlusion. J Thorac Cardiovasc Surg 54:65, 1967

24. Cheng TO, Adkins P: Traumatic aneurysm of left anterior descending coronary artery with fistulous opening into left ventricle and left ventricular aneurysm after stab wound of chest. Am J Cardiol 31:384, 1973

25. Clark TA, et al: Early repair of traumatic ventricular septal defect. J Thorac Cardiovasc Surg 67:121, 1974

26. Cooley DA, et al: Treatment of penetrating wounds of the heart. Experimental and clinical observations. Surgery 37:882, 1955

27. Cooper FW Jr, Stead EA Jr, Warren JV: The beneficial effects of intravenous infusion in acute pericardial tamponade. Ann Surg 120:822, 1944

28. Desforges G, Ridder WP, Lenoci RJ: Successful suture of ruptured myocardium after non-penetrating injury. N Engl J Med 252:567, 1955

29. Desser KB, et al: Traumatic VSD, aortic insufficiency and sinus aneurysm. J Thorac Cardiovasc Surg 62:830, 1971

30. Doty DB, et al: Cardiac trauma: Clinical and experimental correlations of myocardial contusion. Ann Surg 180:452, 1973

31. Forker AD, Morgan JR: Acquired coronary artery fistula from non-penetrating chest injuries. JAMA 215:90, 1971

32. Gerami S, Cousar JE III, Moseley TM: Management of stab and bullet wounds of the heart. J Trauma 8:291, 1968

33. Glancy DL, et al: Successful operative correction of intrapulmonary rupture of a post-traumatic left ventricular aneurysm. Am J Cardiol 30:914, 1972

34. Goldstein S, Yu PN: Constrictive pericarditis after blunt trauma. Am Heart J 69:544, 1963

35. Harris LK: Transient right bundle branch block following blunt trauma. Am J Cardiol 23:884, 1969

36. Heyndricks G, et al: Rupture of the right coronary artery due to non-penetrating cardiac trauma. Chest 65:577, 1974

37. Holdefer WF, Lyons C, Edwards WS: Indications for removal of intracardiac foreign bodies with review and report of 4 cases. Ann Surg 163:239, 1966

38. Huller T, Bazini Y: Blast injuries of the chest and abdomen. Arch Surg 100:24, 1970

39. Hutchinson JE, et al: The surgical management of intracardiac defects due to penetrating trauma. J Thorac Cardiovasc Surg 65:103, 1973

40. Issacs JP: Sixty penetrating wounds of the heart. Surgery 45:696, 1959

41. Jahnke EJ, et al: Tricuspid insufficiency. The result of non-penetrating cardiac trauma. Arch Surg 95:880, 1967

42. Kanber GJ, et al: Left ventricular-right atrial canal with aortic incompetence of probable traumatic origin. Am J Cardiol 20:879, 1967

43. Kemmerer WT, et al: Pattern of thoracic injuries of fatal traffic accidents. J Trauma 1:595, 1961

44. Kerber RE, Ridges JD, Harrison DC: Electrocardiographic indications of atrial puncture during pericardiocentesis. N Engl J Med 282:1142, 1970

45. Killen DA, et al: Post-traumatic aneurysms of the left ventricle. Circulation 39:101, 1969

46. Kirsh MM, et al: Post-pericardiotomy syndromes. Ann Thorac Surg 9:158, 1970

47. Kissane RW, Koons RA, Clark TE: Traumatic rupture of aortic valve. Am J Med 4:606, 1948

48. Lawler MR, Jr, Killen DA, Collins HA: Traumatic aortico-right ventricular fistula with aortic valve insufficiency. South Med J 64:715, 1971

49. Leonard JJ, Harvey WP, Hufnagel CA: Rupture of aortic valve: A therapeutic approach. N Engl J Med 252:208, 1955

50. Levitsky S: New insights in cardiac trauma. Surg Clin North Am 55:43, 1975

51. Liberthson RR, et al: Traumatic coronary arterial fistula. A case report and review of the literature. Am Heart J 86:817, 1973

52. Liedke AJ, DeMuth WE: Non-penetrating cardiac injuries: A collective review. Am Heart J 86:687, 1973

53. Madoff IM, Desforges G: Cardiac injuries due to non-penetrating thoracic trauma. Ann Thorac Surg 14:504, 1972

54. Martin JW, Schenk WG: Pericardial tamponade. Newer dynamic concepts. Am J Surg 99:782, 1960

55. Mary DA, et al: Isolated tricuspid incompetence after penetrating trauma. Am J Cardiol 311:792, 1973

56. Mattox KL, et al: Cardiorrhaphy in the emergency center. J Thorac Cardiovasc Surg 68:886, 1974

57. McLaughlin JS, et al: Mitral valve disease from blunt trauma. J Thorac Cardiovasc Surg 48:261, 1964

58. Morgan BC, Guntheroth WG, Dillard DH: The effect of blood volume on venous pressure in cardiac tamponade. J Thorac Cardiovasc Surg 51:575, 1966

59. Morton JR, et al: Bullet embolus to the right ventricle: Report of three cases. Am J Surg 122:584, 1971

60. Munchow OBG, et al: Cardiac arrest due to ventricular herniation: Report of a case of two successful cardiac resuscitations. JAMA 173:1350, 1960

61. Naclerio EA: Penetrating wounds of the heart. Experience with 249 patients. Dis Chest 46:1, 1964

62. Noon GP, Boulafendis E, Beall AC Jr: Rupture of the heart secondary to blunt trauma. J Trauma 11:122, 1971

63. Parmley LF, Manion WC, Mattingly TW: Nonpenetrating traumatic injury of the heart. Circulation 18:371, 1958

64. Parmley LF, Manion WC, Mattingly TW: Penetrating wounds of the heart and aorta. Circulation 17:953, 1958

65. Pate JW, Richardson RL Jr: Penetrating wounds of cardiac valves. JAMA 207:309, 1969

66. Patterson LT, Schmitt HJ, Armstrong RG: Intermediate care of war wounds of the chest. J Thorac Cardiovasc Surg 1:16, 1968

67. Payne DD, et al: Surgical treatment of traumatic rupture of the normal aortic valve. Ann Thorac Surg 17:223, 1974

68. Pomerantz M, Delgado F, Eiseman B: Unsuspected depressed cardiac output following blunt thoracic or abdominal trauma. Surgery 70:865, 1971

69. Pomerantz M, Hutchinson D: Traumatic wounds of the heart. J Trauma 9:135, 1969

70. Price AC, et al: Post-traumatic left ventricular myocardial infarction and rupture in infants. J Pediatr 72:656, 1968

71. Rea WJ, et al: Coronary artery laceration—an analysis of 22 patients. Ann Thorac Surg 7:518, 1969

72. Reul JG, et al: Recent advances in the operative management of massive chest trauma. Ann Thorac Surg 16:50, 1973

73. Rotman M, et al: Traumatic ventricular septal defect secondary to non-penetrating chest trauma. Am J Med 48:127, 1970

74. Samson PC: Battle wounds and injuries of the heart and pericardium: Experiences in forward hospitals. Ann Surg 127:1127, 1948

75. Scheinman JI, et al: Early repair of ventricular septal defect due to non-penetrating trauma. J Pediatr 74:405, 1969

76. Shoemaker WC, et al: Hemodynamic alterations in acute cardiac tamponade after penetrating injuries of the heart. Surgery 67:754, 1970

77. Sigler LH: Traumatic injury of the heart. Am Heart J 30:459, 1945

78. Stinson EB, Rowles DF, Shumway NE: Repair of right ventricular aneurysm and ventricular septal defect caused by non-penetrating cardiac trauma. Surgery 64:1022, 1968

79. Sugg WL, et al: Penetrating wounds of the heart. An analysis of 459 cases. J Thorac Cardiovasc Surg 56:531, 1968

80. Symbas PN: Traumatic Injuries of the Heart and Great Vessels. Springfield, Ill, Thomas, 1972

81. Tabatznik B, Issacs JP: Postpericardiotomy syndrome following traumatic hemopericardium. Am J Cardiol 7:83, 1961

82. Tector AJ, et al: Coronary artery wounds treated with saphenous vein bypass graft. JAMA 225:282, 1973

83. Thomas TV: Management of cardiac and intrathoracic great vessel injuries. Surg Gynecol Obstet 125:997, 1967

84. Trinkle JK, et al: Management of the wounded heart. Ann Thorac Surg 17:230, 1974

85. Trueblood HW, Wuerflein RD, Angell WW: Blunt trauma rupture of the heart. Surgery 177:66, 1973

86. Valle AR: War injuries of the heart and mediastinum. AMA Arch Surg 70:398, 1955

87. Villareal R, et al: Traumatic aortic-right ventricular fistula. A case with delayed appearance and successful repair. Ann Thorac Surg 5:36, 1968

88. Warburg E: Myocardial and pericardial lesions due to non-penetrating injury. Br Heart J 2:271, 1940

89. Watson JH, Bartholomae WM: Cardiac injury due to non-penetrating chest trauma. Ann Intern Med 52:871, 1960

90. Yao ST, et al: Penetrating wounds of the heart: A review of 80 cases. Ann Surg 168:67, 1968

12. TRAUMA TO THE ESOPHAGUS

Hawley H. Seiler
James W. Brooks

The most serious perforation of any part of the gastrointestinal tract is rupture of the esophagus. If not recognized and treated early, the condition is usually fatal.

Anatomically, the esophagus lies in close proximity to loose connective tissue in the neck and mediastinum. For this reason rapid spread of infection throughout the entire mediastinum may occur once the esophageal wall has been perforated. Because of its close relationship to the trachea, aorta, pleural cavities, and lungs, esophageal perforation or rupture can lead to such severe complications as mediastinitis, empyema, lung abscess, aortic hemorrhage due to erosion, and even tracheoesophageal or esophagobronchial fistula.

The frequently catastrophic results of esophageal injury are readily understood when one recalls the classic description of the organ by Terracol and Sweet [27]:

It is a contaminated tract containing a bacterial flora rich in harmful forms, above all the anaerobes. Its walls are thin and fragile. It has no serous coat, its blood supply is often tenuous. Furthermore, it occupies the middle of the mediastinum, where in case of perforation, dissemination of infection throughout the mediastinal connective tissue is the inevitable and often fatal result. Finally, the retrovisceral (prevertebral) fascial space in the neck communicates directly with the cellular tissue of the posterior mediastinum, and an infection, once it has spread downward, meets no obstacle capable of preventing its widespread diffusion.

Damage to the esophagus may follow: (1) external trauma such as might be caused by a bullet or stab wound; (2) internal injuries, which occur most frequently after instrumentation or foreign body perforation; and (3) postemetic (spontaneous) rupture. Perforation may also be attributable to preexisting disease such as carcinoma, caustic burns, esophagitis, or stricture. Esophageal rupture from blunt trauma has been described, and surgical procedures within the thorax may cause injury to the esophagus, especially when the lesion being treated is close by. A sudden rapid increase in intraluminal pressure may be another cause of esophageal rupture. Table 12-1 gives a comprehensive classification of injuries to the esophagus.

PERFORATION DUE TO EXTERNAL TRAUMA

Because of its well-protected position deep within the neck and mediastinum, injuries to the esophagus from an external source are fortunately quite rare. They usually occur in association with multiple injuries involving the lungs, heart, aorta, or other structures within the chest. This makes early recognition of the esophageal injury more difficult, and such associated trauma to vital structures may result in the rapid death of the patient before esophageal perforation can even be recognized. It is highly important, therefore, that such injuries be recognized and treated immediately if a fatal outcome is to be avoided. Unfortunately, the magnitude of associated injuries is often so great that the initial examining physician will be unaware of the esophageal damage. Nonetheless, such damage should constantly be kept in mind in the presence of any extensive trauma to the thorax.

Injury to the esophagus from an external source is seen more frequently during wartime as the result of gunshot and missile wounds. Even so, such wounds are not common. In the 1364 thoracic and 903 thoracoabdominal wounds cared for by the surgeons of the 2nd Auxillary Surgical Group in World War II [6], there were only 6 such cases. In one of these the diagnosis was doubtful, and the surgeon who removed the missile from the esophageal wall noted that he could not be sure that the lumen had been penetrated. In the 2 patients who had operation, the outcome was fatal. The 3 remaining cases were diagnosed only at postmortem examination. Diagnostic difficulties were related to the fact that many of the symptoms present were due to wounds of associated structures, particularly large sucking wounds and massive hemothoraces, and tended to overshadow whatever clinical picture might have been pro-

Table 12-1. Classification of
Injuries to the Esophagus

Injuries from without (external trauma)

1. Projectile: bullets, shrapnel, stab wounds
2. Blunt or crushing injuries: auto accidents and industrial injuries
3. Injury secondary to thoracic surgical procedures:
right pneumonectomy, excision of mediastinal tumors, repair of hiatus hernia

Injuries from within (internal trauma)

1. During instrumentation procedures:
Diagnostic esophagoscopy and gastroscopy
Dilatation, bouginage, and intubation
2. Foreign body perforation and injuries resulting
from attempted endoscopic removal of foreign
bodies
3. Sudden rapid increase in intraluminal pressure
(pneumatic rupture or blast injuries)

Postemetic (spontaneous) rupture

1. In a previously normal esophagus
2. In a previously diseased esophagus (esophagitis,
peptic ulceration)

*Perforations secondary to preexisting esophageal
lesions*

1. Neoplasms: malignant and benign
2. Caustic burns and corrosives
3. Inflammatory lesions

duced by laceration of the esophagus. Thus, the
examining physician's suspicions were frequently
not aroused until serious complications had occurred.

Worman and associates [35] presented three
patients with rupture of the esophagus from external blunt trauma, two of whom survived following appropriate treatment. One patient required almost total esophagectomy due to the
extensive damage and devascularization. They
were able to document 30 cases of esophageal injury due to external blunt trauma, excluding rupture due to blast injuries, published in the English
literature since 1900. Of the 30 patients referred
to, 12 had developed tracheoesophageal fistula
and 3 had a localized abscess. Of these 15, 12 survived, indicating a better prognosis in this group.
Of the remaining 15 patients with esophageal
trauma due to blunt injury, only 3 survived. Death
was most frequently due to fulminating mediastinitis and empyema.

The emergency room physician is seeing patients with multiple chest injuries due to automobile accidents in increasing numbers. Hence, he
should constantly keep in mind the possibility of
associated esophageal rupture. The importance of
this is illustrated by the report of Randolph and
associates [22] who describe a patient in whom
operation was performed for extensive left diaphragmatic avulsion with the unexpected additional discovery of rupture of the lower esophagus.

Chapman and Braun [7] recently reviewed the
world literature on traumatic tracheoesophageal
fistula caused by blunt chest trauma and assembled
28 such cases. The first of these was described by
Vinson [31] in 1936. Of the 28 cases 23 were
caused by automobile accidents and nearly all were
due to steering wheel injuries. Associated trauma
included rib fractures or pneumothorax but these
were uncommon. Twenty-three of the 28 patients
survived. These authors concluded that a fistula
must be anticipated when a young male patient
has sustained blunt thoracic trauma, usually in an
automobile accident, and develops dysphagia associated with coughing and aspiration several days
after the accident. Early primary repair of the fistula was recommended.

Tsuji and co-workers [28] have described a
stenosis involving the upper esophagus following
blunt chest trauma that required surgical repair in
the form of esophagoplasty. They stress the extreme rarity of such an occurrence because the
esophagus is well protected, pliable, and rarely
filled with fluid. Siebel [25] reported a case of
simultaneous rupture of the intrathoracic trachea
and esophagus from blunt trauma. In this instance, it was possible to do a primary repair of
the trachea, but the esophagus was so severely
damaged that esophageal resection, with subsequent substernal transplantation of the right colon, was required.

In addition to the rare cases of perforation due
to crushing injuries and blunt trauma, esophageal
rupture caused by air under pressure has also been
reported. Sometimes this is the result of a practical
joke, e.g., when a compressed air tube has been
placed directly within the patient's mouth. Crushing injuries and compressed air rupture are both
the result of a sudden increase in pressure within
the esophageal lumen. Kerr, Sloan, and O'Brien
[14] have reported esophageal rupture in a child
with a history of having bitten the projecting
bleb of a rubber inner tube which contained air

under a pressure of 25 to 30 pounds per square inch. There was immediate development of subcutaneous emphysema of the neck, face, and upper thorax, dyspnea, and left pneumothorax. An almost identical case in a 2-year old boy was later reported by Randolph, Melick, and Grant [22]. Volk and associates [32] reported esophageal rupture following explosion of an improvised compressed air tank, the tremendous air blast forcibly distending the esophagus and causing the tear. Cole and Burcher [8] have described accidental pneumatic rupture of the esophagus when a fire extinguisher valve discharged close to the face of a healthy 39-year-old man while he was talking. This resulted in a 9 cm vertical rent in the lower esophageal segment. These authors stress the fact that oxygen administration by oral or nasal catheter to newborn infants can result in esophageal or stomach rupture. Hood [13] has reported rupture of the esophagus by compressed carbon dioxide, and Webster and Taylor [34] have also documented traumatic rupture by compressed air.

Hyperextension injury of the cervical spine with rupture of the esophagus, mediastinitis, and terminal bronchopneumonia has been reported by Morrison [21]. Although the injury seemed relatively trivial at the time it occurred, this author stresses the vulnerability of elderly subjects with cervical osteoarthritis to hyperextension injuries.

Lundberg and associates [15] have reported gastroesophageal lacerations as the second most frequently encountered complication (10 percent) following closed chest cardiac massage. Because of its close proximity to other structures within the thorax, the esophagus is prone to injury during many thoracic operations such as right pneumonectomy, repair of hiatus hernia, vagotomy, and excision of certain large pulmonary and mediastinal tumors [19, 26].

Although injuries to the esophagus from an external source such as bullet or stab wounds do not have any significant predilection regarding the site of injury, such trauma is more commonly encountered in the neck depending, of course, upon the path of the projectile. Traumatic rupture of the cervical esophagus was known even in ancient times and was described in the Edwin Smith Papyrus [5] in 1800 BC, the laceration being closed by suturing. As a general rule, cervical esophageal injuries are less severe and cause less shock and infection than do injuries involving the thoracic or abdominal esophagus.

Diagnosis of esophageal perforation can usually be made on the basis of the type of injury, and a history of rapid onset of substernal or epigastric pain, dysphagia, circulatory collapse, and shock. Cervical subcutaneous emphysema is frequently present. Roentgenograms of the chest may or may not show mediastinal emphysema and may or may not show associated pneumothorax on the side on which the laceration occurs. Effusion may or may not be present. Roentgenograms of the esophagus using contrast media usually reveal the site of perforation unless this is extremely small and will also disclose whether the laceration is on the right or left side and whether or not there is pleural involvement.

Esophagoscopy usually will reveal the location and extent of the laceration although this procedure is frequently unnecessary and not indicated. Once the diagnosis of esophageal injury has been made, it must be considered a surgical emergency and immediate thoracotomy and repair performed. Injuries to the cervical esophagus, unless extensive, do not always require surgical intervention. Depending on the extent of such an injury, the lesion may be treated conservatively, either with antibiotic therapy and close observation or by drainage procedures by way of the cervical approach. If recognition of thoracic and abdominal esophageal perforation is delayed until mediastinitis or empyema occur, primary repair of the esophageal injury may then be impossible and compromise measures such as closed thoracotomy and drainage will be required.

PERFORATION DUE TO INTERNAL TRAUMA

Esophageal injuries are most often associated with internal trauma due to perforations occurring during routine diagnostic esophagoscopy, following ingestion of foreign bodies and the endoscopic procedures required for their removal, as a result of biopsy, and during dilatation of strictures or intubation procedures (Fig 12-1). The character and location of the pain from such an injury are determined to a large degree by the location and size of the perforation and the extent of the resultant inflammatory process. Perforation should be suspected in any patient with a recent history of endoscopy or ingestion of a foreign body or caustic agent when there is a complaint of any degree of pain.

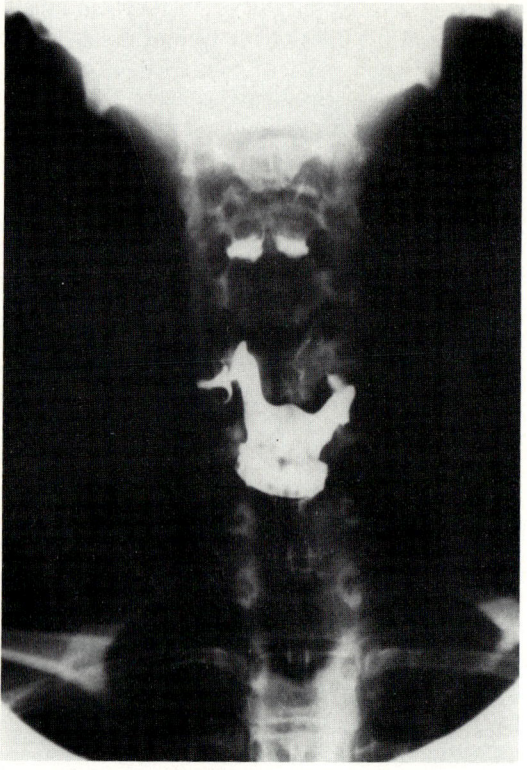

Fig 12-1. Impacted dental plate in cervical esophagus. The resulting minor perforation was treated by conservative measures.

The intrinsic anatomy of the thorax determines to a large extent the site of internal injury to the esophagus that has resulted from instrumentation. There are three areas of narrowing as the esophagus traverses the neck and mediastinum. The narrowest of these, and the site most commonly perforated at the time of esophagoscopy, is at the esophageal introitus just distal to the cricopharyngeal sphincter at the level of the cricoid cartilage. Fortunately, injuries in this area do not have the morbidity and mortality associated with perforations and lacerations involving the thoracic esophagus. The second area of narrowing, and least commonly injured, is at the level of the aortic arch as it crosses the left main stem bronchus. Finally, the esophagus again becomes slightly narrowed at the cardia and deviates toward the left as it approaches and passes through the diaphragm. This area represents the second most frequently perforated site at which the perforation is attributable to instrumentation, although it is by

far the most common location for postemetic rupture of the esophagus. Esophageal rupture in the distal segment (Fig 12-2) is particularly catastrophic and represents one of the true surgical emergencies in the field of thoracic surgery. Perforation in this area is in many instances associated with preexisting disease such as obstructive lesions from a carcinoma or stricture, or perhaps inflammatory conditions such as ulceration or esophagitis.

Perforations during routine diagnostic esophagoscopy are uncommon in the hands of an experienced endoscopist. When such an injury does occur, it is usually in the patient whose esophagus is abnormal, or in a situation in which the procedure may be technically difficult. Pressure of the rigid esophagoscope against the anterior aspect of prominent hypertrophic cervical vertebrae exaggerated by the hyperextended head may lead to an injury of the cervical esophagus. Davidson [9] has reported perforation of the esophagus by a spur arising from the cervical spine during the performance of gastroscopy, with subsequent mediastinal abscess formation. Cure was affected by means of cervical drainage, antibiotics, and the use of a nasogastric tube for feeding. In poorly nourished or debilitated patients, especially elderly individuals, the esophagus is certainly more fragile than is ordinarily the case and thus the hazard of esophagoscopy is increased. This also applies to the patient who is excessively overweight, and such dangers are accentuated when local rather than general anesthesia is employed. Use of the flexible esophagoscope is gaining in popularity and is the preferred technique of many. When one is investigating trauma, especially in the elderly or critically ill, this scope is more easily used and general anesthesia is not necessary.

Edentulous, aged persons are prone to develop esophageal obstruction in the distal esophagus as the result of an impacted food bolus. Endoscopic removal of the bolus is indicated in such cases but can be hazardous especially in the face of preexisting disease such as esophagitis, stricture, ulceration, or carcinoma. Anderson, Bernatz, and Grindlay [2] have reported perforation of the esophagus after use of a digestant agent.

Rupture of the esophagus has been reported following the use of the Sengstaken-Blakemore tube to control hemorrhage from varices [11]. The injury followed forcible withdrawal of the inflated tube. Warden and Mucha [33] reported esopha-

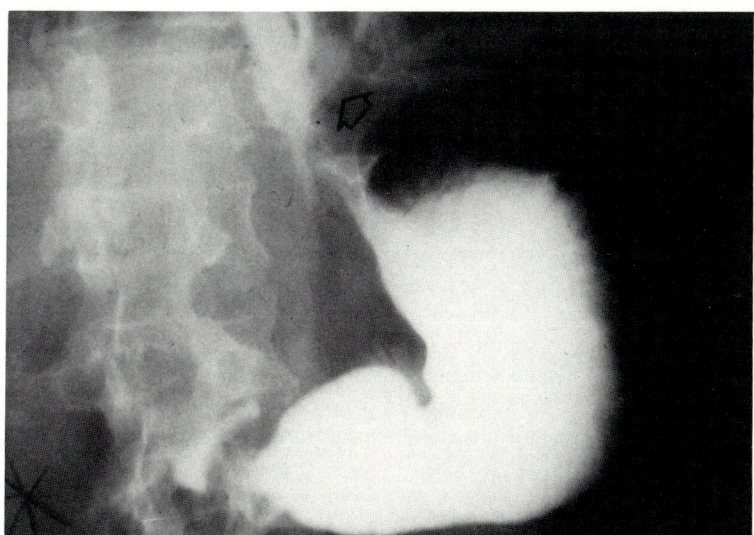

Fig 12-2. Instrumental perforation occurred during biopsy of obstructing carcinoma of lower esophageal segment. Arrow *shows Gastrograffin escaping through the area of perforation.*

geal perforation in the newborn due to trauma. As a result of vigorous aspiration with a stiff rubber catheter at birth, a laceration was produced on the right wall of the midthoracic esophagus.

Perforations occurring in connection with foreign bodies may follow a tearing action or pressure necrosis from a sharp edge, or as the result of manipulation at the time of esophagoscopy when an attempt was made to remove such an object. These injuries tend to occur in the cervical esophagus; the second most common site is the distal esophageal segment just proximal to the gastroesophageal junction. Fatal hemorrhage from esophagoaortic fistula caused by an ingested bone fragment has been reported by Verhage [30]. The terminal episode occurred less than 2 weeks after the patient swallowed a chicken bone.

The wall of an esophagus that has been subjected to continuous regurgitation of acid gastric contents and has thus become inflamed may become the site of ulceration and is therefore particularly susceptible to perforation following biopsy. Perforation occurring during dilatation of strictures is seen most frequently in the distal esophagus, the most common site of stricture or narrowed esophagus. Corrosive strictures (as from lye) are an exception to this rule and may occur in any area of the esophagus or indeed throughout

its entire length. Perforation may occur from hydrostatic dilatation or from bouginage, particularly the former, and it has also been reported from simple intubation, nearly always in the case of a previously diseased esophagus.

POSTEMETIC RUPTURE OF THE ESOPHAGUS

Anderson [1] has pointed out that so-called spontaneous ruptures of the esophagus may be divided into three groups: (1) those due to esophagitis with ulceration, (2) those due to increased intraluminal pressure within the esophagus, and (3) those truly spontaneous cases in which there is no obvious cause. This type of injury, was formerly referred to as *spontaneous rupture of the esophagus,* but it is now known to result most often from a sudden increase in intraesophageal pressure transmitted from a full stomach and associated with severe vomiting. The term *postemetic rupture,* therefore, seems more accurate and descriptive. The weakest point in the esophagus is just above the cardia where it deviates to the left as it approaches the diaphragm. Thus pressure from below, as in forceful vomiting, predisposes to rupture of this vulnerable area, an area so exposed to the forceful, regurgitant jet of vomitus or severe pressure from a distended stomach.

This type of esophageal perforation is potentially the most lethal. It may remain unrecognized for many hours or days and is misdiagnosed as coronary disease, perforated duodenal ulcer, or some other intra-abdominal condition. This delay in diagnosis allows time for gastric contents to gain access to the mediastinum and pleural cavity, which in turn results in the rapid development of overwhelming mediastinitis, pleural effusion, and empyema. As has been stressed by Sealy [24], rupture of the esophagus swiftly leads to the triad of cardiorespiratory embarrassment, major fluid loss, and overwhelming infection. He further points out that these events are easily explained because of the fragile environment of the esophagus and the dangerous potential of infection and corrosion from the fluids within its lumen.

The original, classic description of spontaneous rupture of the esophagus was by Boerhaave [4] in 1724. His patient, the Grand Admiral of the Dutch Fleet, experienced complete transverse disruption of the lower esophagus, and because of the unusual manner of his death an autopsy was performed. The two ends of the severed esophagus appeared to be normal, without evidence of preexisting disease. Despite these findings, the patient had a long clinical history of indigestion and dysphagia. Such a history, it is now known, can frequently be obtained from these individuals with postemetic rupture, as well as a background of overeating and excessive indulgence in alcoholic drinks, usually beer. The earliest review of this subject was by Fitz [10] in 1877, and it was his opinion that sudden muscular violence such as that associated with vomiting could rupture a previously healthy esophagus.

Although vomiting in the immediate postoperative or postanesthetic period is often considered an innocent and normal physiological process, Meagher and associates [20] have described esophageal rupture occurring as a result of such vomiting. They urge a high index of suspicion for esophageal injury in the postoperative patient who develops chest pain and cardiovascular collapse following an episode of vomiting. This is especially true in the chronically ill individual and, in general, the prognosis is poor unless early diagnosis is made and appropriate treatment instituted. Such esophageal perforation would certainly fall into the category of postemetic rupture.

Only a few years ago this catastrophe was inevitably fatal. Today it is being recognized more frequently, being seen probably several times a year in an average busy thoracic surgical clinic. As its symptoms are recognized, the diagnosis made more often, and treatment instituted early, the number of survivors increases to an impressive figure. Diagnosis depends on comprehension and evaluation of the clinical picture along with roentgenographic studies. These patients have severe epigastric and substernal pain, dyspnea, rapid development of prostration and shock, and not infrequently, cervical crepitation due to subcutaneous emphysema. Cyanosis may also be present. Samson [23] has emphasized changes in the quality of the voice in the presence of cervical or mediastinal emphysema. The classic picture of postemetic rupture is rapid onset of symptoms precipitated by vomiting after ingestion of a large meal or following intake of large amounts of beer. The degree of pain experienced by the patient may vary from none at all, in the case of minor perforations, to the severe pain associated with larger lacerations.

Postemetic ruptures are usually large, measuring 1 to 3 cm in length, and are accompanied by sudden excruciating pain simulating that of perforated duodenal ulcer or coronary occlusion. Dysphagia and inability to take food without vomiting may occur but do not necessarily have to be present. If an effort is made to ingest food, it may merely enter the pleural cavity through the lacerated area. Postemetic ruptures occur predominantly in the left posterolateral wall of the lower esophagus, although rare cases of right-sided rupture have been reported. Roentgenographic studies may show pleural effusion, some degree of pneumothorax (nearly always on the left side), and varying degrees of mediastinal and cervical emphysema. A barium swallow will reveal the precise location of the defect in the left lower wall of the esophagus. Although esophagoscopy in most instances will reveal the location and extent of the laceration, it is rarely necessary or indicated in the diagnosis of this condition. A true postemetic rupture constitutes a real surgical emergency and immediate primary repair is mandatory, the condition of the patient permitting.

Complications of esophageal perforation are common and are to be expected because of the usual delay in diagnosis and institution of proper treatment. Such complications include pneumothorax; emphysema (cervical, mediastinal, and subcutaneous); effusion, which is usually on the side involved but may be bilateral; infection in the form of mediastinitis and empyema; fistula formation; and stricture.

TREATMENT

The treatment of choice in esophageal perforation is immediate operative repair combined with the use of large doses of antibiotics. Drainage procedures alone and in conjunction with drug therapy were used formerly but such therapy is currently considered only in rare instances. It may be used as a compromise measure in those patients in whom there has been considerable delay in diagnosis and severe infection or abscess formation has already occurred, or in patients so debilitated that more definitive procedures cannot be undertaken.

Perforations in the cervical area are less hazardous than those in the distal esophagus. Minor leaks may seal spontaneously and be treated safely with conservative measures, including close observation and intensive antimicrobial therapy. Vandever, Ellis, and Hayles [29] have discussed suppurative mediastinitis secondary to external traumatic perforation of the cervical esophagus based on experience in the treatment of a 6-year-old boy with such a condition. Although esophagomediastinocutaneous fistula developed because of the injury, cure was eventually accomplished following cervical mediastinotomy, antibiotic therapy, and nasogastric tube feedings. When cervical drainage is indicated, it is preferable to expose the esophagus completely, close the perforation, and drain the periesophageal space. This procedure is best carried out through a left vertical incision in the neck along the anterior border of the sternocleidomastoid muscle (Fig 12-3). Dissection is carried down to the retrovisceral space with retraction of the carotid sheath laterally and the thyroid gland and trachea medially to expose the esophagus.

On the other hand, perforations involving the thoracic and abdominal esophagus require immediate operative repair. Preoperative roentgenographic studies with barium will usually localize the perforation and indicate whether it is on the left or right side and which approach should be used. Pneumothorax, pleural reaction, and effusion are not infrequent and also indicate the side of proper approach. The cure rate in such cases is in direct proportion to the time that elapses before repair. Good results can nearly always be anticipated if the injury is recognized immediately and repaired within a few hours.

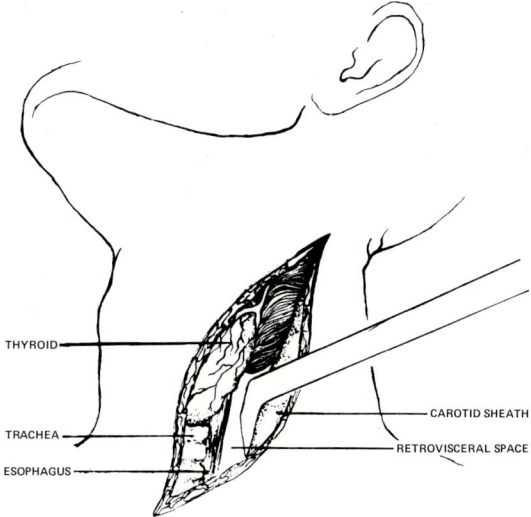

Fig 12-3. Exposure of cervical esophagus.

Once the diagnosis is confirmed, immediate thoracotomy is usually indicated. The pleural cavity and mediastinum are completely lavaged and debrided of foreign material and the esophageal laceration identified. If operation is performed early, the edges of the laceration will probably be in a state of preservation adequate for primary repair and good healing. If diagnosis is delayed, however, there is always the possibility of autolysis and degeneration of the esophageal defect as a result of the corrosive action of regurgitated gastric juice. In such a situation, although primary repair is difficult, it should nevertheless be attempted after debridement and freshening of the edges. The repair should be a two-layer one, using mucosal sutures of fine chromic catgut or silk and fine silk sutures for the muscular wall of the esophagus. The area should then be reinforced with a flap of pericardium, pleura, or omentum to protect the suture line. Thoracic drainage is required of course because of the infected pleural space, and massive doses of antibiotics are indicated. Feeding should be done by means of a nasogastric tube until confidence in the repair is established.

If the perforation remains unrecognized and there is development of mediastinitis, deterioration of the esophageal wall in the area of perforation, abscess formation, or development of empyema, the chances for cure diminish rapidly.

Only in those cases in which the patient is so aged, debilitated, and toxic that primary repair would not be tolerated is a drainage procedure alone acceptable. Massive doses of antibiotics, of course, must be employed in all such cases and alimentation carried out by a nasogastric tube or gastrostomy. If the patient survives, one must be prepared for a prolonged and arduous course of therapy.

Mayer and associates [17] have recently described treatment of patients with esophageal perforation in whom there was delayed recognition and continuing sepsis. Of their group of 5 patients, 4 survived and now have no dietary restrictions. Treatment of these "late" perforations was individualized for each patient and ranged from suture closure of the perforation to esophagectomy. These authors stated that the goals of treatment should be: (1) elimination of sources of chemical and bacterial soilage, (2) drainage of infected areas, (3) augmentation of host defenses by antibiotics, and (4) provision of adequate nutrition. Several treatment adjuncts, alone or in combination, may be used to accomplish these goals. The selection of treatment methods should be influenced by the site of perforation, the extent of local inflammation, the status of the residual esophagus, the overall status of the patient, and the age of the perforation. As the risk of uncontrolled sepsis increases, the surgeon should take more aggressive and definitive steps, up to and including esophagectomy in certain cases, to prevent further soilage.

Lyons and co-workers [16] discuss the place of conservative management in patients with perforations and ruptures of the esophagus. In their total experience with 54 patients, 8 patients with involvement of the lower third of the esophagus were treated conservatively and none died. This group comprised the very ill patients, and it was the belief of these authors that experience demonstrates that with proper supportive therapy, ruptures and perforations of the esophagus can close readily without operative repair. They believe that conservative management should be applied more frequently in the most seriously ill patients.

In the treatment of a persistent fistula that fails to heal following the usual tube drainage method and there is rapid deterioration in the patient's condition, Sealy [24] suggests division of the esophagus at the esophagogastric junction, with turning in of the two ends and performance of gastrostomy. This may well be a lifesaving procedure, and esophageal continuity can be reestablished at a later time.

In rare instances, immediate esophagectomy for instrumental perforation is warranted when this occurs in the presence of preexisting extensive esophageal disease. McBurney and associates [19] carried out one-stage esophagogastrectomy for perforated carcinoma in the presence of mediastinitis. Blalock [3] also performed primary esophagogastrectomy for instrumental perforation of the esophagus. Hendren and Henderson [12] have reported 5 such cases in which immediate esophagectomy was performed (from 8 to 30 hours after perforation); gastrointestinal continuity was reestablished by means of esophagogastrostomy, colon or jejunal interposition, and segmental esophagectomy with end-to-end anastomosis. The pathological changes in the esophagus before perforation included one carcinoma of the midesophagus, one caustic burn with stricture of the lower esophagus, two cases of peptic esophagitis from gastroesophageal reflux, and one stricture of the upper thoracic esophagus following repair of esophageal atresia.

REFERENCES

1. Anderson, HA, Bernatz PE, Grindlay JH: Perforation of the esophagus after use of a digestant agent: Report of case and experimental study. Ann Otol Rhinol Laryngol 68:890, 1959

2. Anderson RL: Spontaneous rupture of the esophagus. Am J Surg 93:282, 1957

3. Blalock J: Primary esophagogastrectomy for instrumental perforation of the esophagus. Am J Surg 94:393, 1957

4. Boerhaave H: Atrocis, nec descripti prius morbi history. Secundum medicae artis leges conscripti. Lugd Boutesteniana, 1724. English translation, Bull Med Libr Assoc 43:217, 1955

5. Breasted J: The Edwin Smith Papyrus. University of Chicago Press, 1930

6. Brewer LA III, Burford TH: Special types of thoracic wounds, Surgery in World War II, Vol. II, Thoracic Surgery. Washington, DC, Office of the Surgeon General, Department of the Army, 1965

7. Chapman ND, Braun RA: The management of traumatic tracheo-esophageal fistula caused by blunt chest trauma. Arch Surg 100:681, 1970

8. Cole DS, Burcher SK: Accidental pneumatic rup-

ture of esophagus and stomach. Lancet 1:24, 1961

9. Davidson JH: Esophageal perforation by cervical spur during gastroscopy. Gastrointest Endosc 15: 79, 1968

10. Fitz RH: Rupture of the healthy esophagus. Am J Med Sci 13:17, 1877

11. Francis PN, Perkins KW, Pain MCF: Rupture of the esophagus following use of the Sengstaken-Blakemore tube. Med J Aust 50:582, 1963

12. Hendren WH, Henderson BM: Immediate esophagectomy for instrumental perforation of the thoracic esophagus. Ann Surg 168:997, 1968

13. Hood RM: Rupture of esophagus by compressed carbon dioxide. US Armed Forces Med J 8:587, 1957

14. Kerr, HH, Sloan H, O'Brien CL: Rupture of the esophagus by compressed air. Surgery 33:417, 1953

15. Lundberg GD, Mattei IR, Davis CJ, et al: Hemorrhage from gastroesophageal lacerations following closed-chest cardiac massage. JAMA 202:123, 1967

16. Lyons WS, Peabody JW, Jr., deGuzman VC, et al: Perforations and ruptures of the esophagus—report of 54 cases. The place of conservative management. Ann Thorac Surg (in press)

17. Mayer JE Jr, Murray CA III, Varco RL: The treatment of esophageal perforation with delayed recognition and continuing sepsis. Ann Thorac Surg 23:568, 1977

18. McBurney RP: Perforation of the esophagus: A complication of vagotomy or hiatal hernia repair. Ann Surg 169:851, 1969

19. McBurney RP, Kirklin JW, Hood RT Jr, et al: One-stage esophagogastrectomy for perforated carcinoma in the presence of mediastinitis. Proc Staff Meet Mayo Clin 28:281, 1953

20. Meagher RP, Lupien J, Albert SN: Postoperative rupture of the esophagus. Surg Gynecol Obstet 115:677, 1962

21. Morrison A: Hyperextension injury of the cervical spine with rupture of the esophagus. J Bone Joint Surg [Br] 42:356, 1960

22. Randolph H, Melick DW, Grant AR: Perforation of the esophagus from external trauma or blast injuries. Dis Chest 51:121, 1967

23. Samson PC: Postemetic rupture of the esophagus. Surg Gynecol Obstet 93:221, 1951

24. Sealy WC: Rupture of the esophagus. Am J Surg 105:505, 1963

25. Siebel EK: Simultaneous rupture of intrathoracic trachea and esophagus from blunt trauma. Tex J Med 58:14, 1962

26. Takaro T, Walkup HE, Okano T: Esophagopleural fistula as a complication of thoracic surgery. J Thorac Cardiovasc Surg 40:179, 1960

27. Terracol J, Sweet RH: Disease of the Esophagus. Philadelphia, Saunders, 1958, p. 443

28. Tsuji HK, Redington JV, Kay JH: Esophageal stenosis secondary to blunt chest trauma. J Thorac Cardiovasc Surg 57:289, 1969

29. Vandever HW, Ellis RH, Hayles AB: Suppurative mediastinitis secondary to traumatic perforation of the esophagus. Proc Staff Meet Mayo Clin 30:288, 1955

30. Verhage JC: Fatal hemorrhage from an esophago-aortic fistula caused by a swallowed bone fragment. Arch Chir Neerl 20:301, 1968

31. Vinson PP: External trauma as a cause of lesions of the esophagus. Am J Dig Dis 3:457, 1936

32. Volk H, Storey CF, Marrangoni AG: Tracheoesophageal fistula due to blast injury. Ann Surg 141:98, 1955

33. Warden HD, Mucha SJ: Esophageal perforation due to trauma in the newborn. Arch Surg 83:813, 1961

34. Webster PD III, Taylor JR: Traumatic rupture of esophagus by compressed air; report of cases with review of 110 cases of esophageal rupture. NC Med J 18:305, 1957

35. Worman LW, Hurley JD, Pemberton AH, et al: Rupture of the esophagus from external blunt trauma. Arch Surg 85:333, 1962

ADDITIONAL READING

Adkins PC: The diagnosis and management of esophageal perforations. Am Surg 21:759, 1955

Anderson RL: Rupture of the esophagus. J Thorac Surg 24:369, 1952

Barrett NR: Spontaneous perforation of the esophagus. Thorax 1:48, 1946

Barrett NR: Report of a case of spontaneous perforation of the esophagus successfully treated by operation. Br J Surg 32:216, 1947

Barrett NR: Perforations of the esophagus and of the pharynx. Proc R Soc Med 49:529, 1956

Bernatz PE: Management of esophageal perforations. Proc Staff Meet Mayo Clin 31:671, 1956

Chamberlain JM, Byerly WG: Rupture of the esophagus. Am J Surg 93:271, 1957

DeBakey ME, Heaney JP: Tracheoesophageal fistula due to non-penetrating injury. Am Surg 19:87, 1953

Eliason EL, Welty RF: Spontaneous rupture of the esophagus. Surg Gynecol Obstet 83:234, 1946

Foster JH, Jolly PC, Sawyers JL, et al: Esophageal perforation: Diagnosis and treatment. Ann Surg 161:701, 1965

Jemerin EE: Results of treatment of perforation of the esophagus. Ann Surg 128:971, 1948

Kernan JD: Perforation of the esophagus as a surgical emergency. Surg Clin North Am 30:405, 1950

Loop FD, Groves LK: Esophageal perforations. Ann Thorac Surg 10:571, 1970

Mallory GK, Weiss S: Hemorrhages from lacerations of the cardiac orifice of the stomach due to vomiting. Am J Med Sci 178:506, 1929

Mathewson C Jr, Schaupp WC, Dimond FC, et al: Traumatic rupture of the esophagus. Am J Surg 93:616, 1957

Nealon TF Jr., Templeton JY III, Cuddy VD, et al: Instrumental perforation of the esophagus. J Thorac Cardiovasc Surg 41:75, 1961

Olsen AM, Clagett OT: Spontaneous rupture of the esophagus: Report of a case with immediate diagnosis and successful surgical repair. Postgrad Med J 2:417, 1947

Overstreet JW, Ochsner A: Traumatic rupture of the esophagus. J Thorac Surg 30:164, 1955

Pate JW, Hughes FA, Patton TB: Spontaneous rupture of the esophagus. Am Surg 24:385, 1958

Paulson DL, Shaw RR, Kee JL: Recognition and treatment of esophageal perforations. Ann Surg 152:13, 1960

Seybold WD, Johnson MA, Leary WV: Perforation of the esophagus. Surg Clin North Am 30:1155, 1950

Thal AP, Hatafuku T: Improved operation for esophageal rupture. JAMA 188:826, 1964

Weisel W, Raine F: Surgical treatment of traumatic esophageal perforation. Surg Gynecol Obstet 94:337, 1952

Wychulis AR, Fontana RS, Payne WS: Instrumental perforation of the esophagus. Dis Chest 55:184, 1969

Wychulis AR, Fontana RS, Payne WS: Noninstrumental perforation of the esophagus. Dis Chest 55:190, 1969

13. FOREIGN BODIES IN THE AIR AND FOOD PASSAGES

James W. Brooks

At the Medical College of Virginia Hospitals, 251 patients with 261 foreign bodies in either the air or food passages were seen over a 10-year period [4, 8, 11, 15, 16, 23, 39]. This group, which included 155 pediatric patients, comprised 137 males and 114 females. There were 200 individuals with foreign bodies in the esophagus and 51 with foreign bodies in the airway. The vast majority of foreign objects in both passages were seen in children between birth and the age of 5. There was a relatively even yearly incidence over the 10-year span of the study.

FOREIGN BODIES IN THE ESOPHAGUS

A total of 116 foreign bodies were seen in the esophagus in children and 94 in adults [18, 25, 30, 41]. For simplicity of discussion, the esophagus has been divided into three parts: (1) the upper one-third, that part extending from the pharyngoesophageal junction to the lower level of the aortic arch; (2) the middle one-third, that portion between the lower level of the aortic arch and the approximate level of the inferior pulmonary vein; and (3) the lower one-third, that section from the level of the inferior pulmonary vein to the esophagogastric junction. The majority of foreign bodies in both children and adults lodged in the upper third of the organ (Table 13-1).

Among the younger patients, the most common offending foreign body was a coin [42]; next came pieces of meat, bones, buttons and tacks (Table 13-2), making a total of 78 percent of the foreign bodies seen in children. In the adults, on the other hand, meat and bones were the predominant agents—a total of 90 percent. The remaining objects, found in 25 children, were springs, jack rocks, safety pins, earring and chain clasps, keychain link, rings, lead slug, toy bell, key, washer, cross, tinfoil, rock, piece of plastic, and gum. Those objects found in the esophagus in 8 adult patients were a safety pin, dental prosthesis, oranges, rubber feeding tube, and a wooden tongue blade.

Of the 200 patients being reviewed, 178 (89 percent) presented no evidence of previous or subsequent intrinsic esophageal disease. Table 13-3 shows the type of disease that can predispose to foreign body retention and did in our patients. It is interesting that during this 10-year span, no patient with a retained foreign body had malignant disease of the esophagus.

Diagnosis

The diagnosis of foreign bodies in the esophagus is relatively easy. With a child a parent usually provides a history of the child ingesting some foreign material. The child then complains of chest or throat discomfort, possibly some gagging, vomiting, or excessive salivation and dysphagia.

In any patient, excessive salivation and gagging, along with respiratory distress, are sometimes evident because of regurgitation and aspiration of saliva from the esophagus. Large foreign bodies, when lodged in the cervical portion of the esophagus, may lead to signs of airway obstruction with wheezing due to partial pressure on the airway [17, 29].

In the adult there is a frequent history of alcoholic intake during the consumption and improper chewing of meat. Occasionally there is an association between a patient trying to eat meat and improper positioning of his or her dentures.

It is interesting that fish bones were not frequently seen except in the tonsils, at the base of the tongue, and in the hypopharynx.

In patients in whom a bone causes an abrasion and then passes on, the pain is usually not quite as severe and is likely to decrease in intensity. However, many such abrasions cannot be differentiated from an actual foreign body except by esophagoscopy.

If all bones lodged in the esophagus could be visualized on roentgenograms, the problem of diagnosis would be simple. As it is, about a quarter of such foreign bodies escape roentgenographic examination, and one must rely upon the clinical picture to determine whether or not esophagoscopy is indicated. Any person who gives a history of having swallowed a bone or who develops pain

Table 13-1. Foreign Body Lodgement in Esophagus in 200 Patients Seen Over 10 Years

Part of Esophagus	Children	Adults
Upper one-third	82	56
Middle one-third	18	15
Lower one-third	16	23
Total	116	94

Table 13-2. Foreign Bodies Most Frequently Found in Esophagus in 200 Patients

Object	Children	Adults
Coin	69	1
Meat	6	51
Bone	5	34
Button	6	0
Tack	5	0
Total	91 (78%)	86 (91%)

Table 13-3. Types of Esophageal Disease Present in 200 Patients with Lodgement of Foreign Bodies

None	178 (89%)
Old stricture	4
Hiatus hernia	6
Congenital web	2
Lye stricture	4
Lye stricture with small bowel anastomosis	1
Corrected tracheoesophageal fistula	3
Diverticula	1
Diverticula with stricture	1

spasm from reflux can initiate the lodging of such a foreign body in the esophagus. The patient is unable to eat or drink anything without regurgitating it. The inability to swallow even saliva is a most uncomfortable symptom. Often these patients complain more bitterly than those with an impacted bone despite the fact that they experience little or no pain. The clinical picture is usually obvious, but the diagnosis of complete esophageal obstruction may be verified by having the patient swallow about an ounce of water, which is promptly regurgitated (free of gastric contents); or, a small quantity of barium may be used to establish partial or complete obstruction.

Whenever a history of foreign body ingestion seems to indicate its retention, the pharynx should first be examined with a mirror to see if anything has lodged there. Removal from this site is easily accomplished without further diagnostic procedures. Following local intraoral examination, it is important to examine carefully the neck and throat externally to check for tenderness, masses, or a possible subcutaneous emphysema, all of which can result from penetration of the esophageal wall and leakage of air and saliva into the surrounding esophageal area. Auscultation of the neck and chest is important to check for air in the subcutaneous tissues.

Roentgenographic Examinations

The taking of routine posteroanterior and lateral chest as well as neck roentgenograms is extremely

Fig 13-1. Small piece of bone lodged obliquely in cervical esophagus. Air in esophagus and trachea is clearly seen in this lateral projection. Symptoms—left neck pain and exacerbation at time of swallowing—were constant.

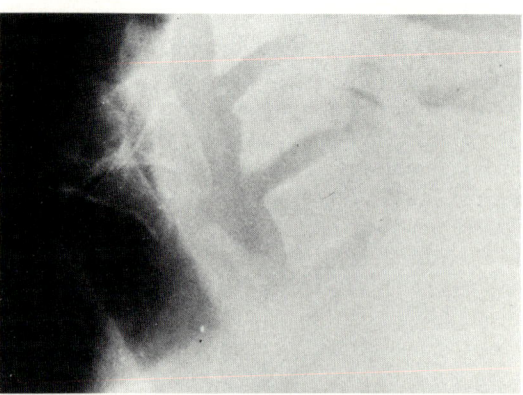

on swallowing during a meal should undergo esophagoscopy unless the pain rapidly disappears, regardless of roentgenographic findings.

The circumstances are quite different when a swallowed bolus of meat—most often beef or chicken—lodges in the esophagus. In such instances there is a history of sudden esophageal obstruction while the person is eating. These patients, when questioned carefully, may give a history of some previous dysphagia although the symptoms had been mild and not bothersome enough to have caused them to seek medical advice. Small hiatus hernias with proximal muscle important to establish whether the retained foreign material is radiopaque. In some cases in which the foreign material is not sufficiently radiopaque, it becomes visible with adequate roentgenograms, particularly if taken in the lateral projection so that the vertebrae will not obscure its recognition. Figure 13-1 shows a radiopaque bone spicule in the esophagus at the pharyngoesophageal junction. There is no evidence of air accumulation in the soft tissues that would suggest perforation. The clearly filled air passages anterior to the foreign body are easily defined. If an obstruction has occurred in the esophagus, an air fluid level may indicate its presence even though the foreign body itself cannot be visualized.

Roentgenograms will show subcutaneous or mediastinal emphysema, or both, caused by penetration of the esophageal wall by a suspected foreign body. Aspiration pneumonitis brought about by regurgitation and aspiration of esophageal contents can also be visualized and evaluated.

Figure 13-2 shows excellent visualization of a radiopaque child's jack in the esophagus. The lateral film on the right shows the anterior air col-

Fig 13-2. Child's metal jack in the upper one-third of the esophagus clearly visualized. Dysphagia, neck pain, dyspnea, and mild stridor were present.

umn of the trachea separate from the jack posteriorly located in the esophagus. Figure 13-3 illustrates another well-defined radiopaque foreign body, a finger ring, in the midesophagus. The lateral film on the right shows the air column of the trachea anteriorly with the foreign body lodged posteriorly in the middle one-third of the esophagus. Figure 13-4 shows a coin in the lower part of the esophagus with air proximal to the obstruction and the air-filled trachea anteriorly. Figure 13-5 shows two coins, one on top of the other, in the upper part of the esophagus at the site of the esophageal aortic indentation. Again, the lateral film (on the right) illustrates the posterior position of the foreign body with the air-filled trachea anterior.

Figure 13-6 illustrates a large bolus of steak in the lower one-third of the esophagus of a previously asymptomatic male. Swallowed barium outlined the typical appearance of such an obstruction. It is our feeling that those patients in whom retained foreign bodies of meat are suspected should be given a small amount of thin barium to outline the location of the obstructing agent and thus provide some idea as to whether obstruction is total or partial. We prefer barium because of its excellent contrast. Also, if one cannot see a foreign body by routine examination and roent-

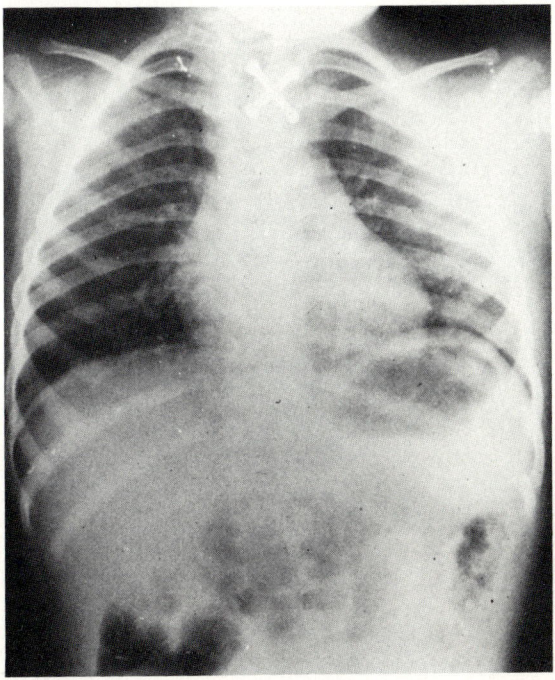

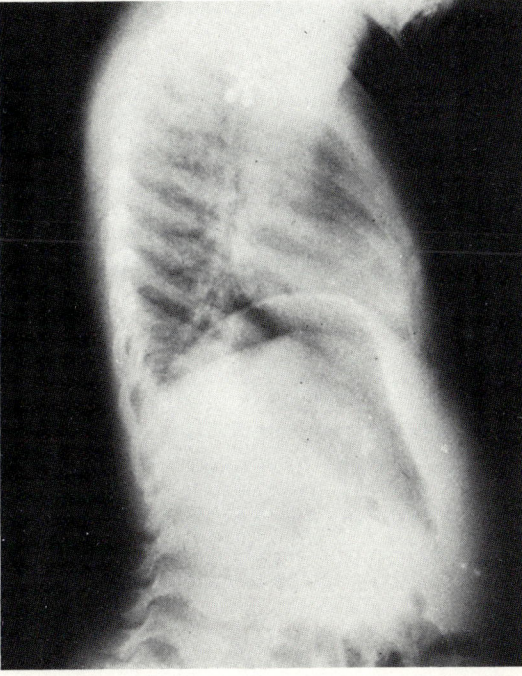

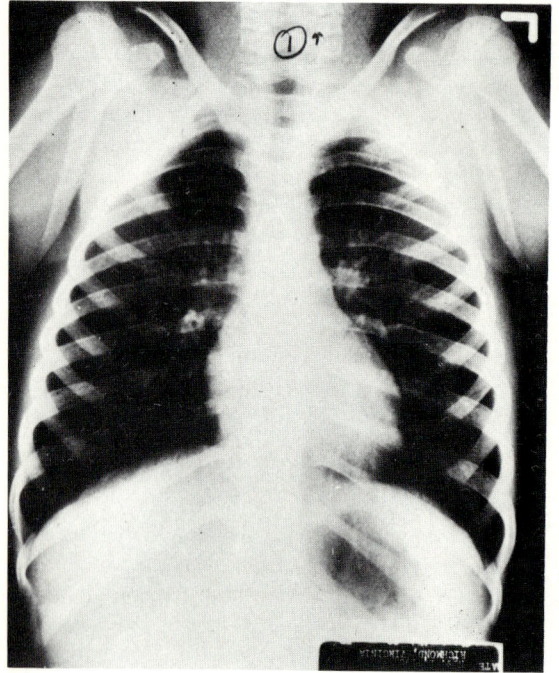
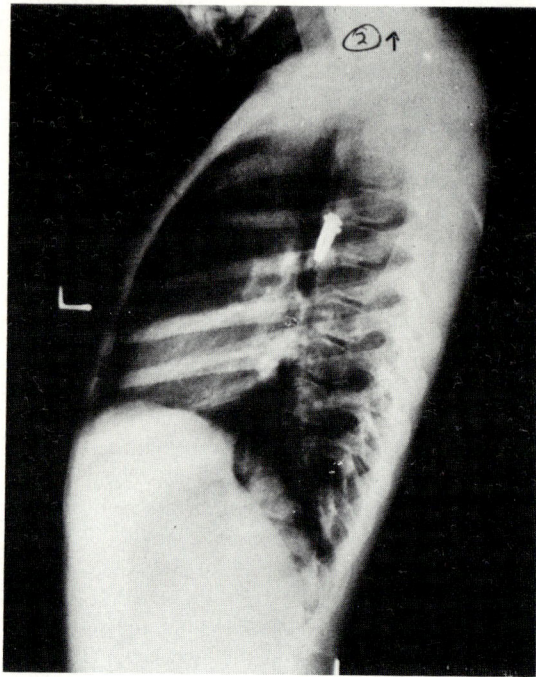

Fig 13-3. Ring foreign body seen in the middle one-third of the esophagus. The only symptom was mild discomfort on swallowing liquids. She would not take solids.

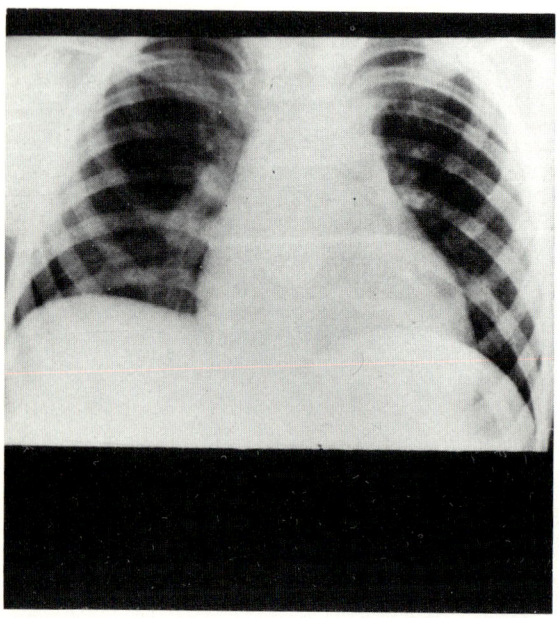
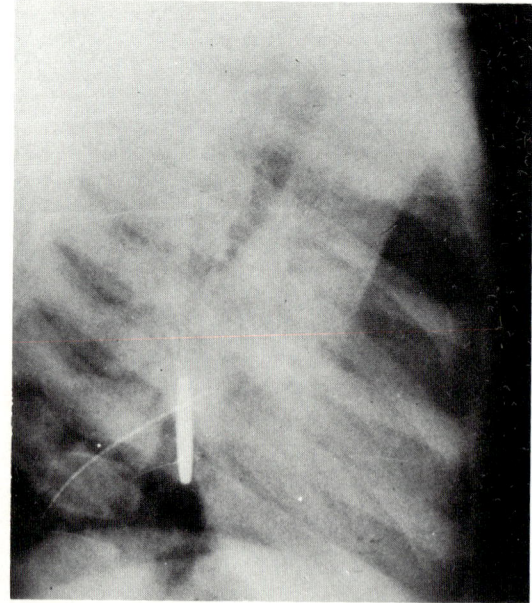

Fig 13-4. Coin seen in lower one-third of esophagus. Note the typical flat lie of the coin in the esophagus.

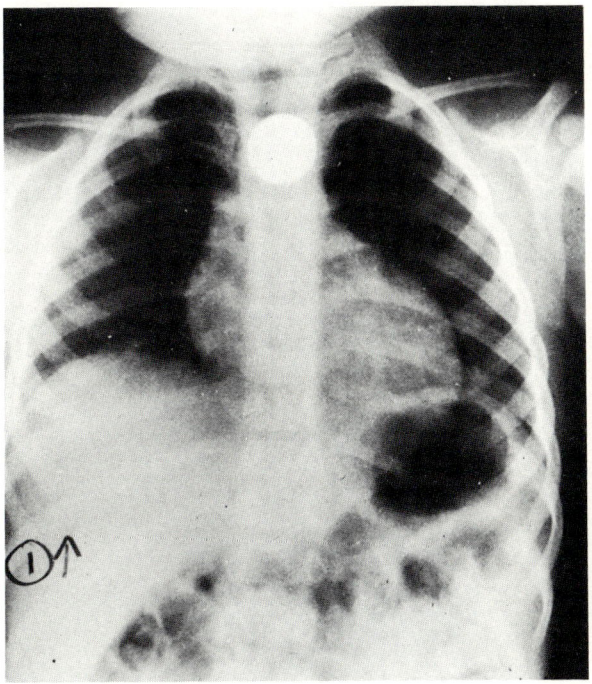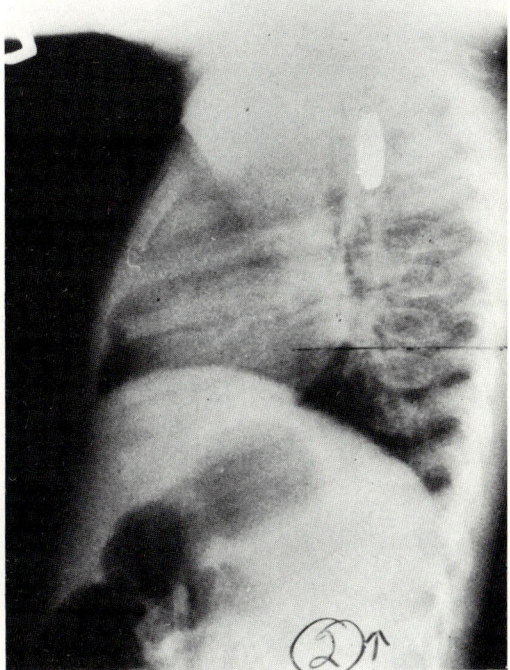

Fig 13-5. Two coins in the upper one-third of esophagus lie one immediately on top of the other.

genograms, the ingestion of a small amount of barium by the patient with subsequent careful study can help locate it. The plastic ring outlined by a barium swallow in Figure 13-7 is a clear example of this type of identification.

Esophagoscopy may be necessary for diagnosis when all other methods fail to identify a possible retained object in a patient with persistent symptoms.

Treatment

The treatment of foreign bodies in the esophagus is removal by esophagoscopy. Once confirmation of the object's presence has been obtained, except in the case of meat without a bone, we feel esophagoscopy carried out under general anesthesia is the treatment of choice [5, 38]. It is our preference that the patient have nothing by mouth for 8 hours prior to the induction of general anesthesia. Vomiting followed by aspiration before, during, or after general anesthesia may be most harmful to a patient with anything in his stomach. General anesthesia should be used with all procedures of foreign body removal that require esophagoscopy

because of the importance of total relaxation on the patient's part.

It is most important that a preoperative roentgenogram be obtained just prior to the induction of anesthesia. Figure 13-8A shows a coin lodged in the proximal esophagus of a child brought to the emergency room. Two hours later, just before the induction of general anesthesia, a repeat roentgenogram (Fig 13-8B) showed the coin in the stomach. Such precautions are important because in many cases, after a short period in hospital the patient's esophagus will relax sufficiently for a smooth object to pass on. Having reached the stomach it is rare for the foreign body not to pass through the intestinal tract.

At the time of esophagoscopy, careful attention should be paid to the character of the esophageal wall and to the possible presence of blood or a tear in the mucosa. It is important that the esophagoscope be inserted gently into the esophagus and that the foreign body be grasped firmly before its withdrawal is attempted. Many foreign bodies cannot be brought out through the esophagoscope because of their size, and it is necessary

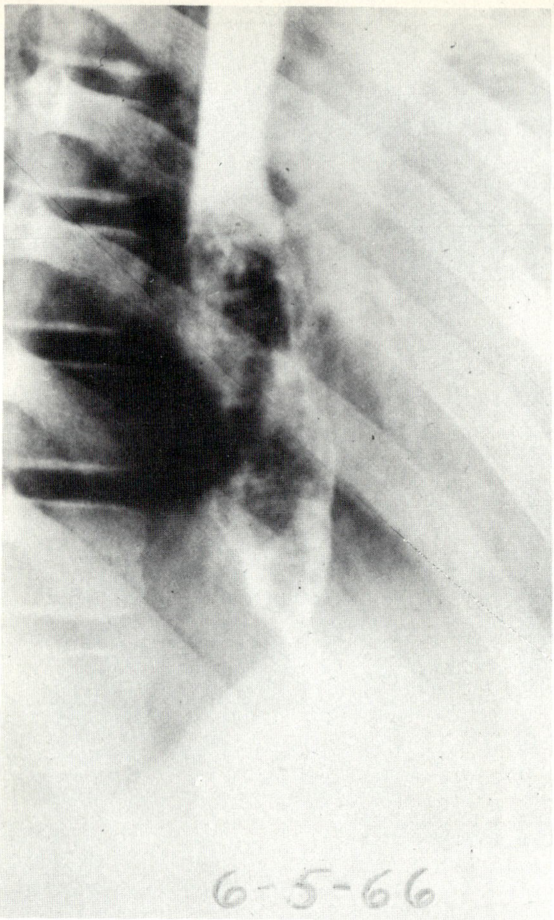

6-5-66

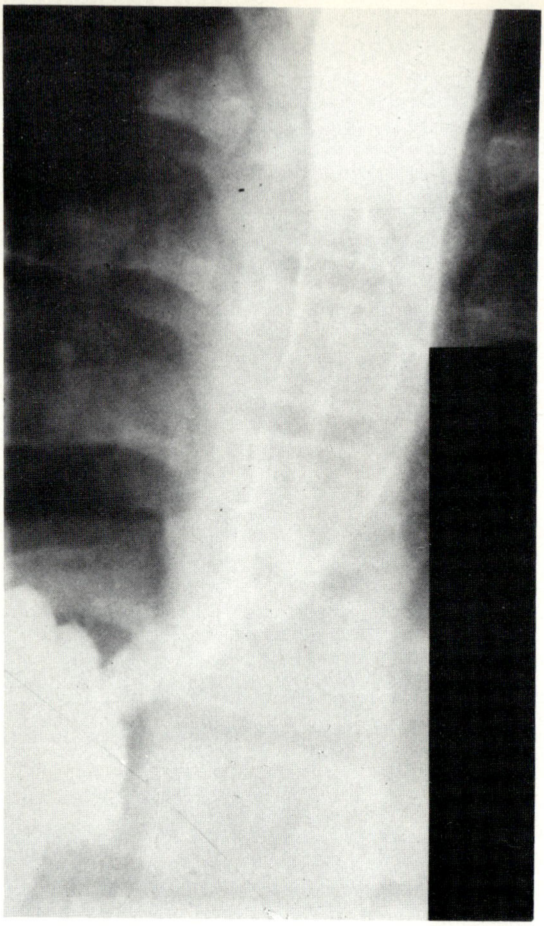

Fig 13-6. Large bolus of steak in lower one-third of esophagus is outlined as a filling defect in this barium swallow esophagogram. Obstruction is not complete.

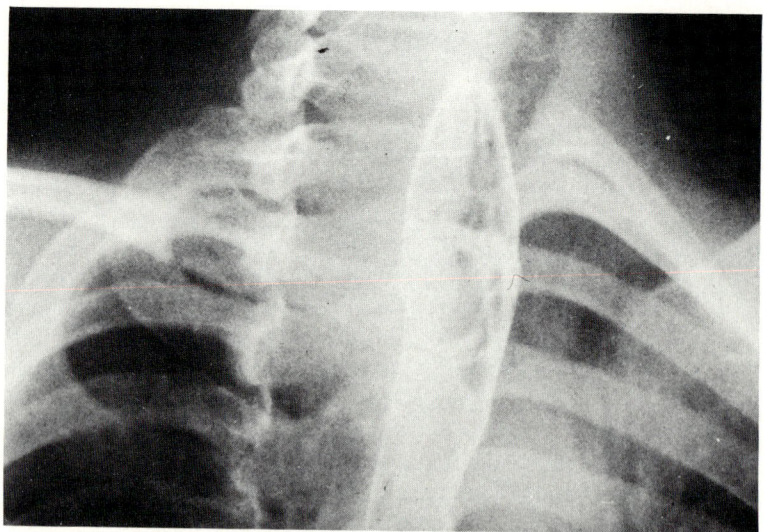

Fig 13-7. Plastic ring in upper one-third of esophagus is visualized as a negative shadow at the time the esophagogram with thin barium was done.

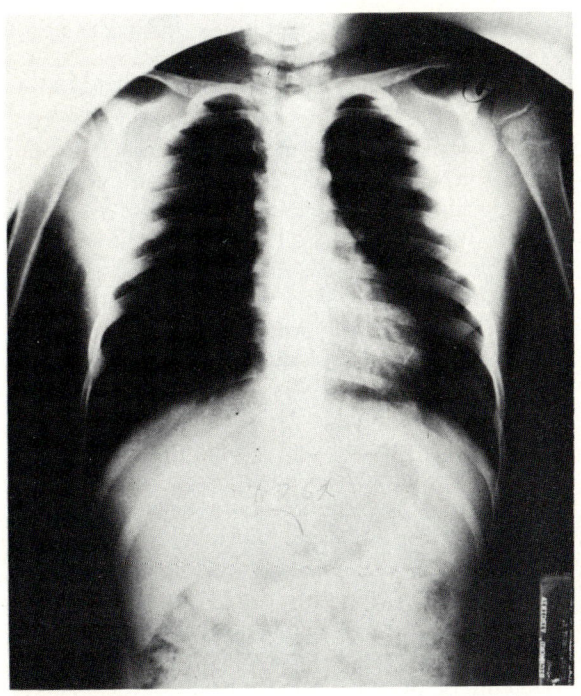

A

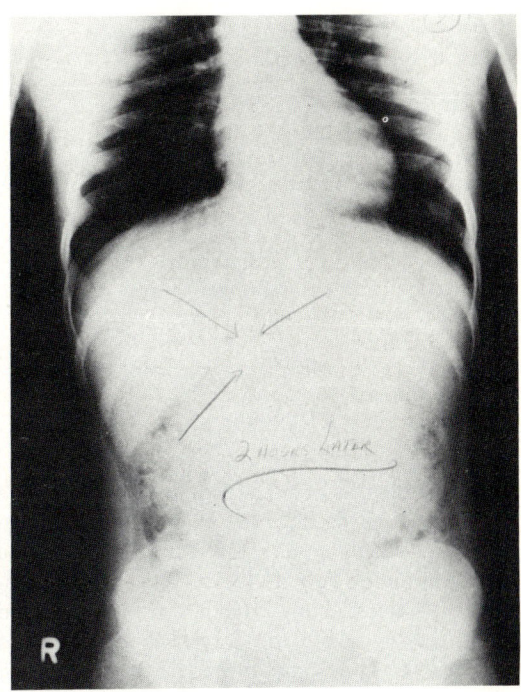

B

Fig 13-8. (A) Coin seen in upper one-third of the esophagus. (B) A repeat roentgenogram taken 2 hours later just prior to induction of anesthesia shows the coin in the stomach. Passage through the gastrointestinal tract from this point is virtually routine.

to simultaneously remove the foreign body and esophagoscope [10]. Care must be taken to prevent any sharp edges from penetrating the esophagus during withdrawal. Should the object become impacted when removal is attempted, it may become advisable to push the foreign body down into the stomach.

It has been suggested that for smooth, round, radiopaque foreign bodies in the esophagus, e.g., a coin in children, one may be able to carry out treatment by inserting a Foley catheter into the esophagus and, under fluoroscopy, inflating the bag after the catheter has been passed distal to the foreign body. The Foley catheter should then be withdrawn slowly, bringing the foreign body up with it [2, 40]. I have not used this technique because of the possibility that the foreign body may be lodged across the epiglottis at the time of withdrawal and cause asphyxiation.

If a reliable patient gives a history of meat ingestion followed by prompt obstruction, and if roentgenograms show no bone in the meat, it is our feeling that the best treatment is enzymatic. We use a 20% papain in water solution; 5 ml of this mixture is ingested every 5 minutes for 1 hour. The action of the enzyme on the meat usually softens it enough to allow it to pass into the stomach without difficulty. Before using it, however, we insert a Levin tube and gently wash the proximal esophagus with saline so that the enzyme will come into direct contact with the meat. The papain solution must be freshly prepared for proper enzymatic activity [12, 31, 33].

Over the past 10 years, we have removed meat by means of an esophagoscope in 26 patients (Table 13-4). Perforations caused by manipulations with the esophagoscope or foreign body forceps occurred in 3 patients. One died because of a fulminating mediastinitis that did not respond to prompt drainage. Another death occurred because of the patient's reaction to the local anesthetic. However, in another group of 25 patients treated by the papain enzymatic technique, all responded without complications. Because of the hazards presented by removing meat through an esophagoscope, it is our feeling that only enzymatic de-

Table 13-4. Treatment of Meat Obstruction
in Esophagus in 56 Patients

Treatment	Number of Patients
Esophagoscopy	26
Perforations	3
Deaths: fulminating mediastinitis (1); reaction to local anesthesia (1)[a]	2
Papain enzymatic technique	25
Passed unassisted	5

[a] One percent mortality.

bridement should be used. On the other hand, 2 cases have been documented in which the esophageal wall was digested by the enzymes, leading to the mediastinitis and death. If the enzyme technique (commercial meat tenderizer) is not used in patients in whom the foreign body has been impacted for some time or who have experienced hematemesis or an evident elevation of temperature, we feel that it is a safe procedure.

Three patients in our series (1.5%) had a sharp foreign body in the esophagus with resultant perforation and abscess formation. Recognition of such perforation is most important (Table 13-5) [1, 7, 21, 26, 28, 34–36, 44]. The majority of these patients give a clear history of increasing pain located either substernally, in the neck, in the epigastrium, or in the back. A combination of pain of all these locations may be present in lower esophageal perforation. There also is evidence of toxicity, with an elevated temperature, rapid pulse, rapid respirations, and a feeling of impending danger. In those patients with a perforation of the cervical esophagus, there may be a mass with increased tenderness and pain as well as palpable subcutaneous emphysema, also visible on roentgenogram. Lower esophageal perforation may in turn be accompanied by mediastinal emphysema,

Table 13-5. Symptoms of Esophageal Perforation

Pain (substernal, neck, epigastric, back)
Systemic toxicity
Neck mass
Subcutaneous emphysema
Appearance on roentgenogram after contrast studies

with or without air fluid levels and widening of the mediastinum.

The best method for diagnosing mediastinal disease secondary to esophageal perforation is a contrast swallow. Our contrast preference is barium because it shows excellent detail and because of the small quantity necessary to visualize a perforation. Whenever a perforation is demonstrated, we prefer to expose the area surgically and remove the foreign body, either through the exposed incision or concurrently with an esophagoscope. The esophagus should subsequently be closed in two layers and the area drained. If, as occasionally happens, the foreign body has been present for some time, it may be advisable to perform only a drainage procedure and foreign body removal without primary closure of the esophagus. Perforations of the esophagus above the fourth thoracic vertebra are best drained through the right side of the neck. On the other hand, those in the lower esophagus may be drained posteriorly through the mediastinal route or transthoracic opening with closure of the esophagus and subsequent drainage into the pleural space. Obviously, whenever esophageal perforation is present, antibiotic therapy is important; if perforation is not an established fact, antibiotic therapy may still be necessary while the patient remains under observation.

In the adult patient with meat or other foreign bodies lodged in the esophagus, it is our feeling that repeat contrast studies of the esophagus, after the obstruction is removed, are important to pick up any underlying esophageal disease, although as noted earlier seldom does organic esophageal disease lead to the retention of foreign material within the organ. Due to the edematous reaction within the wall when there is a foreign body, however, repeat contrast studies of the esophagus are best carried out 14 to 21 days after removing any obstruction. At this time, local edema or spasm, or both, brought about by the foreign body will be relieved and one will have a better idea as to the organic or intrinsic esophageal disease that may be present.

If dilatation of the esophagus is necessary, as in cases of stricture, it is best to wait until this 14- to 21-day period has elapsed because there will be less danger of esophageal perforation at that time. When the contrast studies are repeated, they may indicate a condition needing operative repair, such as hiatus hernia with stricture or esophagitis, or both.

Recurrence of the same foreign bodies in the esophagus of a given individual is unusual. In our series of 200 patients, for example, only 3 males (2 children and 1 adult) and 3 females (all adults) were repeaters. In 4 patients, there were 2 obstructions; in 1 patient, obstruction occurred 3 times; and in 1 patient, it occurred 5 times. There were also 3 strictures.

FOREIGN BODIES IN THE AIR PASSAGES

During the 10-year period of study foreign bodies in the air passages occurred in 51 patients [3, 20]. It is interesting that none of these subjects had the experience twice and that only one foreign body occurred per individual. Table 13-6 illustrates the area of the tracheobronchial tree involved in both children and adults. Children predominated in this group—45 of the total of 51. It was a little unusual that the left main stem bronchus was implicated more often than any other single area of the tracheobronchial tree. Table 13-7 shows the types of foreign material most often found in the tracheobronchial tree, particularly in children. Other objects found in the air passages of 16 children were: picture hook, bone, pinto bean, ballpen top, chestnut, crayon, tacks, soybean, popcorn kernel, eggshell, tooth, marble, hatpin, bean, and a rubber balloon. The objects found in 4 adults were: bones, toothpick, and a hypodermic needle.

Diagnosis

The symptoms following the entry of a foreign body into the air passages are usually described vividly by the parents of the child or by the adult

Table 13-6. Foreign Body Lodgement in Air Passages in 51 Patients Seen Over 10 Years (1960–1970)

Part of Tracheobronchial Tree	Children	Adults
Trachea	9	—
Right main bronchus	9	1
Right upper lobe	—	1
Right intermediate bronchus	6	2
Right lower lobe	4	1
Left main bronchus	11	—
Left upper lobe	2	—
Left lower lobe	4	1
Total	45	6

Table 13-7. Foreign Bodies Most Frequently Found in Airway Passages in 51 Patients

Object	Children	Adults
Peanut	19	1
Plastic bullet	6	0
Safety pin	1	1
Screw	2	0
Sewing needle	1	0
Total	29 (64%)	2 (33%)

involved. Gagging, cyanosis, wheezing, and sometimes near respiratory arrest occur because of the irritation, obstruction, and violent coughing as the foreign body passes through the glottis to the trachea. Vomiting is not unusual. After the initial episode during which the foreign material becomes lodged in a bronchus, the patients have a persistently annoying cough that may or may not be, but usually is, accompanied by an audible wheeze. When the impacted object has been present for several hours, the cough may become minimal or nonexistent because of a deadening of the cough reflex, although the wheeze remains in most instances.

Physical examination at the time of foreign body aspiration frequently reveals a child or an adult with minimal to no respiratory distress. As a matter of fact, they frequently tend to breathe quietly and easily in order not to aggravate the troublesome cough. An audible wheeze may be heard at the bedside; this is also often heard on auscultation, being more intense during expiration. The wheeze may become more obvious if one can get the patient to cough or perhaps breathe forcibly, which latter action also helps to stimulate the cough. Very frequently one notices a definite diminution of breath sounds over the area of lung whose bronchus is partially or totally occluded by the foreign body. This may be a more prominent finding than the wheeze.

Roentgenographic examination is most important. If the foreign body is radiopaque, the diagnosis is rapidly confirmed. Again, posteroanterior and lateral films are necessary in this type of investigation.

The most reliable roentgenographic finding in a patient with a recently aspirated nonopaque foreign body in the bronchus is evidence of obstructive emphysema ("air trapping"). This sign is

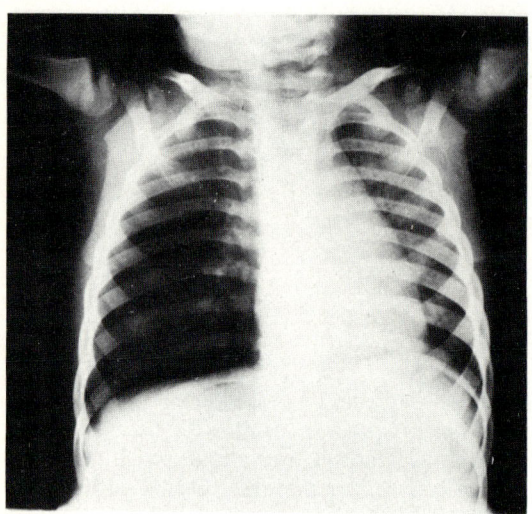

Fig 13-9. Expiratory film shows obstructive emphysema ("air trapping") in the right lung in a patient with a peanut as a foreign body in the right main bronchus. Note (1) the clear right lung; (2) the depressed right diaphragm that is widened in the right intercostal spaces; and (3) the mediastinal shift to the left.

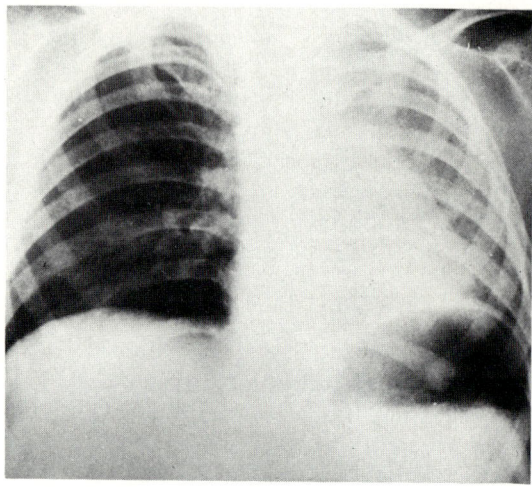

Fig 13-10. Start of atelectasis shown in a roentgenogram of a child in whom a peanut has been in left main bronchus for over 24 hours.

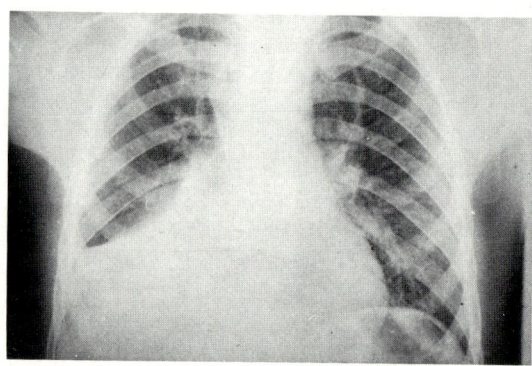

Fig 13-11. Complete atelectasis of the right lower lobe is seen in a child with a peanut that has obstructed a right lower lobe bronchus for 3 days.

most obvious when films taken during inspiration and expiration are compared. With expiration, the area of obstructive emphysema does not deflate as in the contralateral normal lung (Fig 13-9).

The result of a peanut embedded in the left main bronchus for over 24 hours is shown roentgenographically in Figure 13-10. There is marked obstruction on the left side with signs of a beginning atelectasis. Figure 13-11 demonstrates the more clearly established atelectasis and some pneumonitis in the right lower lobe of another child with a peanut in the right lower lobe bronchus for 3 days. Figure 13-12 shows a beginning atelectasis of the right lung due to a peanut lodged in the right main bronchus for over 2 days [24, 37].

In a few patients with bronchial foreign bodies there may be a "silent" period following the aspiration, with pneumonia distal to the obstruction occurring several days or weeks later. Therefore, in any child who has pulmonary signs and symptoms such as unilateral wheeze, hemoptysis, recurrent pneumonia in the same area of the lung, isolated lung abscess, or a combination of these, a careful history should be taken dating back over several weeks to determine whether there is reason to suspect an aspirated foreign body [9, 13, 14].

This is especially true if there is clinical evidence of bronchial obstruction as manifested primarily by suppression of breath sounds or by roentgenographic signs of atelectasis.

Treatment

Retained foreign objects within the lumen of bronchi cause a reaction in the mucosa leading to edema and varying degrees of bronchial spasm. Drainage distal to the foreign body is impaired. Atelectasis and infection, both bronchial and pneumonic, are enhanced. With the passage of time, bronchiectasis, bronchial stenosis, lung abscess, empyema, and

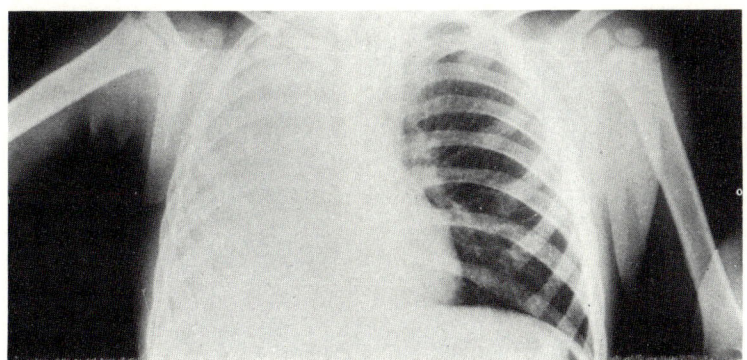

Fig 13-12. Early atelectasis in the right lung is seen in a child with a peanut in the right main bronchus for 2 days.

occasionally bronchopleural fistula may develop [22]. These changes can result in loss of functional lung tissue because of subsequent operative resection. Severe hemoptysis caused by erosion from infection or the foreign body itself has been reported. Foreign bodies in the tracheobronchial tree may migrate to other areas of the thorax.

With the confirmation of a foreign body in the tracheobronchial tree, the treatment of choice is its extraction by bronchoscopy [19, 27, 32]. If the patient is not in acute distress, the bronchoscopy should be delayed until at least 8 hours following the last meal. Should distress be present, bronchoscopy must be initiated promptly. We prefer employing general anesthesia with relaxing drugs as well as using the rigid ventilating Jackson bronchoscope in the adult and the ventilating Storz-Hopkins telescopic bronchoscope in children. In same cases, however, the air jet provided by these instruments may force small particles deeper into the respiratory tree and make them more difficult to manage. The flexible fiberoptic bronchoscope is only occasionally helpful in the management of foreign bodies in the air passages.

In the absence of a ventilating bronchoscope we advocate a general anesthetic, e.g., ether, that allows the patient to be well anesthetized but still continue an adequate respiratory effort. This lessens the haste with which the surgeon must work and allows more prolonged exploration of the tracheobronchial tree for the extraction of multiple pieces of peanut or similar foreign material. If one cannot definitely establish the presence of a foreign body in the tracheobronchial tree, it is safer to proceed with bronchoscopic inspection rather

than to keep the patient around the hospital for prolonged periods of examination.

Most extraneous particles can be extracted with a foreign body forceps and minimal trauma. An additional tool for removing foreign bodies in the air passages is the Fogarty catheter, which was originally designed for emboli and clot evacuation from blood vessels [43]. After visualization of the foreign body by bronchoscopy, the Fogarty catheter may be introduced through the bronchoscope and passed beyond the foreign body. The balloon is next inflated and the catheter withdrawn, carrying the foreign body with it.

Complications following instrumental removal of foreign bodies from the tracheobronchial tree are usually confined to vocal cord edema for which steroid therapy for 12 hours is often sufficient. Occasionally tracheostomy may be lifesaving in cases of, for example, tracheal occlusion from within or at the level of the epiglottis (2 cases in our study). Pneumothorax or pneumomediastinum, or both, may be noted occasionally after endoscopy and foreign body removal. Prompt tube drainage for the pneumothorax then becomes necessary.

Figure 13-13 illustrates a screw in the right intermediate bronchus of a child, three efforts at removal of which were unsuccessful. This child later underwent a thoracotomy. By opening longitudinally the membranous portion of the right intermediate bronchus, the foreign body was easily extracted, the bronchus repaired, and complete expansion of the lower and middle lobes regained without evidence of damage in those lobes from infection [6].

Bronchoscopic removal of the foreign bodies was successful in all but 4 patients (8%). These patients were treated by thoracotomy. One patient developed empyema secondary to pneumonia distal

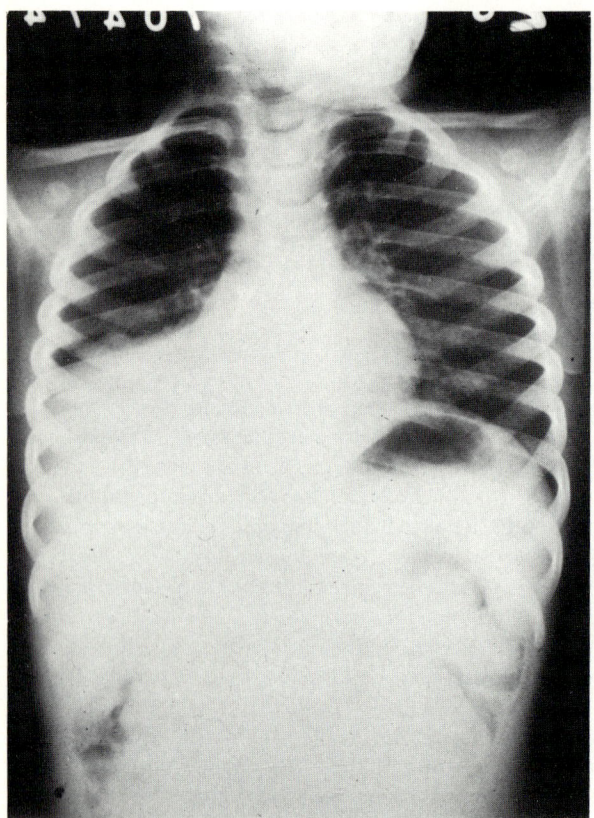
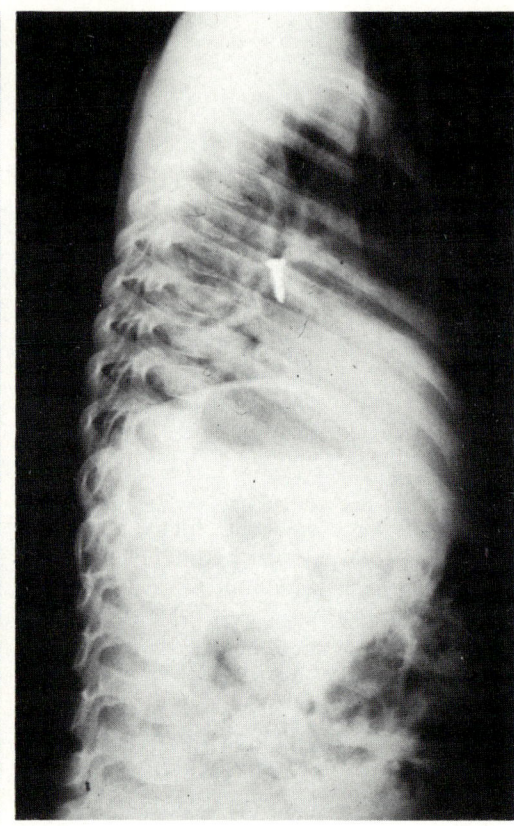

Fig 13-13. A screw in the right intermediate bronchus required thoracotomy for removal.

to the point of foreign body obstruction. Drainage of the empyema was carried out with complete recovery of the patient.

The 1 death in our series occurred in a small child who had attempted to blow up a toy balloon. It exploded and he aspirated the rubber material into his trachea. He was dead on arrival in the emergency room.

Two of our patients (4%) had cardiac arrest because of tracheal foreign bodies. The obstructions were promptly extracted in the emergency room and in both instances resuscitative efforts were successful.

REFERENCES

1. Barker GN: Oesophageal abscess. J Laryngol 57: 491, 1962
2. Bigler FC: The use of a Foley catheter for removal of blunt foreign bodies from the esophagus. J Thorac Cardiovasc Surg 51:759, 1966
3. Brown BSJ: Foreign bodies in the tracheobronchial tree in childhood. J Can Assoc Radiol 14: 158, 1963
4. Bunker PG: Unrecognized foreign bodies in the air and food passages. GP 29:78, 1964
5. Camarata SJ, Salyer JM: Management of foreign bodies in air passages and esophagus under general anesthesia. Am J Surg 31:725, 1965
6. Carter R: Bronchotomy: The safe solution for an infarcted foreign body. Ann Surg 10:93, 1970
7. Clark JV: A case of submucous abscess of the esophagus. J Laryngol 62:461, 1948
8. Clerf LH: Foreign bodies in the air and food passages. Surg Gynecol Obstet 70:328, 1940
9. Clery AP, Ellis FH, Schmidt HW: Problems associated with aspiration of grass heads (inflorescences). JAMA 171:1478, 1959
10. Equen MS: The alnico magnet: An aid to bronchoscopy and esophagoscopy. Ann Otol Rhinol Laryngol 54:178, 1948
11. Graham EA, Singer JJ, Ballon HC: Surgical Diseases of the Chest. Philadelphia, Lea & Febiger, 1935

12. Hargrove MD Jr, Shreveport LA, Worth Boyce, LTD, H Jr: Meat impaction of the esophagus. Arch Intern Med 125:277, 1970
13. Hays DM, Huberty GT, O'Laughlin BJ: Radiopaque grass heads in the lungs. Dis Chest 33:38, 1958
14. Jackson C: Grasses as foreign bodies in bronchus and lung. Laryngoscope 62:897, 1952
15. Jackson C, Jackson CL: Bronchoesophagology. Philadelphia, Saunders, 1950
16. Jackson C, Jackson CL: Disease of the Nose, Throat, and Ear. Philadelphia, Saunders, 1959
17. Jackson C, Jackson CL: Pulmonary symptoms due to esophageal disease. Arch Otolaryngol 18:731, 1933
18. Jackson CL: Foreign body in the esophagus. Am J Surg 93:308, 1957
19. Kassay D: Management of bronchial foreign bodies. Eye Ear Nose Throat Mon 42:54, 1963
20. Kassay D: Observations on 100 cases of bronchial foreign bodies. Arch Otolaryngol 71:42, 1960
21. Kramer R: Endoscopic treatment of esophageal suppuration. Laryngoscope 39:97, 1929
22. Laurance B: Hemoptysis, bronchiectasis and foreign body in lung. Br Med J 1:125, 1954
23. Le Roux BT: Intrathoracic foreign bodies. J R Coll Surg Edinb 9:220, 1964
24. Linton JSA: Long-standing intrabronchial foreign bodies. Thorax 12:164, 1957
25. Matheson I: Foreign bodies in the esophagus. A review of 602 cases. J Laryngol Otol 63:435, 1949
26. McLaughlin RT, Morris JD, Haight C: The morbid nature of the migrating foreign body in the esophagus. J Thorac Cardiovasc Surg 55:188, 1968
27. Neematallah F, Nassar H: Extraction of a globular, hard, slippery foreign body inhaled in the bronchial tree by postural dislodgement and direct laryngoscopy. Br J Anaesth 37:547, 1965
28. Overstreet JW, Ochsner A: Traumatic rupture of the esophagus. J Thorac Cardiovasc Surg 30:164, 1955
29. Pimpinelli RJ: Airway obstruction due to a foreign body in the esophagus. Arch Otolaryngol 79:606, 1964
30. Ray ES, Vinson PP: 584 foreign bodies removed from the esophagus; a statistical study. Va Med Mon 85:61, 1958
31. Richardson JR: A new treatment for esophageal obstruction due to meat impaction. Arch Otolaryngol 54:328, 1945
32. Roach GS, Majoras M: Removal of a toy bullet from the lung with a new instrument. Arch Otolaryngol 82:403, 1965
33. Robinson AS: Meat impaction in the esophagus treated by enzymatic digestion. JAMA 181:1141, 1961
34. Sanborn EB: Intramural abscesses of the esophagus: A complication of foreign bodies. J Thorac Surg 39:586, 1960
35. Schechter DC, Gilbert L: Injuries of the heart and great vessels due to pins and needles. Thorax 24:246, 1969
36. Seybold WD, Johnson MA III, Leary WV: Perforation of the esophagus. Surg Clin North Am 30:1155, 1950
37. Slim MS, Yacoubian HD: Complications of foreign bodies in the tracheobronchial tree. Arch Surg 92:388, 1966
38. Smith COMS, Shroff PF, Steele JD: General anesthesia for bronchoscopy. Ann Thorac Surg 8:348, 1969
39. Stein L: Foreign bodies of the tracheobronchial tree and esophagus. Ann Thorac Surg 9:382, 1970
40. Symbas PN: Indirect method of extraction of foreign body from the esophagus. Ann Surg 167:78, 1967
41. Terracol J, Sweet RH: Disease of the Esophagus. Philadelphia, Saunders, 1958
42. Tucker GF: The age of incidence of lodgement of single coins in the esophagus. Ann Otol Rhinol Laryngol 73:1116, 1964
43. Ullyot DG, Norman JC: The Fogarty catheter: An aid to bronchoscopic removal of foreign bodies. Ann Thorac Surg 6:185, 1968
44. Vistreich F: Two cases of esophageal foreign body with complications. Laryngoscope 50:1178, 1940

14. TRAUMATIC HERNIA OF THE DIAPHRAGM

James W. Brooks
Hawley H. Seiler

Traumatic diaphragmatic hernia [35, 41, 43, 53, 71, 72] may follow injury to the diaphragm from stab and bullet wounds [21, 27, 37, 39], indirect blunt violence, postoperative diaphragmatic dehiscence [14, 24, 30, 55], diaphragmatic erosion from infection, be spontaneous [75, 80], or occur through previous congenital weaknesses.

When disruption of the continuity of either side of the diaphragm occurs from any cause, physiological disturbances are prone to occur because the abdominal contents (omentum, stomach, spleen, small and large intestines, liver) may enter the thoracic cavity. Negative intrapleural pressure facilitates herniation of visceral contents into this cavity due to the positive pressure of the abdominal cavity. The contents of the latter may plug the hole in the diaphragm or pass into the cavity with oscillation between both cavities. The size and location of the diaphragmatic disruption determines what organs enter the thorax and, to some extent, the potential for incarceration or strangulation [82]. As the abdominal contents enter the thorax pulmonary tissue is compressed, and, depending on the quantity of material compressing the pulmonary tissue, various degrees of respiratory embarrassment occur. When a large mass passes upward, compression of the lung is extensive and the heart and mediastinum are displaced toward the contralateral side, causing further respiratory embarrassment. Distortion of the great veins in the mediastinum by such displacement will cause decreased venous emptying into the atria of the heart, decreased cardiac output, and lowering of systemic blood pressure. If the disruption of the diaphragm is extensive, the diaphragmatic contractions will be ineffectual and the hole will act much as a "flail" portion of the chest wall. This flail causes the same physiological alterations of ventilation and cardiovascular function as does the flail rib cage. Thus the initial symptoms and signs of a ruptured diaphragm are focused on the respiratory mechanism.

If the intestinal contents become inflated with gas upon entering the thorax and do not empty properly, the gastric or bowel expansion, or both, will further adversely affect respiratory and cardiovascular function. Such distention also favors incarceration and possible advancement to strangulation (Fig 14-1). Vomiting would then be apt to occur and lead to possible aspiration of gastric contents into the respiratory passages.

Blood loss from the edges of the torn diaphragm always occurs and may be large in amount. This further complicates the adverse cardiovascular and respiratory response to the injury.

Traumatic disruption of the diaphragm may remain undiagnosed for an extended period of time because of the absence of symptoms or perhaps the presence of only vague, poorly understood signs [2, 45]. After a delay of several months or years in the diagnosis of diaphragmatic disruption, the predominant symptomatology quite frequently is associated with obstruction in the gastrointestinal tract (Fig 14-2). The effects on the respiratory system at this stage of development may be less obvious and partially compensated for by a natural avoidance of stressful activity. Respiratory trouble will become apparent if a careful history is taken.

STAB, BULLET, AND GUNSHOT WOUNDS

When the track of a bullet or stab wound suggests involvement of either side of the diaphragm, careful investigation of the patient's symptoms and signs and roentgenographic evidence of pleural or peritoneal injury, or both, must be carried out. Positive identifications include such things as hemothorax, pneumothorax, or hemopneumothorax with a rigid abdomen or rebound abdominal tenderness, or both; omentum protruding from a thoracic wound site; or intestinal contents draining from a thoracic wound. In our institution all bullet and stab wounds of the abdomen are explored in the operating room under general anesthesia. Careful inspection of the whole diaphragm is always a part of the abdominal investigation at the time of laparotomy. Admittedly such wounds may be easily missed if the abdominal approach is used

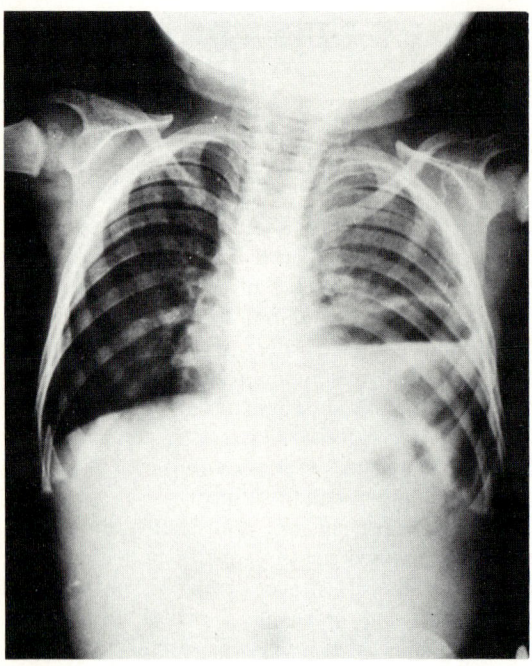

Fig 14-1. Posteroanterior chest roentgenogram of a 2-year-old boy hit by an auto. Sudden death occurred 45 minutes later. No use had been made of a nasogastric suction tube. Postmortem examination revealed massive gastric dilatation with total collapse of the left lung and marked mediastinal shift.

when they are looked for. Wounds so discovered are closed with interrupted, nonabsorbable sutures.

Since all wounds within the thoracic area (bullet or stab wounds) need not necessarily be explored, careful attention is directed to the level of the diaphragm after complete lung reexpansion and chest tube insertion. Tube insertion is indicated when either air or fluid (blood) or both are seen roentgenographically in the hemothorax after these injuries. Generally the patient with a bullet or stab wound who has a perforation of the diaphragm has problems in the chest or abdomen of a much more urgent nature than that of the diaphragm. These lesions can include such things as bleeding from the intercostal arteries, bleeding from the internal mammary artery, spleen or liver bleeding, disruption of the intestinal tract (esophagus, stomach, small and large bowel), injuries to the genitourinary system, and injuries to the lung or major vessels within the thoracic cavity. Obviously these more pressing problems must be dealt with, and although closure of the tear in the dia-

phragm made by the bullet or stab wound is usually incidental, it is nonetheless important at the completion of the primary procedure. If an opening in the diaphragm secondary to a bullet or stab wound is neglected or not visualized and properly closed, later difficulties with herniation of intestinal organs may lead to incarceration, obstruction, or strangulation of these organs (Fig 14-3).

When one is in doubt concerning the possibility of diaphragmatic injury, the best nonoperative method to use to investigate possible damage with perforation is the performance of a diagnostic pneumoperitoneum [33, 79] of 500 to 700 ml (Fig 14-4). The appearance of a pneumothorax following this diagnostic procedure confirms a communication between the pleural and peritoneal cavities. If there is a congenital defect, which is rare, there may be a false positive result. However, this problem has not arisen in our experience to confuse interpretation of the diagnostic pneumoperitoneum at the time of injury. (The use of a diagnostic pneumoperitoneum was initially described by Hollander and Dugan [46] and by Clay and Hanlon [22].)

In carrying out a diagnostic pneumoperitoneum we do a four-quadrant abdominal tap using a plastic needle. The procedure is completed in the left lower quadrant where the air is then inserted, provided the abdominal tap has yielded no blood or intestinal fluid. Should the abdominal tap be positive no air is inserted because exploration of the abdomen would already be indicated and the diaphragm would then be explored at the same time. If trauma to the lung includes air leakage and a torn diaphragm, air under the diaphragm may be seen on a roentgenogram because of its escape through the diaphragm into the abdomen. Conversely a perforated viscus can give rise to a pneumothorax through a defect in the diaphragm without lung injury. In this instance, air would also be seen under the diaphragm. In either case, operative exploration is indicated. Other than the infrequent but well-known complications that follow the induction of a therapeutic pneumoperitoneum, this procedure has two obvious disadvantages in the posttraumatic patient undergoing evaluation in the emergency ward:

1. With the placement of air in the peritoneal cavity abdominal symptoms and shoulder pain are intensified. The procedure will thus mask or possibly give false impressions regarding fu-

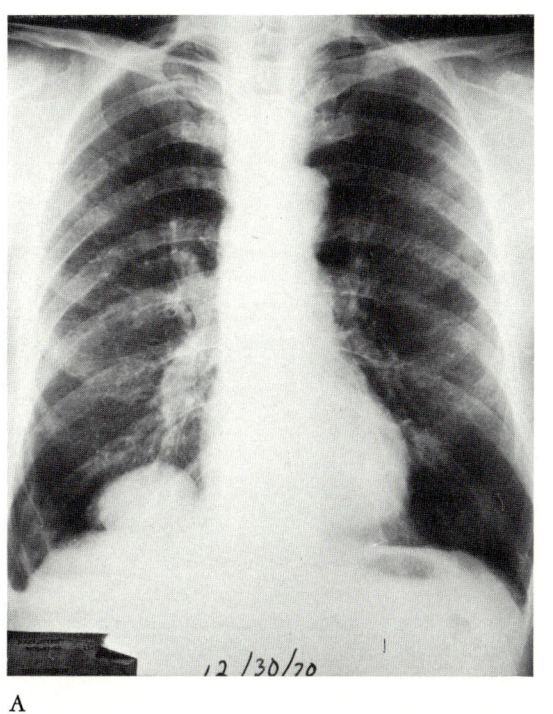

A

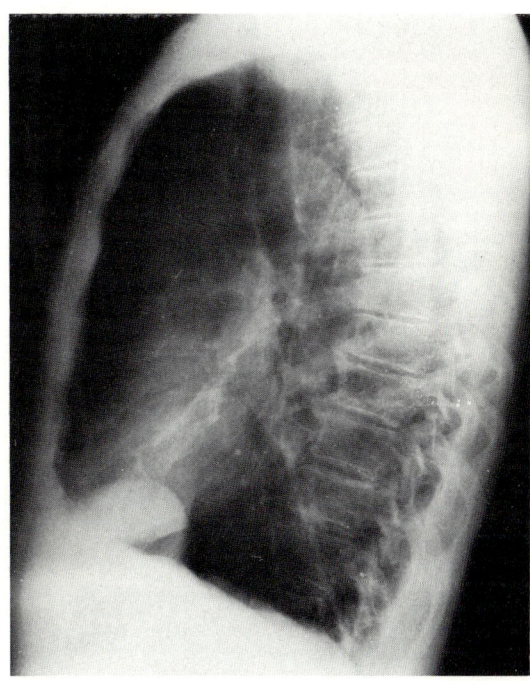

B

C

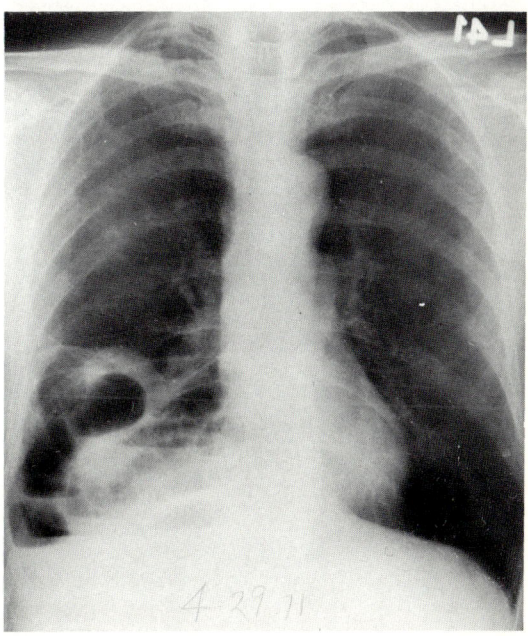

D

Fig 14-2. Posteroanterior (A) and right lateral (B) chest roentgenogram of a 60-year-old male who had been in an auto accident 15 years previously. Diagnostic pneumoperitoneum (C) reveals air in right pleural space with no outlining of the mass. (D)

Posteroanterior chest roentgenogram taken 4 months later when he was admitted with acute intestinal obstruction. At operation a gangrenous terminal ileum was resected. There was no hernia sac, and the patient recovered.

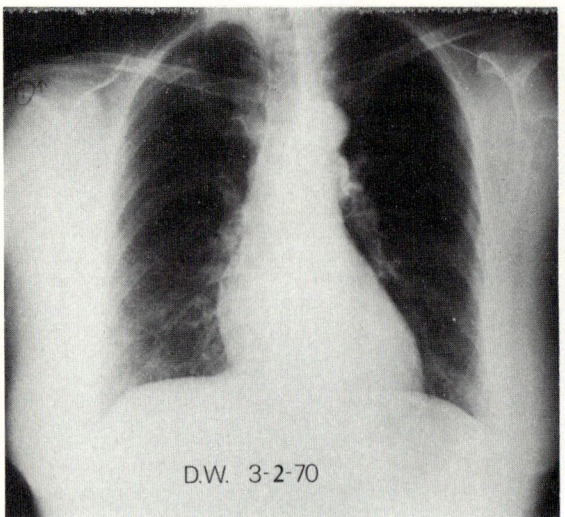

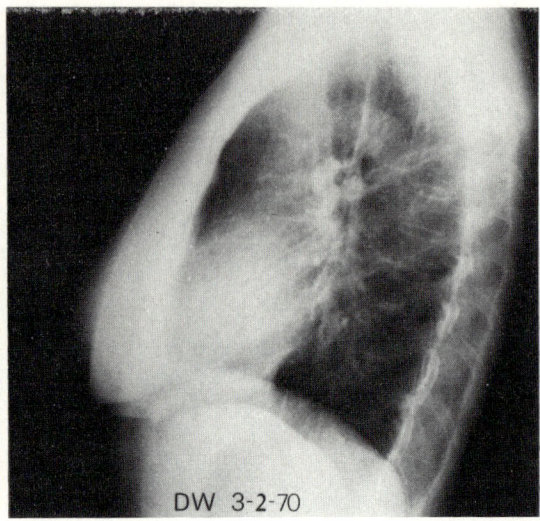

A

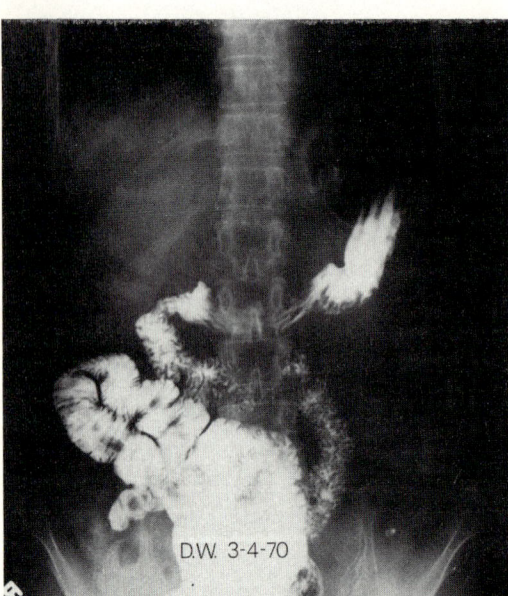

B

Fig 14-3. (A) Posteroanterior and lateral roentgeno-
grams of 60-year-old female who sustained a self-
inflicted bullet wound in the left chest 2 months pre-
viously. (B) Gastrointestinal series on the same
patient. (C) Gastrointestinal series 1 year later shows
massive gastric herniation through the diaphragm.
At thoracotomy a laceration 2 inches long from the
bullet was found in the diaphragm.

ture developments in the abdomen should exploration not be carried out.
2. The pneumothorax that results will further enhance pulmonary restrictive problems and
   should therefore be aspirated rapidly.

BLUNT TRAUMATIC RUPTURE
OF THE DIAPHRAGM

A diagnosis of blunt traumatic rupture of the diaphragm should be constantly kept in mind because
of the number of present-day auto accidents occurring at high speeds. In patients with multiple
system injuries the procedures taken to diagnose
them tend to draw the physician's attention away
from the more subtle diaphragmatic injuries [17,
63, 68, 84]. A high index of suspicion is the most
important factor in making the diagnosis of blunt
traumatic rupture of the diaphragm.

Physical findings in these patients are frequently
atypical for any given patient. When conscious the
patient may complain of pain and tenderness, or
show guarding in the epigastrium or either upper
quadrant of the abdomen. At the time of initial

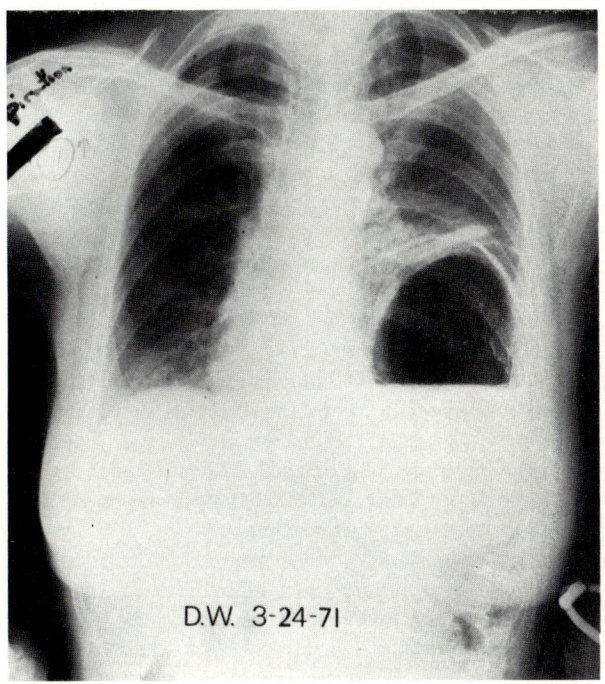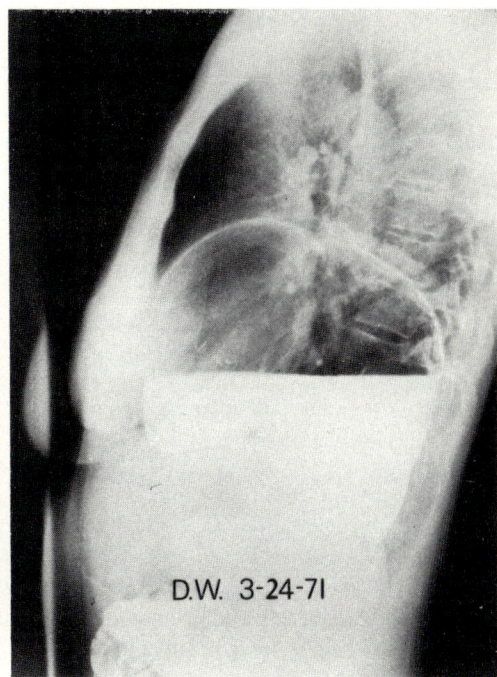

C

abdominal examination, bowel sounds may be present and unremarkable, or markedly reduced to absent, depending on the amount of peritoneal irritation. Chest examination may reveal obvious tenderness. If such tenderness is present, it is usually associated with fractured ribs and bony crepitation may therefore be felt. If the lung has been injured one may notice subcutaneous emphysema. All of these findings point to chest injury but obviously are not diagnostic of diaphragmatic injury.

With intestinal contents in the thoracic cavity, or with the liver in the thoracic cavity as seen with right diaphragmatic rupture, there may be dullness to percussion, diminished to absent fremitus, and diminished to absent breath sounds. All of these physical signs denote the presence of abnormal tissue between the examining physician's stethoscope and the lung parenchyma. Auscultation of intestinal sounds high in the axilla tends to arouse suspicion as to the presence of intestinal contents in the pleural cavity, but such sounds may be transmitted there from normal bowel below the diaphragm.

A preoperative diagnosis of blunt traumatic rupture of the diaphragm is most frequently suspected on or confirmed by observations made of chest roentgenograms. In general, any patient who has sustained a traumatic injury and in whom a chest film shows an obscure or abnormal diaphragmatic shadow is a suspected victim of blunt traumatic rupture of the diaphragm. Further studies must then be made promptly to establish the true state of the patient's diaphragm.

At the Medical College of Virginia Hospitals from 1952 to 1977 we have seen a total of 42 patients with blunt traumatic ruptures of the diaphragm. Of these, 38 (90%) occurred on the left side and 4 (10%) on the right [10, 44, 50, 65, 78, 88]. Thirty-six (86%) occurred in males and 6 (14%) in females. The mortality rate was 14% (6 patients). All deaths except one (tracheostomy complication) were caused by other injuries sustained during the same accident; the other 5 deaths occurred from thermal burns, perforated stomach, ruptured aorta, tension pneumothorax (gastric), and heart failure. Reference to Figure 14-5 reveals that the greatest number of blunt traumatic injuries of the diaphragm occur between the ages of 20 and 30 years [61]. This age group corresponds to that most frequently incurring massive trauma due to automobile accidents. Figure 14-6 suggests that there has not been an increased yearly

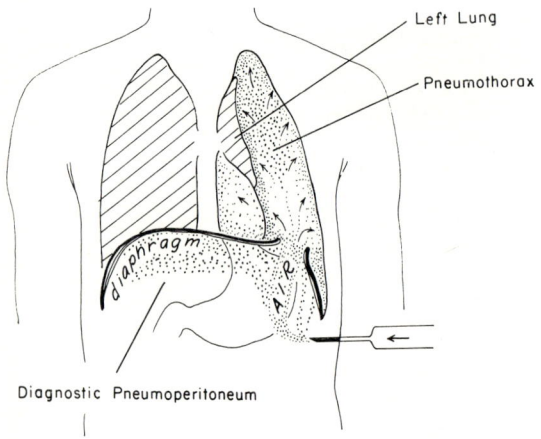

Fig 14-4. Illustration of diagnostic pneumoperitoneum.

incidence of traumatic rupture of the diaphragm since 1952. In our institution recognition of this injury is currently quicker because of a higher index of suspicion [73].

Blunt traumatic rupture of the diaphragm should be recognized at the time the workup is carried out after an accident. However, some diagnoses are delayed for several weeks because of the multiplicity and gravity of the patient's other injuries as well as the lack of definite signs or symptoms alerting one to the possibility of such a rupture. Unfortunately, some cases are not diagnosed until many years after the actual injury, and then are frequently brought to light only because of obstruction to the gastrointestinal tract secondary to herniation of intestinal contents into the chest cavity [3, 4, 8, 18, 20, 28, 47, 62, 86]. In our series of 42, immediate recognition was accomplished in 29, an interval of 4 to 47 days intervened before recognition in 7, and in 5 patients the diagnosis was delayed between 5 months and 12 years (Table 14-1). Diagnosis was made in 1 at postmortem examination.

Recognition of blunt traumatic rupture of the diaphragm hinges on a high index of suspicion. Any patient involved in trauma in whom there is evidence of chest injury should be examined carefully, both physically and by roentgenogram. All of our patients with blunt traumatic rupture of

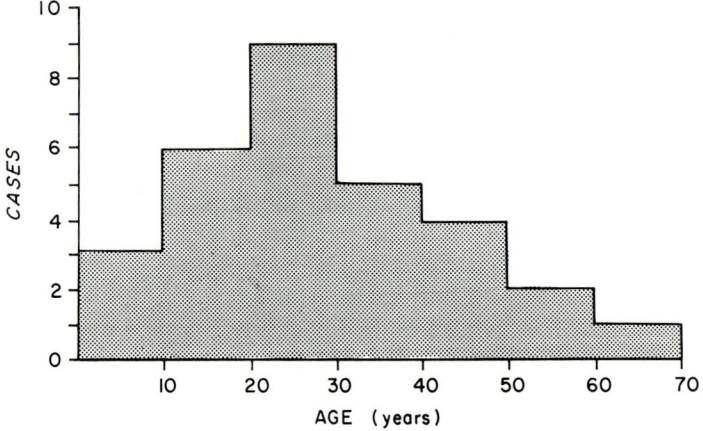

Fig 14-5. Occurrence of blunt traumatic injuries of the diaphragm by age.

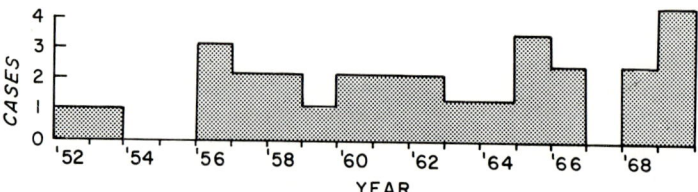

Fig 14-6. Incidence of blunt traumatic injuries of the diaphragm by years (1952–1970).

Table 14-1. Interval Between Injury and Diagnosis
of Blunt Trauma Diaphragmatic Rupture

Immediate recognition	29	
Interval (4–47 days)	7	
Delayed	5	
5 months		1
11 months		1
18 months		1
12 years		2
At postmortem examination		1

the diaphragm also had associated severe injury of multiple systems. Fractured ribs, fracture of long bones, fractured pelvis, head injuries, kidney contusion, and ruptured spleen were present concomitantly in many of our patients. In such circumstances any evidence of an obscured diaphragmatic shadow should lead to further investigation.

Roentgenographic evidence of an atypical pneumothorax [12] or mediastinal shift should arouse suspicion regarding the possibility of ruptured diaphragm. Figure 14-7 shows a large air space in the left lower hemithorax. Differentiation between this as a low trapped pneumothorax or a high gastric bubble under an eventration of the diaphragm is necessary.

Confirmation of the presence of the stomach in the left hemithorax can be obtained by inserting a Levin tube as illustrated in Figures 14-8 and 14-9. An abnormal left hemithorax, air in the left lower chest, and a barium swallow outlining the stomach confirm the presence of the stomach in the area (Fig 14-10). Figure 14-11 shows an abnormal left diaphragmatic contour with intestines in the left hemithorax and displacement of the mediastinum to the right. Barium has not entered the intrathoracic portion of the stomach. Diagnostic pneumoperitoneum has produced pneumothorax, proving a ruptured left diaphragm.

Figure 14-12 shows that intestines are present in the left lower chest through a ruptured diaphragm. There is displacement of the mediastinum toward the right side.

In Figure 14-13 there is a 3-week-old rupture of the right diaphragm, obscured lower right chest, hemothorax, and fractured lower ribs. (A diagnostic pneumoperitoneum with air in the right chest through the ruptured diaphragm still occurs even after this interval after injury.) At opera-

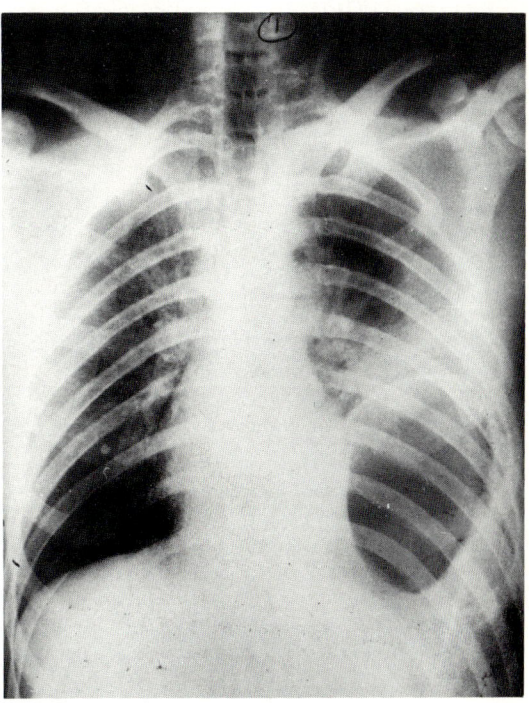

Fig 14-7. Posteroanterior chest roentgenogram showing a gas bubble in stomach that herniated through the ruptured left diaphragm into left hemithorax.

tion in this patient the liver was seen through the ruptured diaphragm (Fig 14-14).

Should one suspect the presence of a ruptured diaphragm, fluoroscopy may reveal other signs strongly suggestive of such rupture. These are: (1) invisibility of the injured dome, (2) intermittent twitching movements in the area of the diaphragm, and (3) changing density with change of position and respiratory movements (Fig 14-15A). Pneumoperitoneum (Fig 14-15B) gives positive diagnosis.

TREATMENT

When traumatic rupture of the diaphragm is evident, operation should be carried out at a time permitted by the patient's general condition [54, 64], since often there will be severe concurrent injuries and these will tend to preclude immediate operation. It is our feeling that there should be no delay if there is (1) uncontrolled blood loss, either in the abdomen or in the thorax; (2) altered cardiopulmonary physiology interfering with

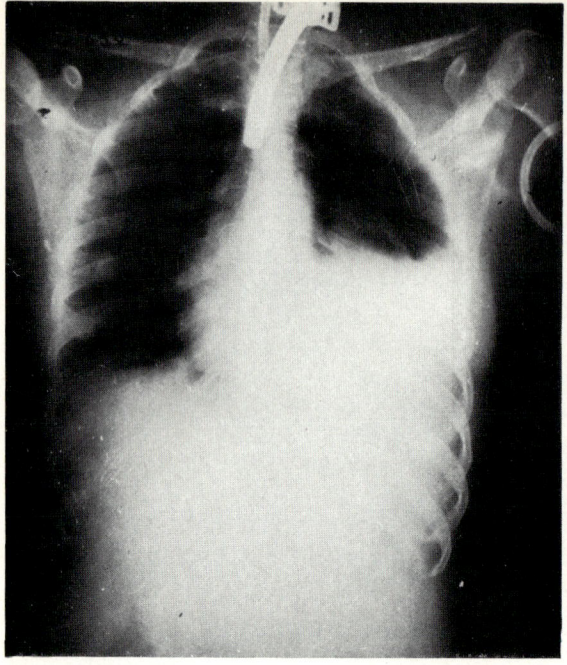

A

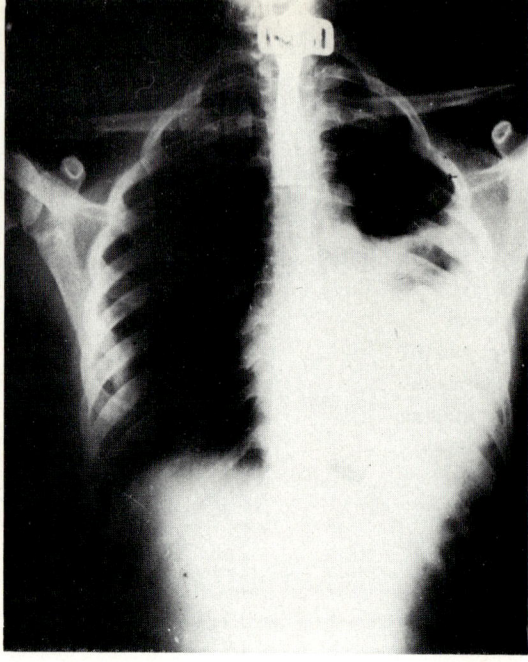

B

Fig 14-8. This patient suffered multiple systems injury. (A) Posteroanterior chest roentgenogram shows obscured left diaphragm, density in the left lower hemithorax, fractured ribs, and mediastinal displace-

ment to right side. (B) Levin tube is seen in the stomach, which is high in the left chest; also seen is an air bubble in stomach.

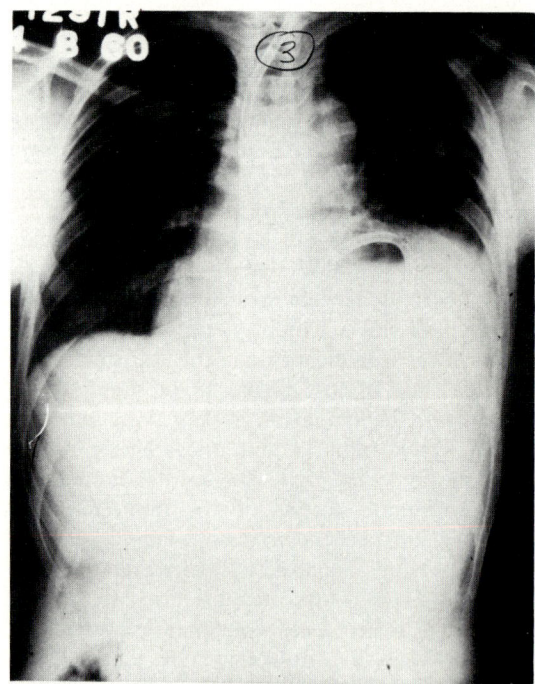

Fig 14-9. This patient suffered acute multiple systems injury. Shown here is an obscured left diaphragm, density in the lower one-third of the left chest, Levin tube deviation toward right side in upper thoracic aorta (ruptured aorta hematoma), and stomach partially decompressed by Levin tube in left hemithorax.

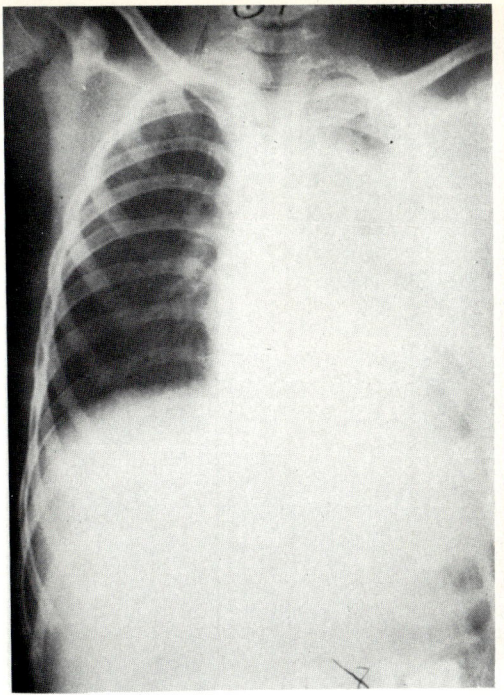

A

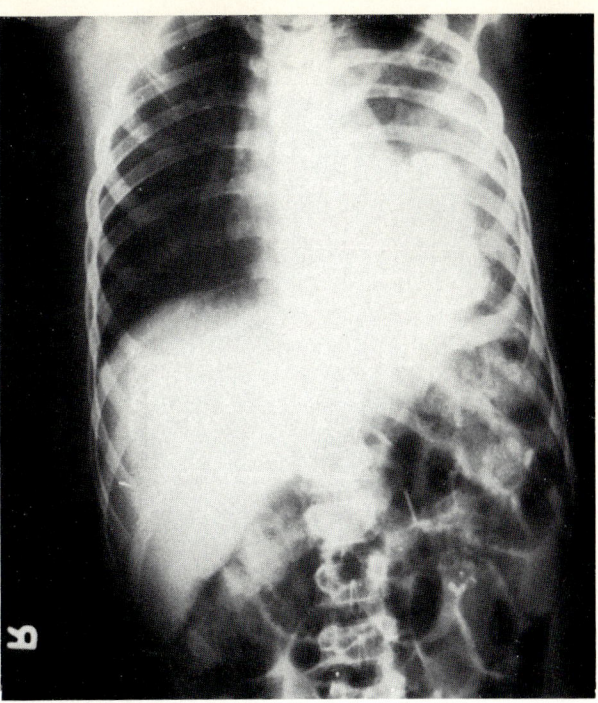

B

Fig 14-10. *Posteroanterior chest roentgenograms show fluid in the left hemithorax and an abnormal pneumothorax on left side. (A) After barium swallow.*

(B) Stomach is outlined by the barium in the left hemithorax adjacent to the cardiac border.

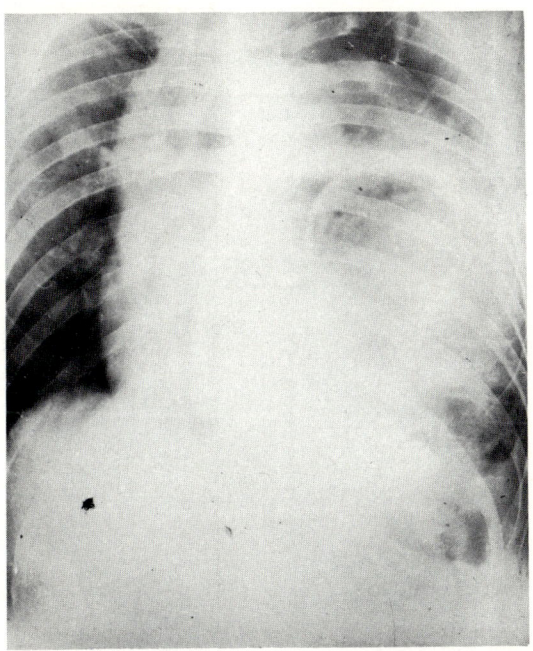

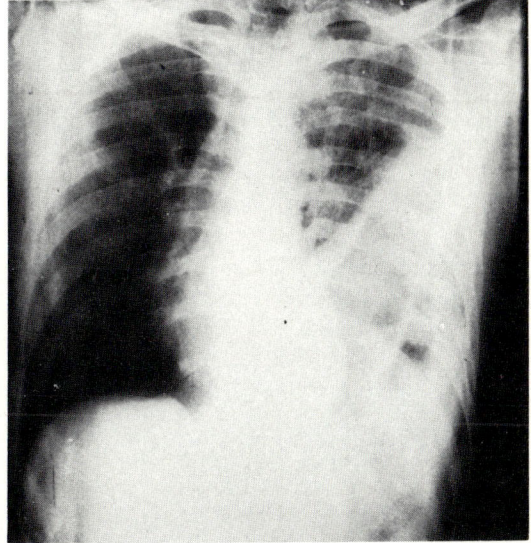

Fig 14-12. *Abnormal left diaphragm shadow with stomach, intestines, traumatic pneumothorax, all on left, displacing mediastinum to the right.*

Fig 14-11. *Posteroanterior chest roentgenogram shows: stomach and intestines in left hemithorax; abnormal or absent left diaphragm shadow; mediastinal shift to contralateral side; barium has not entered intrathoracic portion of stomach; diagnostic pneumoperitoneum produced ipsilateral pneumothorax, proving ruptured left diaphragm.*

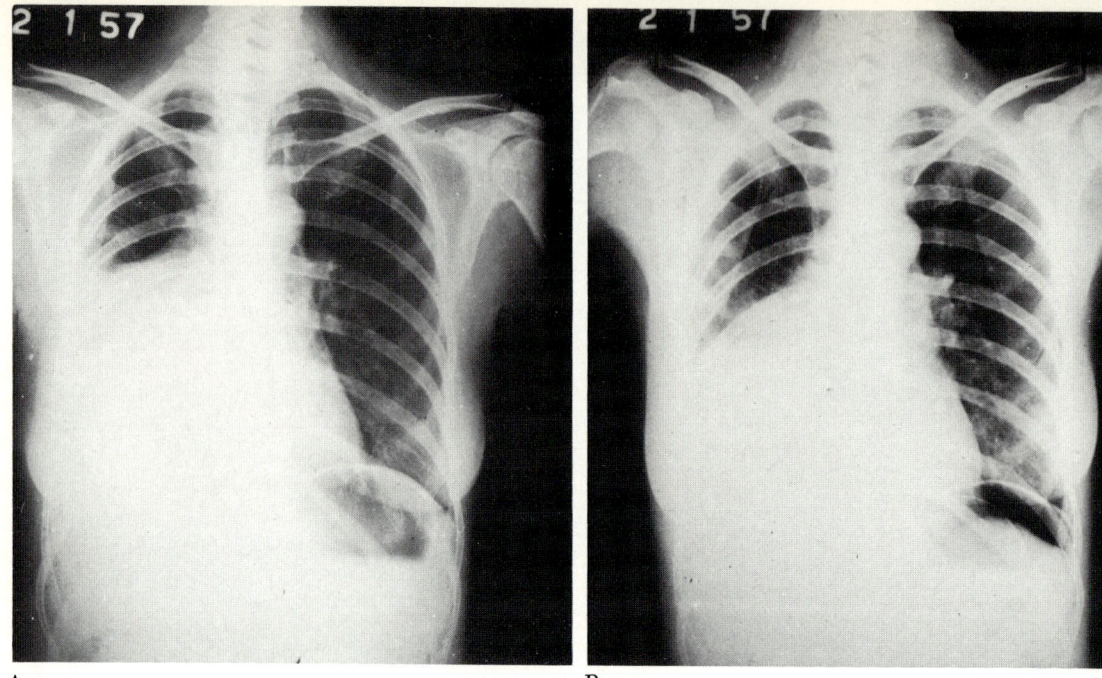

A   B

Fig 14-13. Positive diagnostic pneumoperitoneum 3
weeks after rupture of right diaphragm with liver
pushed into the chest.

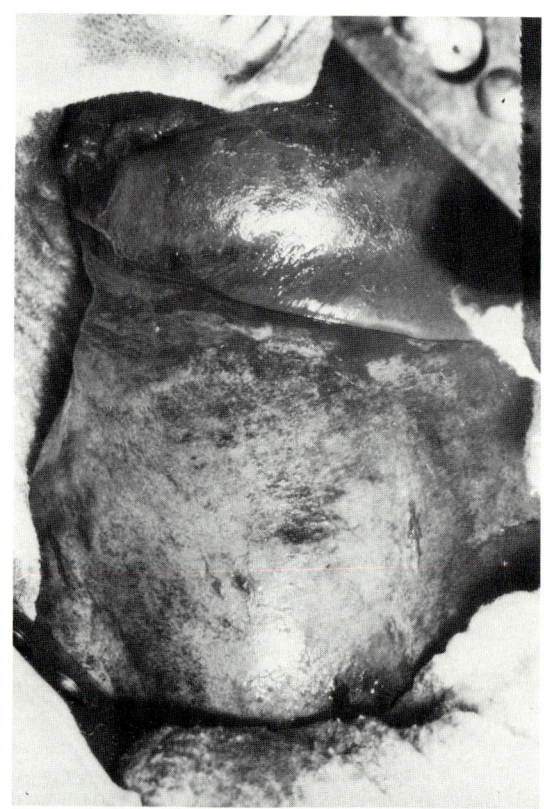

Fig 14-14. Same patient as in Figure 14-13. At operation liver is in the right hemothorax, seen through
the diaphragm.

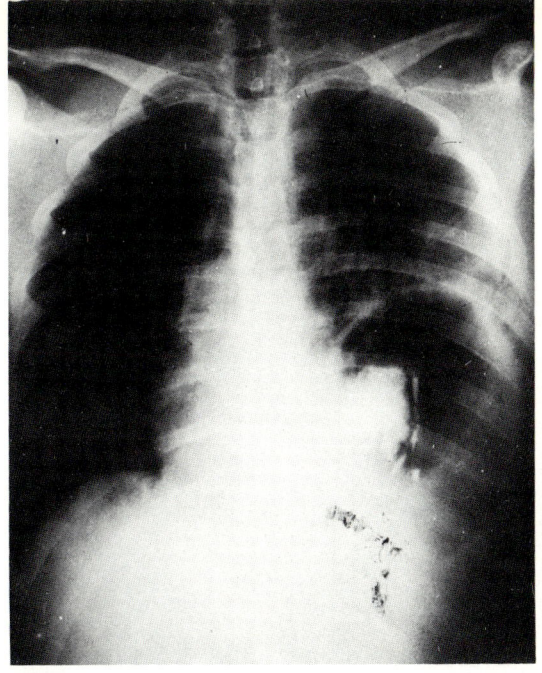

A

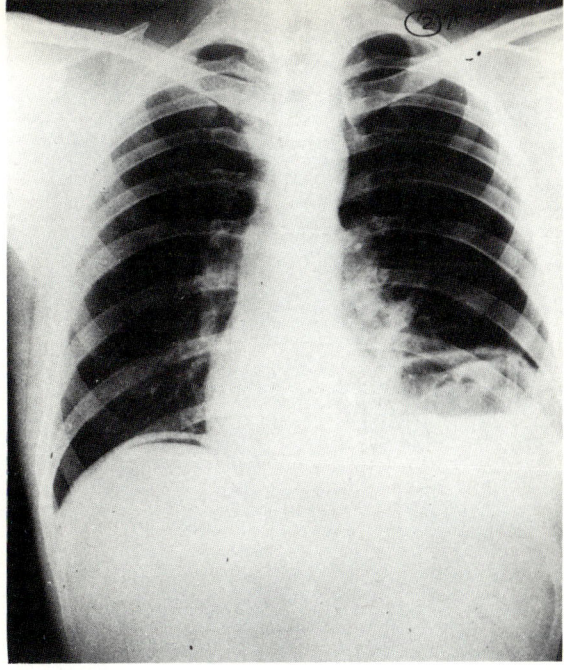

B

Fig 14-15. Ruptured diaphragm. (A) Absent left diaphragm shadow; abnormal left lower hemithorax air density; compressed and/or contused left lung; barium in intrathoracic stomach; mediastinum displaced to right; end fractured ribs. (B) Positive diagnosis on pneumoperitoneum.

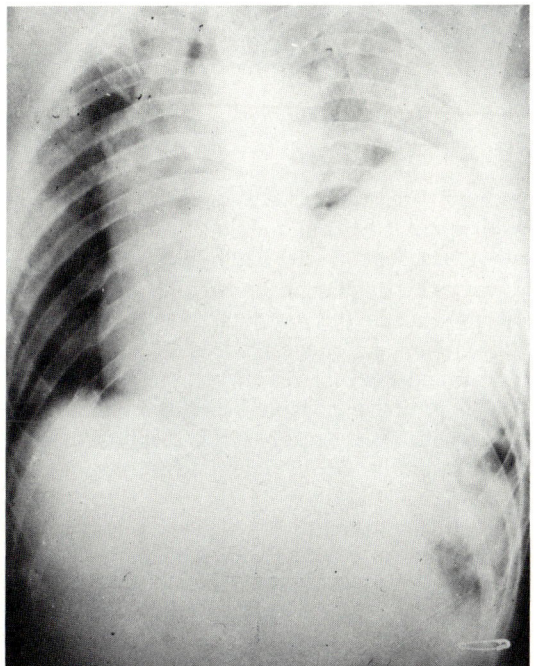

Fig 14-16. Ruptured left hemidiaphragm with marked and rapid deterioration of cardiopulmonary function in an older male giving a history of previous pulmonary and cardiac chronic illness.

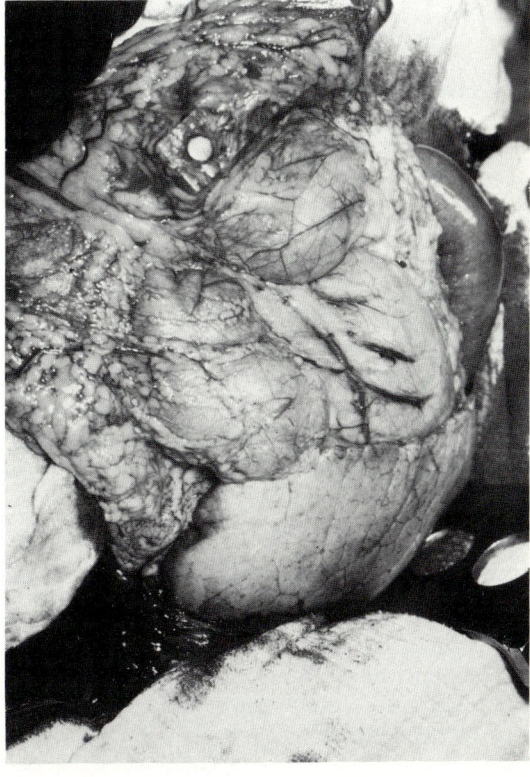

Fig 14-17. Abdominal contents in left hemithorax as seen at time of thoracotomy in 1 of 34 patients with injury to the left diaphragm.

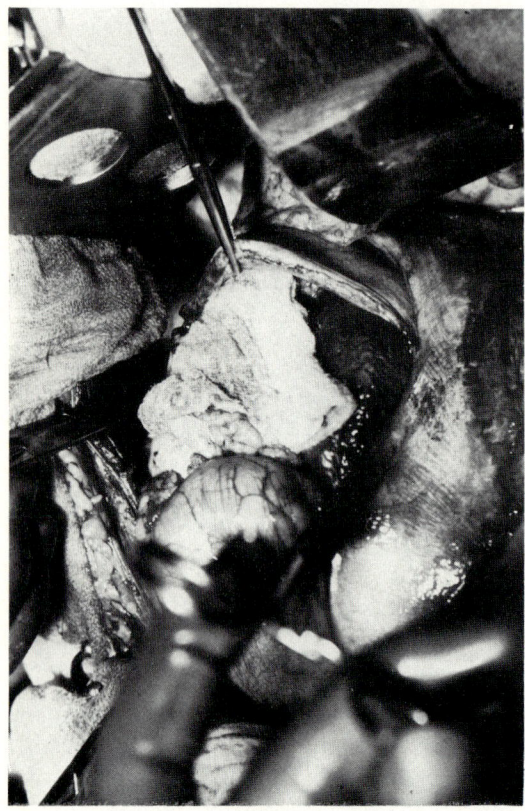

Fig 14-18. Abdominal contents replaced through the ruptured diaphragm. Note clean edges of the diaphragm.

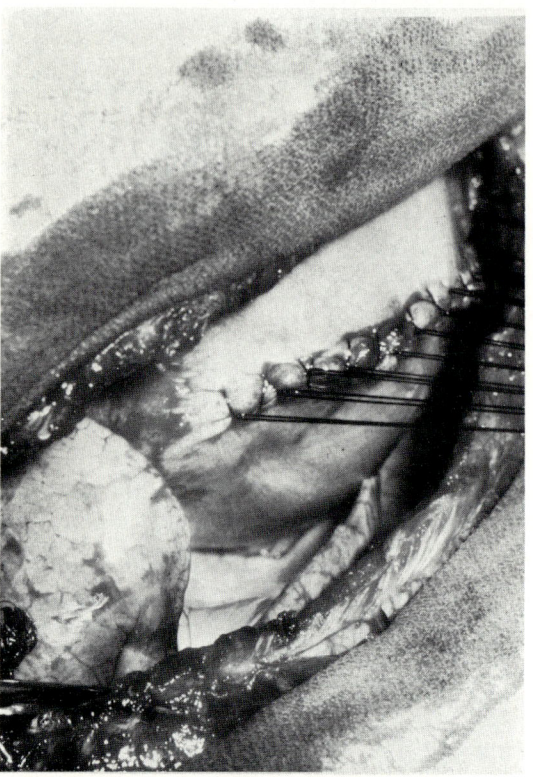

Fig 14-19. Repaired diaphragm.

the patient's survival (Fig 14-16); (3) undiagnosed internal injury of an operative nature; and (4) if there are no contraindications to surgery. The thoracic approach is the one of choice when repairing a traumatic rupture of the diaphragm. The field is best exposed in this fashion and intrathoracic injury corrected. If concurrent abdominal trauma is present, the incision, if need be, can be extended across the costal arch to allow exploration of the abdomen.

In all the patients in our group operative repair was carried out through a thoracotomy incision with transection of the seventh rib posteriorly and entrance into the pleural space through the seventh intercostal space (except the rupture seen in Figure 14-2 that was repaired transabdominally). When the hemithorax was opened, 34 of 38 patients who had injury to the left diaphragm had stomach, colon, omentum, small bowel, and spleen in the left chest (Fig 14-17); in 2 patients, only

omentum and colon were present; 1 had only small bowel (ileum); and in 1 patient only the spleen had herniated through the rupture. In 3 patients with diaphragmatic rupture only the liver was present. In this last case the contents were easily returned to the abdominal cavity (Fig 14-18), and the ruptured diaphragm was repaired with interrupted nonabsorbable sutures without imbrication. The edges of the diaphragm were clean and did not require debridement (Fig 14-19).

In only one patient [85] was it necessary to use an artificial prosthesis (Marlex mesh) to repair the hernia. This was associated with a delayed diagnosis—18 months (Fig 14-20).

In 2 patients the diaphragm was disrupted from the chest wall, requiring resuture with horizontal type sutures based upon diaphragm anchorage to the rib.

A rupture of the diaphragm can involve the pericardium with the large bowel entrapped within the pericardial cavity [7, 15, 25, 42, 59, 70, 74, 77, 87, 89]. This occurred in 1 of our patients.

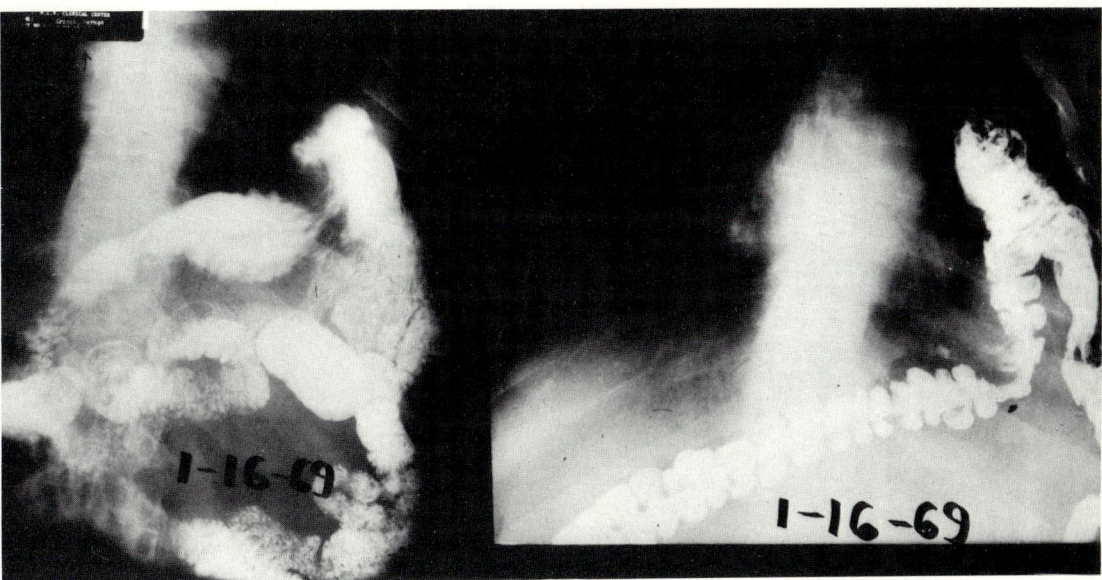

A

Fig 14-20. (A) Barium swallow and enema showing
stomach and small and large bowel in left hemithorax 18 months after previously undiagnosed traumatic rupture of the left diaphragm. (B) Repair
necessitated Marlex mesh to complete closure of the
anterior chest wall disruption site.

He was admitted to the hospital with intestinal
obstruction 3 months after his injury. Reduction
of the colon into the abdominal cavity with repair
of the diaphragm and pericardium resulted in cure
(Fig 14-21).

The patient shown in Figure 14-22 had traumatic rupture of the left diaphragm and cerebral
injury so severe that it was believed she would not
recover. Accordingly, after the diagnosis was made
by barium swallow, decompression of the intestinal tract was carried out by insertion of a Levin
tube. Within 7 days, bowel sounds returned to
normal and she was fed through the tube for a
period of 3 months. At that time, she had made a
total recovery from her central nervous system injury and repair of the damaged left diaphragm
was carried out.

One of our patients sustained in an automobile
accident fractured ribs on the left side together
with a left hemopneumothorax (Fig 14-23). Tubes
were inserted into the left chest on two occasions
before the hemopneumothorax resolved [60]. No
other injury was diagnosed. Two years later, when

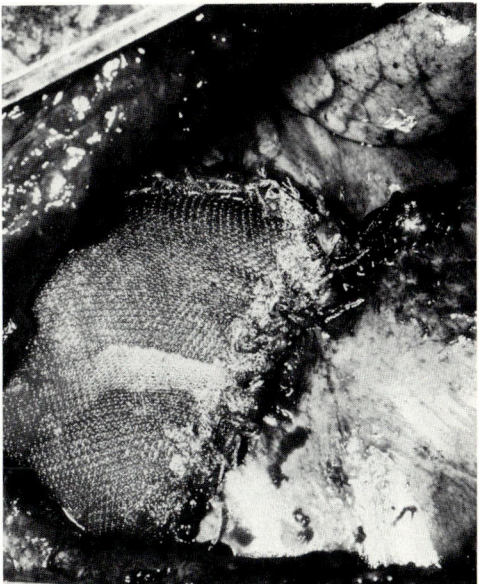

B

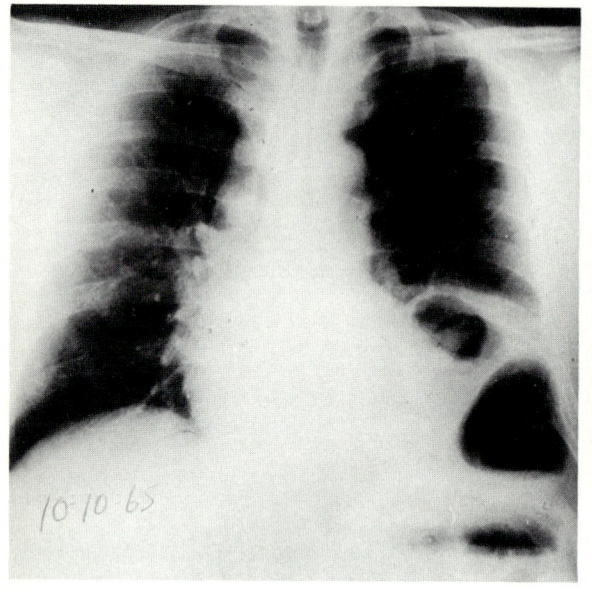
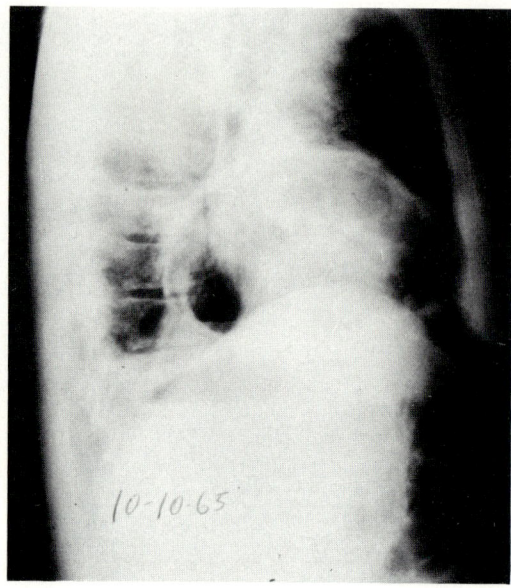

A

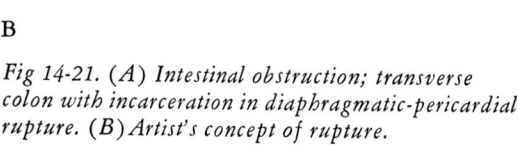

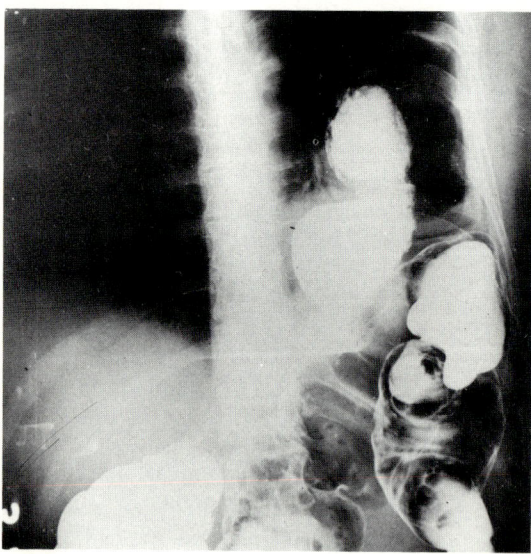

B

Fig 14-21. (A) Intestinal obstruction; transverse colon with incarceration in diaphragmatic-pericardial rupture. (B) Artist's concept of rupture.

Fig 14-22. Traumatic rupture of the left diaphragm with stomach and small bowel in the left chest. Patient was fed by nasogastric tube for 3 months due to severe central nervous system (CNS) injury. Diaphragm was repaired after recovery from CNS injury.

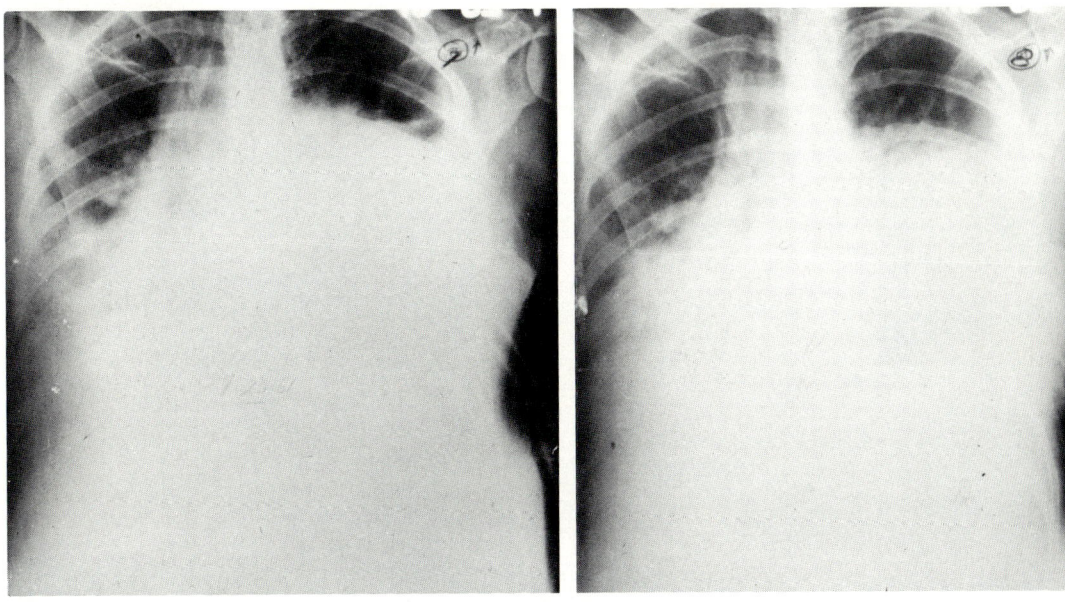

A

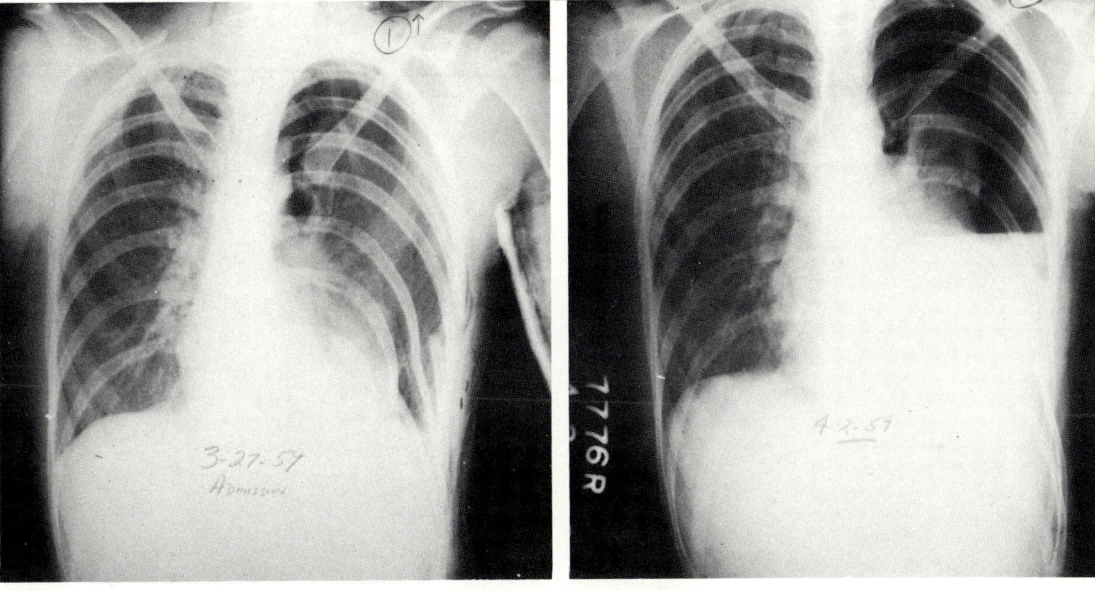

B

Fig 14-23. (A) Traumatic fractured ribs on the left side and hemopneumothorax treated by tube insertion. Patient was discharged. (B) Two years later and 8 months pregnant the patient was admitted with a strangulated, gangrenous stomach herniated through the previously ruptured left diaphragm. Correction was successful, but patient died 2 weeks later when tracheostomy eroded into the innominate artery.

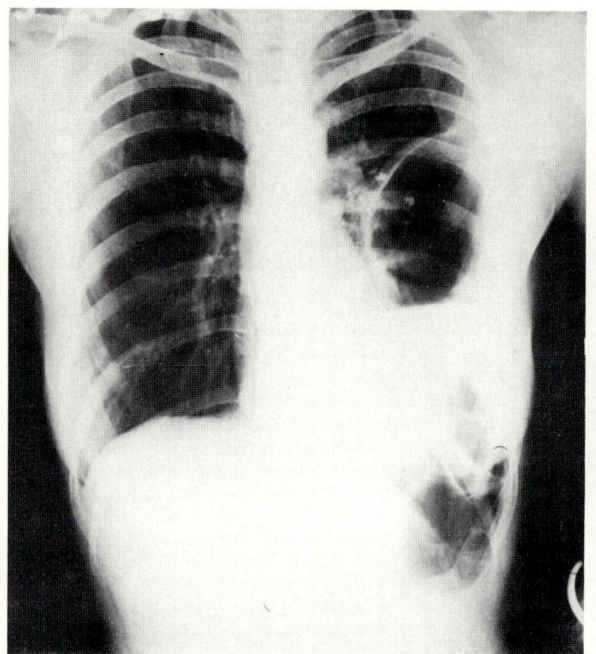 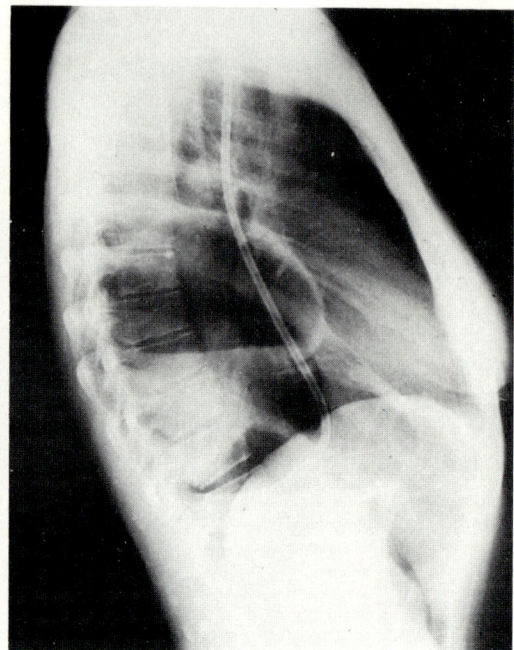

Fig 14-24. Chest roentgenogram shows herniation of stomach and small bowel into the left chest through disruption of diaphragm closure after a thoracoabdominal incision for splenorenal venous shunt.

Signs of intestinal obstruction brought the patient back to the hospital; operative correction was required.

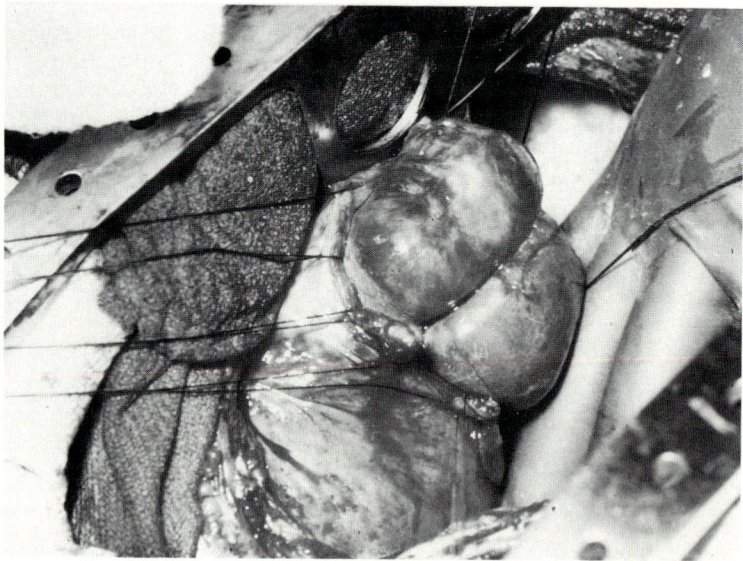

Fig 14-25. Operative photograph of disrupted right diaphragm with liver herniation. Disruption followed previous thoracoabdominal incision for portacaval venous shunt.

eight months pregnant, she was admitted with gangrene of two-thirds of her stomach that had herniated through a ruptured left diaphragm into the left hemithorax. Correction was successful, but death occurred 2 weeks after operation from tracheostomy erosion into the innominate artery and sudden exsanguination.

POSTOPERATIVE DIAPHRAGMATIC HERNIA

Following operative procedures involving incisions through the diaphragm with subsequent suture repair, disruption of the suture line in the diaphragm can occur with herniation of intestinal contents through this defect. Operative repair is indicated. Figures 14-24 and 14-25 illustrate such problems.

EROSION OF DIAPHRAGM FROM INFECTION

Although we have not seen disruption of the diaphragm from infection, suspicion of such an occurrence must be kept constantly in mind when infection involves the diaphragm. Establishment of the diagnosis of perforation from infection will follow the same lines as outlined for diagnosis of perforation from trauma.

REFERENCES

1. Alivistos CN, Bonnellos CH, Aulamis GP, et al: Traumatic closed rupture of the diaphragm. Dis Chest 46:435, 1964
2. Arbulie A, Read RC, Berkas EM: Delayed symptomatology in traumatic diaphragmatic hernia with a note on eventration. Dis Chest 47:527, 1965
3. Aries LJ, Hobbins W: Traumatic diaphragmatic hernia with obstruction of the bowel. Q Bull Northwestern Med School 27:6, 1953
4. Arndt JH, Healy MJ, Schonfeld MD: Strangulated Richter's hernia of the stomach. Am J Roentgenol 91:766, 1964
5. Asbury GR: Rupture of the diaphragm from blunt trauma. Arch Surg 97:801, 1968
6. Bailes PM: Traumatic diaphragmatic hernia. Dallas Med J 40:97, 1958
7. Beddingfield GW: Cardiac tamponade due to traumatic hernia of the diaphragm and pericardium. Ann Surg 6:178, 1968
8. Bernardo AA, Marcus WY, Shackelford RI: Incarcerated traumatic diaphragmatic hernia. Arch Surg 83:650, 1961
9. Bernatz P, Burnside AT Jr, Clagett OT: Problems of the ruptured diaphragm. JAMA 168:877, 1958
10. Bjork VO, Hedenstadt S, Nordlund S: Traumatic right diaphragmatic hernia with dislocation of the liver into the right thorax. Acta Chir Scand 128:761, 1964
11. Blades B: Ruptured diaphragm. Am J Surg 105:501, 1963
12. Bosher LH Jr, Tishman L, Webb WR, et al: Strangulated diaphragmatic hernia with gangrene and perforation of the stomach. Dis Chest 37:504, 1960
13. Bowditch H: Diaphragmatic hernia. Buffalo Med J 9:1, 9:65, 1953
14. Boyd DP: The hazards of the counter-incision in the diaphragm in transthoracic repair of hiatus hernia. Lahey Clinic Found Bull 10:109, 1959
15. Brookes US: Intrapericardial diaphragmatic hernia. Br J Surg 40:511, 1953
16. Bugden WT, Chu PT, Delmonico JE: Traumatic diaphragmatic hernia. Ann Surg 142:851, 1955
17. Carlson RI, Diveley WL, Gobbel WG, et al: Dehiscence of the diaphragm associated with fractures of the pelvis or lumbar spine due to nonpenetrating wounds of the chest and abdomen. J Thorac Surg 36:254, 1958
18. Carter BN, Guiseffi J: Strangulated diaphragmatic hernia. Ann Surg 128:210, 1948
19. Carter NB, Guiseffi J, Telson B: Traumatic diaphragmatic hernia. Am J Roentgenol 65:56, 1951
20. Carter R, Brewer LA: Strangulating diaphragmatic hernia. Ann Thorac Surg 12:281, 1971
21. Childress ME, Grimes OT: Immediate and remote sequelae in traumatic diaphragmatic hernias. Surg Gynecol Obstet 113:573, 1961
22. Clay RC, Hanlon CR: Pneumoperitoneum in the differential diagnosis of diaphragmatic hernia. J Thorac Cardiovasc Surg 21:57, 1951
23. Cooley JC, Rogers JCT: Traumatic diaphragmatic hernia. Arch Surg 79:551, 1959
24. Coppinger WR: Rupture of the diaphragm following repair of hiatal hernia. Arch Surg 80:998, 1960
25. Cranshaw GR: Herniation of the stomach, transverse colon, and portion of the jejunum into the pericardium. Br J Surg 39:364, 1962
26. Desforges G, Strieder JW, Lynch JP, et al: Traumatic rupture of the diaphragm. J Thorac Surg 39:779, 1957
27. Drews JA, Mercer EC, Benfield JR: Acute diaphragmatic injuries. Ann Thorac Surg 16:67, 1973

28 Dugan DJ, Samson PC: Strangulation of the stomach and traumatic diaphragmatic hernia. J Thorac Cardiovasc Surg 17:771, 1948

29. Ebert PA, Gaertner RA, Zuidema GD: Traumatic diaphragmatic hernia. Surg Gynecol Obstet 125:59, 1967

30. Effler DB: Allison's repair of hiatal hernia: Late complication of diaphragmatic counter-incision and technique to avoid it. J Thorac Cardiovasc Surg 49:669, 1965

31. Efron G, Hyde I: Non-penetration traumatic rupture of the diaphragm. Clin Radiol 18:394, 1967

32. El Galaini TI: Traumatic diaphragmatic hernia. Br J Clin Pract 20:646, 1966

33. Firestone TM, Taybi H: Bilateral diaphragmatic eventration: Demonstration by pneumoperitoneography. Surgery 62:954, 1967

34. Gerard TP, Sabety AM: Traumatic ruptured diaphragms: Report of a case. Dis Chest 47:340, 1965

35. Gravier L, Treeark RJ: Traumatic diaphragmatic hernia. Arch Surg 86:363, 1963

36. Graze TB, MacLean LD, Campbell GS: Traumatic rupture of the diaphragm: A report of 26 cases. Surgery 46:669, 1959

37. Griffin JA, Pisani JJ, Sheridan P, et al: Traumatic diaphragmatic hernia due to stab wound of the chest. Ill Med J 110:22, 1956

38. Griswold FW, Warden HE, Gardner RJ: Acute diaphragmatic rupture by blunt trauma. Am J Surg 124:359, 1972

39. Gupta RL: Traumatic diaphragmatic hernia due to stab wound of chest. Br Dis Chest 55:159, 1961

40. Hardy KJ: Traumatic rupture of the diaphragm: Report of two cases. Aust NZ J Surg 34:314, 1965

41. Hedblom CA: Diaphragmatic hernia. JAMA 85:947, 1925

42. Herman PG, Goldstein JE: Traumatic intrapericardial diaphragmatic hernia. Br J Radiol 38:631, 1965

43. Hill GC: Some unusual cases of traumatic diaphragmatic hernia. J Natl Med Assoc 56:401, 1964

44. Hill GC: Right-sided traumatic diaphragmatic hernia in paraplegia. Ohio Med J 60:1471, 1963

45. Hofferman M, Breckler IA: Traumatic diaphragmatic hernia; A case simulating phrenic nerve avulsion. Calif Med 86:185, 1957

46. Hollander AG, Dugan DJ: Herniation of the liver. J Thorac Cardiovasc Surg 29:357, 1955

47. Holloway JB: Traumatic diaphragmatic hernia with intestinal obstruction. J Ky Med Assoc 51:62, 1953

48. Hood R: Traumatic diaphragmatic hernia. Ann Thorac Surg 12:311, 1971

49. Hughes T, Kay EB, Meade RH Jr, et al: Traumatic diaphragmatic hernia. J Thorac Surg 17:99, 1948

50. Jallah EM, Trater RWM, Freeman LM: Tension hepatothorax diagnosed by rapid scintiphotography. J Thorac Cardiovasc Surg 59:283, 1970

51. Keats TE: Traumatic trans-diaphragmatic herniation of stomach. Mo Med J 57:444, 1960

52. Kerr H: Closed traumatic rupture of the diaphragm. Br J Surg 50:891, 1963

53. Knight CD, McCook WW: Traumatic diaphragmatic hernia. Am Surg 26:656, 1960

54. Lam CR: Treatment of traumatic hernia of the diaphragm. Arch Surg 60:421, 1950

55. Loitman BS, Hoover WB, Miscall L, et al: Postoperative diaphragmatic hernia: A complication of hiatus hernia repair. Am J Roentgenol 65:56, 1967

56. Lucido JL, Wall CA: Rupture of the diaphragm due to blunt trauma. Arch Surg 86:989, 1963

57. MacLean LD: Traumatic rupture of the diaphragm. Postgrad Med 29:383, 1961

58. Miller JD, Howie PD: Traumatic rupture of the diaphragm after blunt injury. Br J Surg 55:423, 1968

59. Moore TC: Traumatic pericardial diaphragmatic hernia. Arch Surg 79:827, 1959

60. Moos DJ: Traumatic diaphragmatic hernia with strangulation and gangrene of stomach. Minn Med 39:795, 1956

61. Myers MA: Traumatic rupture of the diaphragm in children. Aust NZ J Surg 34:123, 1964

62. Nelson JB Jr, Ziperman HH, Christensen NM, et al: Diaphragmatic injuries and post-traumatic hernia. J Trauma 2:36, 1963

63. Nevins IN: Spontaneous reduction of an incarcerated acute diaphragmatic hernia. JAMA 185:671, 1963

64. Noon GP, Beal AC, DeBakey ME: Surgical management of traumatic rupture of the diaphragm. J Trauma 6:344, 1966

65. Peck WA: Right-sided diaphragmatic liver hernia following trauma. Am J Roentgenol 78:99, 1957

66. Perry T Jr, Francis WW, Lonergan JC: Traumatic diaphragmatic hernia. Arch Surg 75:763, 1957

67. Pomerantz M, Rodgers BM, Sabiston DC Jr: Traumatic diaphragmatic hernia. Surgery 64:529, 1968

68. Pomerantz RM, Twigg HL: Intrathoracic omental herniation. J Thorac Cardiovasc Surg 52:735, 1966

69. Probert WR, Harvard C: Traumatic diaphragmatic hernia. Thorax 16:99, 1961

70. Rabb D: Traumatic diaphragmatic hernia into the pericardium. Br J Surg 50:664, 1963

71. Sanford MC, Stafford ES: Diaphragmatic hernia caused by trauma; diagnosis and treatment. Postgrad Med 19:60, 1956

72. Schneider CT: Traumatic diaphragmatic hernia. Am J Surg 91:290, 1956

73. Schwindt WD, Gale JW: Late recognition and treatment of traumatic diaphragmatic hernia. Arch Surg 94:330, 1967

74. Smith L, Lippert KM: Peritoneo-pericardial diaphragmatic hernia. Ann Surg 148:798, 1958

75. Solomon J, Teller N, Levy MJ: A case of spontaneous rupture of the diaghragm. J Thorac Cardiovasc Surg 58:221, 1969

76. Spann JL, Chingan TA: Traumatic diaphragmatic hernia. J Okla State Med Assoc 58:316, 1965

77. Stein J, Colmore HD, Green RA: Diaphragmatic pericardial tear with intrapericardial herniation of the transverse colon. Radiology 60:417, 1953

78. Sterns LP, Schmidt WR, Jenson NK: Traumatic rupture of the right leaf of the diaphragm. Dis Chest 51:205, 1961

79. Stevens GM, McCort JJ: Abdominal pneumo-peritoneography. Radiology 83:480, 1964

80. Stone AM, Pearson WT, Lansdown FS, et al: Spontaneous rupture of the right diaphragm. Ann Thorac Surg 9:479, 1970

81. Strug B, Noon GP, Beall AC Jr: Traumatic diaphragmatic hernia. Ann Thorac Surg 17:444, 1974

82. Sullivan RE: Strangulation and obstruction in diaphragmatic hernia due to direct trauma: Report of two cases and review of the English literature. J Thorac Cardiovasc Surg 52:725, 1966

83. Sutton JP, Carlisle RB, Stephenson SE Jr: Traumatic diaphragmatic hernia: A review of 25 cases. Ann Thorac Surg 3:136, 1967

84. Thomas V: Congenital eventration of the diaphragm. Ann Surg 10:181, 1970

85. Waldhausen JA, Kilman JW, Helman CH, et al: The diagnosis and management of traumatic injuries of the diaphragm including the use of Marlex prosthesis. J Trauma 6:332, 1966

86. Walker EW: Strangulated hernia through traumatic rupture of the diaphragm; laparotomy; recovery. Int Surg 23:257, 1900

87. Wetrich M, Sawyers TM, Hough GA: Diaphragmatic rupture with pericardial involvement. Ann Thorac Surg 8:361, 1969

88. Wood NE, Stutzman TL: Right diaphragmatic hernia secondary to trauma. Calif Med 91:251, 1959

89. Wren HB, Chapman WS, Pearce CW: Traumatic diaphragmatic intrapericardial hernia. South Med J 56:1043, 1963

90. Wren HB, Tehada PJ, Krementz ET: Traumatic rupture of the diaphragm. J Trauma 2:117, 1962

15. TRAUMA TO THE MEDIASTINUM

DeWitt C. Daughtry
Luiz C. Kuntz
James DeWitt Daughtry

The mediastinum contains such vital organs as the heart, major blood vessels, esophagus, tracheobronchial tree, the thoracic duct, and the vagus and sympathetic nerve trunks. Major injuries to mediastinal structures can occur from blunt or penetrating trauma to the chest, sometimes with minimal evidence of external trauma. Children have a very elastic rib cage, and thus blunt trauma with serious consequences can result from seemingly minor injuries.

During and immediately following the early appraisal in the emergency treatment facility the attending physician must determine the extent of injury. This requires careful evaluation of all the evidence available, which includes previous history; the mechanism of trauma; the external signs of injury; the possible pathways of projectiles or other penetrating forces; and pertinent physical, roentgenographic, and electrocardiographic findings, and others as required in order to determine the extent of mediastinal injury, if any.

Related injuries that can arouse suspicion of mediastinal injury include blunt trauma to or fracture of the sternum, particularly by a steering wheel; fracture of a thoracic vertebra or the first rib; and gunshot wounds or knife and other wounds in which the injuring instrument probably entered or traversed the mediastinum. Differences in the arterial pulses or blood pressures of the extremities are significant. A "crunching" sound heard at auscultation that is synchronous with the respiratory cycle or heartbeat is strong evidence of trauma to the aorta or air-containing structures such as the trachea, bronchi, and esophagus. Severe interscapular pain is a common complaint in aortic rupture. Acute dysphagia is highly suggestive of esophageal trauma. Severe coughing synchronous with or immediately after swallowing suggests tracheoesophageal fistula. Soreness in the neck, pain on manipulation of the larynx, and slight to moderate subcutaneous emphysema confined to the neck provide further confirmatory evidence of a tear or perforation of the upper esophagus. Marked subcutaneous emphysema in the neck, upper thoracic cage, and shoulders, with or without acute airway obstructions suggests injury to the major airways.

Localized hematoma or generalized enlargement of the mediastinal shadow on roentgenogram suggests significant vascular trauma. Free air in the mediastinum or pericardial sac and unusual prominence or displacement of mediastinal structures on roentgenogram indicate the need for additional studies to differentiate and define the thoracic lesion. A normal initial chest film does not exclude injury to the mediastinum. Repeat or serial films are often necessary in order to detect changes that may not become evident until hours or days later. An initial electrocardiogram and blood enzyme measurements followed by serial determinations are necessary for proper cardiac evaluation in these patients. Once a reasonable degree of suspicion of mediastinal injury exists, additional studies such as an aortogram, a venogram, an esophagogram, and an esophagoscopy or bronchoscopy, or both, may be deemed necessary, depending upon initial and subsequent changes.

Patients with penetrating wounds of the mediastinum require especially careful initial studies and subsequent monitoring. In our experience only about 10 percent of those with penetrating injuries to the mediastinum have required operative exploration, whereas operation has been performed in about 25 percent of those in whom a projectile has transversed the mediastinum.

Individuals who still have an object embedded in the mediastinum, especially in the area of the heart or great vessels, should not have it removed in the emergency room but should await transfer to the operating room. Here the wound can be explored and the object removed under direct vision; major hemorrhage may ensue otherwise (Fig 15-1). We have managed objects on which a patient has been impaled in the same manner.

Detailed discussions of the common injuries to the mediastinum are found in Chapters 7 and 9 through 12.

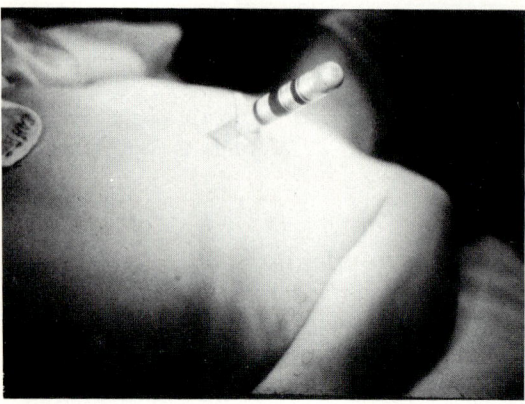

Fig 15-1. Hunting knife embedded into the precordium of the left thorax. The blade would oscillate 1 inch with each heartbeat; the apex of the heart rested on the knife blade. The heart and other mediastinal structures were not injured. The knife was removed under direct vision by thoracotomy.

INJURIES TO THE SUPERIOR VENA CAVA

Its moderately protected location and low intraluminal pressure make the superior vena cava less likely to sustain major injury. Most injuries to the superior vena cava are penetrating in type, though rupture or contusion may occasionally be produced by blunt trauma. Most major vena caval injuries result in severe hemorrhage and the person does not reach the hospital alive. Those who do arrive alive are usually in shock from hemorrhage and require immediate operation. Also a contributing factor in the higher mortality is the association of other major injuries. Ochsner, Crawford, and De-Bakey [8] reported that only 45 percent of 85 patients with vena caval injuries reached the hospital alive and in most of those that could be saved the injuries were of the inferior vena cava. Saha, Goff, and Stephenson [13] reported a mortality of 25 percent in their management of 16 patients with injury to the inferior vena cava, 14 of whom had gunshot type injuries; most also had other major associated injuries. The common factor determining mortality was the amount of blood lost. Statistics could be improved by the use of autotransfusion immediately prior to and during the operative repair.

Damage to the superior vena cava can be suspected when an accident victim develops a right hemothorax from a penetrating injury when there is no other obvious source of the bleeding. The initial treatment for these consists of closed thoracoscopy decompression of the hemothorax. Emergency exploration is indicated for those in shock from blood loss or in whom the bleeding is massive or continuous from the outset. Continuous monitoring of the thoracostomy drainage tube output and repeat roentgenograms of the chest are mandatory. When the diagnosis is in doubt, a venogram, performed through an arm vein, will usually confirm the diagnosis.

Steering wheel or other blunt trauma to the mid- or upper chest may be followed by thrombosis of the superior vena cava. Injury and subsequent propagation thrombosis of the jugular, subclavian [9], and innominate veins may also produce vena caval obstruction. It is surprising that thrombosis can occur from a seemingly minor force, although it does usually require a heavy blow to initiate major thrombosis without evidence of rib or sternal fractures. The rib cage is more resilient in the young, and they are thus more vulnerable to traumatic thrombosis of the superior vena cava without multiple fractures of the rib cage.

Chronic or permanent superior vena caval thrombosis is usually severely incapacitating and is produced by severe contusion of the vena cava or its major tributaries. Thrombosis may extend or propagate in either direction. If there are extensive open collaterals through the azygos and hemiazygos systems, adequate return of venous blood from the upper half of the body may be present and thus severe consequences may not follow. Those people with a major thrombosis of the superior vena cava without adequate venous collateral may not be able to stoop or perform certain types of occupations because of the symptoms produced by the resulting high venous pressure in the upper half of the body, particularly the brain. These patients often have a headache, dizziness, visual disturbances, syncope, and a feeling of tightness or fullness in the head and neck, all due to the venous hypertension and the resulting cerebral congestion. Symptoms are greatly aggravated by exercise, lifting, or stooping. Cyanosis and edema of the conjunctiva and of the upper half of the body are common. Thrombosis of the superior vena cava should be suspected when the neck veins become distended and large superficial veins are seen in the neck, shoulders, chest, and midtrunk areas. Infrared photography (Fig 15-2A) will often show the collateral venous network bet-

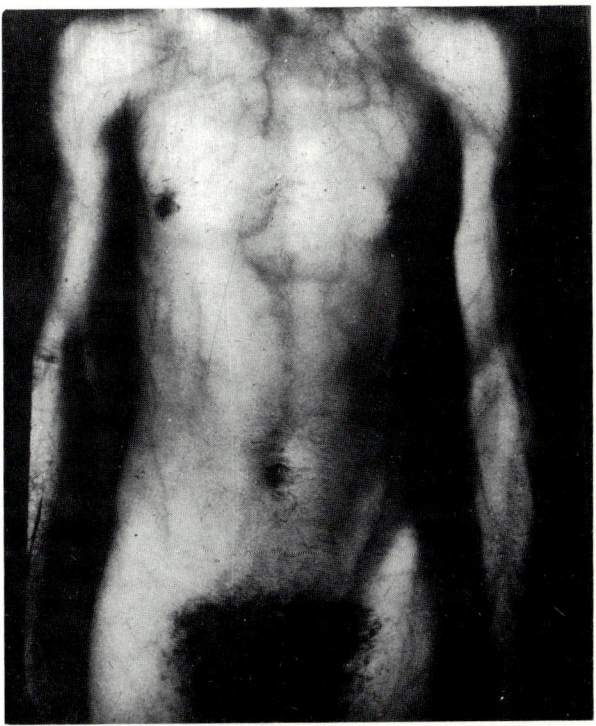

A

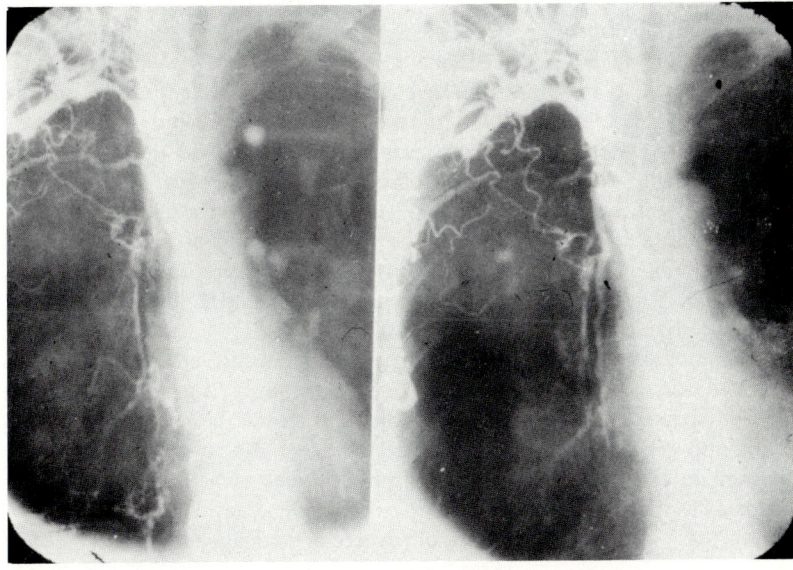

B

Fig 15-2 (A) Infrared photograph shows collateral veins over the thorax, arms, and trunk due to traumatic chronic thrombosis of the superior vena cava. (B) A venous angiogram of an incapacitating superior vena caval thrombosis of 15 years' duration produced by an apparently mild injury to the thorax (sternum) when the patient was young.

ter than can be seen by ordinary inspection of the patient. A venous angiogram (Fig 15-2B) proves the diagnosis and delineates the extent of the obstruction, but additional studies—including tomograms of the chest and mediastinum, an esophagogram, bronchoscopy, and other studies—may be necessary to rule out other causes of superior vena caval obstruction.

In many cases mediastinal exploration may be indicated to establish the etiology, thus eliminating a diagnosis of tumor, fibrosing mediastinitis, and other mechanisms that might require specific treatment. Definitive management by bypass or replacement of the vena cava with vein and prosthetic grafts [4, 7] have often been unsuccessful because of thrombosis and fibrosis, the latter being most extensive at the atrial suture line [5]. If the process is incapacitating, correction may be attempted, but it should be realized that the success rate is not high. Autogenous composite cephalic or saphenous veins opened and sutured to the appropriate size in a spiral manner is the preferred type of graft [2] or bypass conduit to use and seems to increase the long-term patency rate. If grafting is indicated and the grafts do not remain patent, anticoagulant therapy should be given to prevent extension of the thrombotic process. Patients who are treatment failures should be instructed to avoid stooping, lifting, and hard manual labor, all of which further increase the already markedly elevated venous pressure, and they should be rehabilitated to other less demanding occupations. At the outset conservative therapy with anticoagulants is suggested. In many patients the condition subsides in a few weeks to a few months by either recannulization or by the development of adequate collateral venous return.

An extensive review of the literature by Allansmith and Richards [1] found that most cases of vena caval obstruction were associated with a malignancy in the mediastinum. A small percentage, however, were due to mediastinitis and other benign processes, and so it is important to establish the exact etiology of superior mediastinal obstruction prior to making a decision as to the course of management.

TRAUMATIC ASPHYXIA

Traumatic asphyxia is somewhat a nonspecific pathological process and is known by many names, a few of which are:

1. Perthe's syndrome
2. Mediastinal compression syndrome
3. Stasis cyanosis
4. Traumatic vena caval syndrome
5. Thoracic compression syndrome (ecchymotic masque ecchymotique)

Shamblin and McGoon [14] and Fred and Chandler [3] have described the syndrome as being caused by a crushing injury to the thorax and characterized by varying degrees of reddish cyanosis, proceeding to purplish black discoloration of the skin over the upper half of the body, including red discoloration of the conjunctivae (suffusion). We have observed exophthalmos and varying degrees of neck vein distention. The crushing or squeezing type force that causes this syndrome often produces fracture of the ribs, sternum, and spine, and occasionally produces subcutaneous emphysema.

Ollivier [10] first noted the condition in 1837, but it was not until 1900 that Perthe [12] provided a complete clinical description. The syndrome is unforgettable once it has been seen. In our experience, these patients are usually apprehensive at the outset. Mild mental confusion is often present, but this disappears rapidly. There is a gradual clearing of the discoloration of the upper half of the body over a period of 2 to 3 weeks. It is theorized that the marked compression of the column of blood in the heart and central veins produces such a high pressure in the venous system that there is suffusion of blood through the wall of the vessels into the tissues, producing a mild generalized extravasation of blood in the tissues of the upper half of the body. Bright red, confluent conjunctival hemorrhage was present in our patients (Fig 15-3). The extravasated blood produces edema and the usual uncomfortable foreign body reaction in the soft tissues that requires some 2 to 3 weeks to clear. The process disappears without sequelae except for an occasional thrombosis of the superior vena cava. This may progress to a chronic superior vena caval syndrome with a considerable degree of permanent disability.

Treatment of traumatic asphyxia is nonspecific and involves primarily bedrest and observation. It appears that more rapid clearing occurs when the upper half of the body is kept elevated. Because we have seen it produce chronic vena caval thrombosis followed by severe sequelae, the question arises as to whether these patients might profit

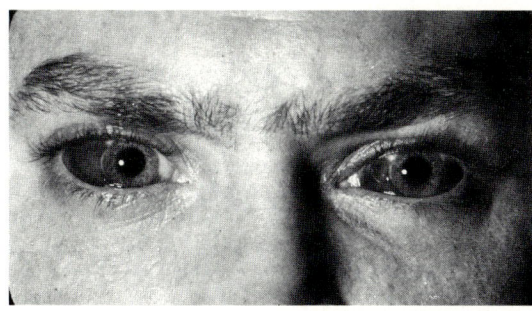

Fig 15-3. Asphyxia syndrome resulting from marked compression of a young man's thorax. Marked suffusion and extravasation of blood into all tissues of the head, neck, and conjunctiva are obvious. It is very impressive when seen in its acute phase.

from being placed on heparin or another anticoagulant 1 or 2 days after the appearance of the acute discoloration of the upper half of the body.

THORACIC DUCT INJURIES

A thorough knowledge of the anatomy of the thoracic duct is necessary for the proper understanding of injuries to this structure and proper management. The thoracic duct arises from the cisterna magna, at the level of the first or second lumbar vertebra. It runs to the right of and behind the aorta, ascending through the aortic hiatus into the thorax. It courses posterior to the aorta, between it and the azygos vein and in close proximity to the esophagus. At the level of the fourth thoracic vertebra it ascends behind the left subclavian vein, then proceeds in front of the scalenus anticus muscle where it curves anteriorly to join the left jugular vein at its junction with the left subclavian vein. Two tributaries join it just before the thoracic duct enters the subclavian vein. Two valves at the termination of the thoracic duct prevent the retrograde flow of blood into the duct. Numerous anatomical variations have been described but this classic pattern occurs in about half the population [15].

The thoracic duct may be injured at any point in its course. Iatrogenic trauma during operation is the most common type of injury to the thoracic duct system [11]. It can occur during resection of the esophagus and is not uncommon during operative therapy of other mediastinal malignancies.

Thoracic duct injury occurs more frequently in small children during operations for coarctation of the aorta, vascular "rings," and correction of patent ductus arteriosus. Twigs or tributaries of the cisterna magna are often divided during resection of an abdominal aorta aneurysm and during the radical periaortic lymph node resection. Milky fluid appears from the cut ends of the tributaries and these are ligated as one would ligate for hemostasis. We have not seen any long-term complications from trauma to the chyle drainage system during abdominal surgery. Blunt and penetrating trauma are rarely responsible for injury to the thoracic duct drainage system, although we have on rare occasions encountered a collection of chyle in the left supraclavicular region following blunt trauma to the left side of the neck and upper thorax.

Two to four liters of lymph per day flow through the thoracic duct to enter the venous system [6]. The occurrence of a fistula with complete diversion of the flow of chyle produces rapid malnutrition, electrolyte imbalance, and dehydration because the concentration of electrolytes in the chyle is identical to that of the blood serum. It is also important to prevent and correct as early as possible any metabolic and nutritional insults [11, 17]. As much as 195 grams of protein per day may be lost through a fistula and 20 to 30 percent of ingested fats pass through the duct in the form of triglycerides. Fibrinogen is lost, which causes slow clotting of chyle from a fistula formation in the neck or diversion of the thoracic duct contents. Marked hyponatremia and hypochloremia also result [6]. Needle aspiration of milk-like fluid from the thorax usually confirms the diagnosis; this fluid can be proved to be chyle by a fat staining technique. It usually does not contain bacteria.

If more than a small amount of pleural fluid is present, a thoracostomy drainage tube should be inserted into the involved pleural cavity so as to bring about complete and continuous evacuation of the free chyle. The leakage of chyle from a chylous fistula is usually self-limited and ceases draining in a few hours to a few days. The patient should also be on a low-fat diet; this minimizes the amount of chyle formation and drainage. Rarely is operative treatment necessary for minor leakage of chyle. If injury to the thoracic duct in the neck occurs during an operation, a small rubber drain in the operative wound allows escape of chyle as it appears in the wound and only rarely will a sizable collection of chyle develop in the soft tissues of the neck. Also a pressure dressing may be of some value in preventing or minimizing the leakage of chyle into the soft tissues of the neck.

The treatment of chylothorax due to trauma is conservative or nonoperative as a rule, but on rare occasions it is necessary to perform ligation of the thoracic duct by way of an open thoracotomy procedure. It is not wise to let any considerable amount of chyle accumulate in a pleural cavity, because it produces a rather severe fibrothorax, even more severe than that resulting from the accumulation of blood clots in the thorax. Decortication may become necessary if the chylothorax is neglected or the chyle has been allowed to accumulate and remain in the pleural cavity for any considerable length of time. Lymphangiography is of assistance in locating the site of injury if it appears that operative intervention is necessary. The administration of a heavy fat such as butter laden with a dye is helpful in locating the area of leakage at the time of operative exploration. Whenever operation is necessary and the location of the tear in the thoracic duct cannot be located, we have been successful with multiple ligations of the soft tissues immediately anterior and to the left of the eighth and ninth thoracic vertebrae, which is the usual location of the thoracic duct in the lower thorax.

REFERENCES

1. Allansmith R, Richards V: Superior vena caval obstruction. Am J Surg 96:353, 1958
2. Doty DB, Baker WH: Bypass of superior vena cava with spiral vein graft. Ann Thorac Surg 22:490, 1976
3. Fred HL, Chandler FW: Traumatic asphyxia. Am J Med 29:508, 1960
4. Gomez MN, Hufnagel CA: Superior vena caval obstruction (by benign disease). Ann Thorac Surg 20:344, 1975
5. Heydorn WH, Zajtchuk R, Miller J, Schuchmann GF: Gore-tex grafts for replacement of the superior vena cava. Ann Thorac Surg 23:539, 1977
6. Keele CA, Neil E: Thoracic duct. Applied Physiology. Edited by S Wright. London, England, Oxford University Press, 1971
7. Miller DB: Palliative surgery for benign superior vena caval syndrome. Am J Surg 129:361, 1975
8. Ochsner JL, Crawford ES, DeBakey ME: Injuries of the vena cava caused by external trauma. Surgery 49:397, 1961
9. Olin R: Primary thrombosis of the subclavian vein. Minn Med 57:93, 1974
10. Ollivier (d'Angers): Relation médicale des évènemens survenus au Champ-de-Mars le 14 juin 1837. Ann Hyg Publique Med Legale 18:485, 1837
11. Penn I: Injuries to the cervical portion of the thoracic duct. Br J Surg 50:19, 1962
12. Perthe G: Uber "Druckstanung." Dtsch Z Chir 55:384, 1900
13. Saha P, Goff RD, Stephenson SE Jr: Management of injuries of the inferior vena cava. J Fla Med Assoc 62:24, 1975
14. Shamblin JR, McGoon DC: Acute traumatic compression with traumatic asphyxia. Arch Surg 87:967, 1963
15. Shieber W: The demonstration of thoracic duct anomalies by lymphangiography. Angiology 25:73, 1974
16. Sterns EE: Current concepts of lymphatic transport. Surg Gynecol Obstet 138:773, 1974
17. Stubbs WK, Tabb HG: Thoracic duct injuries. South Med J 70:1062, 1977

16. CHEST TRAUMA AS AFFECTED BY AGE AND PREEXISTING DISEASE

William E. Bloomer

Whether or not chest trauma results in serious consequences depends on the degree to which it impairs the vital functions of the thoracic organs and structures. Accurate assessment of a given injury must include an appraisal of the actual and potential derangement of each of these vital functions. In some individuals, one or more of these may already have been significantly reduced by reason of age, congenital anomalies, or preexisting disease to an extent that could make even minimal trauma dangerous. For example, consider this possible occurrence: an elderly male sustains a simple fracture of two ribs over the right anterolateral chest. A chest film reveals a mild pneumothorax with a small amount of fluid at the base, and the man is admitted to the hospital for observation. He does not appear to be in respiratory distress but complains of pain; he is given morphine for its relief. During the night, the patient becomes restless and confused and is given nasal oxygen and further sedation. The following morning he is found to be comatose and in shock. Before restorative measures can be instituted, he dies of either cardiac or respiratory arrest.

This course of events can easily occur in an aging, poor-risk patient with a relatively mild closed-chest injury. Such a patient tends to have a reduced cardiac and ventilatory reserve because of associated emphysema or other disease commonly found in the elderly. This makes undertreatment or an error in management a particularly likely source of serious if not fatal complications. It is well, therefore, to consider what type of functional restriction may already be present when such a patient suffers a chest injury.

A detailed history of any prexisting cardiorespiratory disease or malfunction is of vital importance. Prior history of a therapeutic pneumothorax, thoracoplasty, partial pulmonary resection, pulmonary tuberculosis, emphysema, pleural effusion, stroke, aortic aneurysm, complete heart block, or myocardial infarction will assist in devising treatment for the particular patient. More intensive initial management may be necessary for a successful outcome in such individuals. Previous adrenal insufficiency, hypothyroidism, diabetes, chronic steroid therapy, heavy smoking, and obesity may also require special considerations.

ADVANCED AGE

The aged have a more rigid and brittle chest cage and quite often sustain more fractures and more underlying intrathoracic injury than younger people. They have a greater tendency toward multiple level fractures and flail chest. Obviously, the effects produced by flail chest in the elderly are far more dangerous or lethal than those occurring in those who are younger. Those in the latter age group possess a more elastic chest cage, which tends to cushion a blow and thereby reduces the number of fractures and intrathoracic injuries. Even in the absence of disease, older people experience a reduction in cardiorespiratory reserve. Vital capacity in the octogenarian is usually assessed at about 50 percent of what it was at the age of 25. Decreased elasticity in the otherwise healthy lung can be expected to increase the residual volume-total capacity ratio to more than the normal 35 percent after age sixty-five [4]. The increased resistance to air flow increases the work load of breathing with advancing age. Furthermore, there is an increase in susceptibility to the depressant effects of narcotics and sedatives. The tussive force of cough is reduced. There is also an increased tendency for the development of thromboembolization after injury and its resulting immobilization. The cardiac output is reduced because the maximal pulse rate that can be achieved shows a decrease with advancing years. All these factors contribute to increased risk when aged people sustain thoracic trauma [3, 8].

Translated into terms of management, the above considerations call for an underscoring of certain principles. Thus, the use of local anesthesia is indicated to achieve adequate analgesia without depressing the cough reflex or respiratory function. The importance of good tracheobronchial toilet must be emphasized and should include encouragement of coughing and deep breathing, the use of endotracheal aspiration when needed, and the use of nebulized oxygen with an adequate amount of humidity to prevent drying of secretions. Intercostal nerve block is particularly effective in decreasing the amount of sedation necessary to control pain; it also facilitates coughing and self-clearing of secretions from the tracheobronchial tree and is effective in the prevention of atelectasis and the wet lung syndrome. More frequent monitoring of vital signs and arterial blood gases is also indicated in these patients. Use of assisted or controlled ventilation through tracheal intubation is important in many instances. Measures to prevent thromboembolism are also important and should include the use of elastic stockings, early mobilization, avoidance of dehydration, and judicious use of anticoagulants.

Age was reported by Sankaran and Wilson [10] to be an important factor affecting prognosis in patients with flail chest. It may well be that principles outlined by Trinkle and co-workers [12, 13] for the treatment of flail chest and contusion of the lung will be especially important in management of this injury in the aged. These authors have stressed that the contused lung is very sensitive to the administration of noncolloid fluids. They find vigorous pulmonary toilet, intercostal nerve block, fluid restriction, diuretics, methylprednisolone, and albumin to maintain a normal plasma oncotic pressure are often sufficient, and that mechanical ventilation through an endotracheal tube need only be used if the arterial Po_2 cannot be maintained above 60 mm Hg on room air or 80 mm with supplemental oxygen. They found central venous pressure was not an accurate index of crystalloid overload and that contused lungs were especially apt to be worsened with crystalloid overload.

At the other extreme of age, very young individuals with highly elastic chest cages may be the victims of serious functional derangement due to internal injuries masked by minimal apparent trauma to the bony thorax. Torsion of the lung has occurred in a child with little evidence of trauma to the chest wall [6]. It is not rare for a young child to have an avulsion of a main bronchus or a rupture of the esophagus secondary to blunt trauma even though he didn't fracture any ribs. Due to the small airways in infants, laryngospasm associated with chest injury may be life-threatening and may need to be treated intensively with high humidity and steroids on a prophylactic basis.

OBESITY

Marked obesity is usually associated with impaired ventilation and an increased oxygen requirement. The oxygen requirement of very obese patients at rest and during comparable degrees of activity has been found to be greater than those of patients of normal weight [1, 2]. The ventilatory demand in these instances is, therefore, actually greater than normal.

Impairment in ventilation is due to a reduced ability to expand the chest cage except by diaphragmatic activity. In such patients, the maximum voluntary ventilation may average only 60 percent of the value predicted on the basis of ideal body weight [2]. Moreover, the expiratory reserve volume is found to be diminished in excessively obese patients [5]. It should also be noted that when the Pickwickian syndrome is present, one may find alveolar hypoventilation to be a factor, although this is relatively rare.

Management of markedly obese patients with chest trauma should take into account that because of the already reduced ventilatory reserve and the increased work of breathing ventilatory assistance and support will be required much earlier than in nonobese subjects. The need for support may not be evidenced by the usual hyperpnea, and results obtained from arterial blood gas analysis are valuable in pointing out the need for ventilatory support.

PREEXISTING DISEASE OF THE CHEST WALL, PLEURA, AND DIAPHRAGM

Preexisting disease of the chest wall affecting ventilatory function includes kyphosis and kyphoscoliosis, thoracoplasty, eventration of the diaphragm, paralysis of the diaphragm due to localized phrenic nerve injury or to poliomyelitis, and other lesions of the diaphragm such as fibrosis of the costophrenic sinus or posttraumatic hernia of the diaphragm.

Kyphosis has been shown to produce very marked restriction in ventilation because of the enhanced elastic resistance of the thorax and the resultant diminution in compliance, leading to an increase in the work of breathing. In such patients, it has been found that whereas total lung capacity and its subdivisions are decreased somewhat, the timed vital capacity is within the normal percentile range; nevertheless, maximal breathing capacities may be less than 50 percent of normal. This is attributable in part to a reduced lung volume but particularly to fixation of the thoracic cage and loss of musculoskeletal power. The compliance of the total respiratory system in these patients averages one-third of the average normal [11].

Frequent bouts of respiratory infection, to which kyphotic patients are subject, may be important in reducing compliance of the lung. The Hurler syndrome (lipochondrodystrophy or gargoylism) is manifested by pulmonary and chest wall changes such as kyphoscoliosis, restriction of chest motion, upper airway obstruction from changes in cartilage and perichondral tissue, and repeated pulmonary infection and abnormal diffusion [7]. Thus, these patients may be subjected to much more work than might be expected with superimposed chest trauma and therefore may more rapidly succumb to respiratory failure unless this is recognized and treated with proper mechanical assistance.

Deformity due to thoracoplasty is rarely seen today, but may cause a decrease in the dynamic function as well as the static volume, depending upon the degree of collapse, the elasticity of the thoracic wall, the amount of underlying *fibrosis in the lung parenchyma,* and the amount of functional loss of the chest wall. Unilateral diaphragmatic (phrenic) paralysis or eventration of the diaphragm reduces functional breathing and also increases the chances of atelectasis due to a reduced ability to spontaneously clear the tracheobronchial tree of secretions after thoracic injury.

Pleural Effusion

Pleural effusion may be associated with a reduction in lung volume and in pulmonary chest wall compliance, but it ordinarily is not associated with abnormalities of arterial blood gases unless there is some associated parenchymal disease [14]. When possible, pleural fluid should be removed immediately so that the ventilatory mechanics can be restored.

PREEXISTING DISEASE OF THE LUNG

Because of the bronchospasm and excessive secretions that are not seen in the average nonsmoker, smoking can be a real hazard if the smoker sustains a moderate to severe thoracic injury. This is particularly true in the patient who is already dyspneic upon exertion and has a considerable amount of coughing, wheezing, and sputum production.

Chronic Obstructive Bronchopulmonary Disease

The threat to life imposed by chronic obstructive bronchopulmonary disease has been underscored by a cooperative study carried out by the Veteran's Administration in 1966 and reported by Renzetti, McClement, and Litt [9]. In this study, there was a 53 percent mortality in the whole group of patients over a 4-year period. The mortality appeared to correlate highly with the degree of ventilatory disturbance with blood oxygen desaturation and hypercapnia, and with a history of right heart failure. Those incapacitated by a chronic respiratory problem are in great jeopardy when they sustain a thoracic injury, especially if an operative procedure becomes necessary. Thus, even a very small, untreated pneumothorax can prove lethal. This is a situation similar to that encountered by the thoracic surgeon when he has to resect a portion of the lung for malignancy in a patient who has compromised pulmonary function studies and symptoms and findings related to the above. A patient with bullous emphysema is in particular jeopardy because one of the bullae may be ruptured by the impact of the accident and produce a dangerous pneumothorax. This pneumothorax may soon become extensive and of the tension variety due to a large rent or hole in the bullous formation. Also, large bullae may give the impression that the patient has a pneumothorax and a decompression tube may mistakenly be introduced into the corresponding pleural cavity and directly into the bulla, thereby creating serious and unnecessary complications. Under these circumstances it may not be possible to remove the tube without causing a serious pneumothorax. It may then be necessary to perform a thoracotomy to suture the opening in the bullous cyst inadvertently produced at the time the tube was inserted.

Clearly, the margin of safety in such patients may already have been reduced to the point at which the least additional impairment from chest trauma may be lethal. Management in such instances will be dictated by the principles outlined for the treatment of chronic obstructive lung disease; these have been well set forth in the proceedings of the Eighth Aspen Emphysema Conference. Briefly, the therapeutic approach should take cognizance of chronic airway obstruction by removing secretions, using bronchodilators, using a mechanical respirator in some patients, and humidifying inhaled gases. Treatment should also include antibiotics for specific infections. Hypoxemia, hypercapnea, and respiratory acidosis should be corrected by administering adequate amounts of oxygen. Alveolar ventilation should be ensured with a mechanical volume respirator and by correction of any airway obstruction. Adequate oxygen must be used to restore arterial PO_2 to normal or near normal levels (70 to 100 mm Hg). Right ventricular failure is dealt with by the treatment of the hypoxemia and hypercapnea as well as by the use of digitalis, potassium chloride, diuretics, and aminophylline. Any dehydration must be prevented or corrected by proper fluid intake, and the metabolic alkalosis due to hypokalemia or hypochloremia, or both (seen so frequently in these patients) should be properly treated by adequate replacement with potassium chloride.

Pulmonary Fibrosis

Pulmonary fibrosis of either the localized or generalized type may be difficult to recognize in patients presenting with chest trauma. Fibrosis is, of course, secondary to a variety of etiological factors. Extensive pulmonary involvement may be of unknown etiology, although the so-called hypersensitivity reaction may play a part. Its presence is often the result of occupational exposure to damaging agents or acute and chronic infectious processes. In any event, chronic fibrosis tends to reduce pulmonary efficiency, both by its restrictive effect on ventilation and by impairment of diffusing capacity.

Hypoxia occurs in chronic pulmonary fibrosis just as it does in emphysema. However, the PCO_2 is reduced in pulmonary fibrosis rather than elevated as a consequence of the increase in minute ventilation, a characteristic of the disease. Complicating cor pulmonale may occur with the same severity as in emphysema or other types of pulmonary insufficiency.

Management of trauma in patients with chronic pulmonary fibrosis will then make use primarily of oxygen therapy to offset the reduction in diffusing capacity and to reduce the work of breathing. In some instances corticosteroids may be found helpful. Use of a volume type respirator is preferable because of the stiff or less compliant lungs.

Other Preexisting Conditions

A host of conditions such as asbestosis, scleroderma, tuberculosis, leukemic and carcinomatous infiltration, rheumatoid arthritis, and systemic lupus erythematosis produce varying patterns and degrees of pulmonary fibrosis that alter pulmonary function and increase the complexity of the management and possible sequelae with the added burden of thoracic trauma. Chest injury superimposed on asthma, chronic bronchitis, bronchiectasis, acute bacterial or viral pneumonia, and chronic or recurring pneumonitis from reflux aspiration due to a sliding hiatus hernia or some obstructing esophageal disease often presents the attending surgeon with a complex therapeutic problem. The combination of severe thoracic injury, bronchospasm, increased secretions, and preexisting impaired respiratory function may well tax the ingenuity of the most able and experienced physician. Intensive care should be initiated at the outset in anticipation of a rapidly deteriorating status. The barrel-shaped chest, even in the absence of an obvious decrease in lung function, produces more hazards and complications than one without such a deformity. A similar situation may be encountered in the injured patient who has the chest wall deformity of pectus excavatum in which the respiratory volume is reduced and the mechanics of respiration are considerably altered.

The mechanics of respiration seem to be adversely altered on the contralateral side after a pneumonectomy. Injury on the side of a remaining lung is particularly dangerous and difficult to manage. Fractured ribs and a small pneumothorax may well be lethal. Treatment must be meticulous and intensive in order to give such patients the best possible chance for survival.

Proper acid-base equilibrium may be particularly difficult to maintain when a serious injury is superimposed on chronic renal insufficiency. Massive steroid therapy may be of value in reducing the subsequent risks of trauma in the already compromised pulmonary or cardiovascular-renal functions and may help stabilize the acid-base balance.

A variety of pathophysiological circumstances can arise in a patient with carcinoma of the lung, either primary or metastatic. Postresection irradiation can cause a significant injury to the thorax, producing additional altered pulmonary physiology. Preexisting and added diminution in already altered lung function can present a grave problem in management. The same principles of therapy pertain, however, unless the malignancy is terminal or is the overriding problem. A special problem arises when an accident is the factor that first focuses attention on an otherwise unknown carcinoma. The proper management of the tumor and the necessary diagnostic studies may need to be delayed until the patient has made sufficient recovery from the effects of the accident. Pulmonary hematoma may look much like a primary carcinoma of the lung and vice versa.

Rarely the findings are such that one cannot determine whether all the pulmonary changes noted are due to the accident or whether they are superimposed upon carcinoma, tuberculosis, pulmonary emphysema (bullous type), or some other significant pulmonary disease. Often the combination can be treated effectively concomitantly.

Mortality and morbidity in patients with acute respiratory problems are much higher even with the best of care but can be minimized with early and continued intensive management. It is of the utmost importance to have these patients admitted to an acute Respiratory Care Unit. If this type of unit is not available, a fully equipped Intensive Care Unit will meet the requirements reasonably well. In the absence of an acute treatment facility the patient should be transferred to another institution where appropriate care and personnel are available. Given adequate circumstances he may be transferred considerable distances with relative safety and to great ultimate advantage.

Stress ulcer is not uncommon in the elderly following thoracic trauma or in a patient with chronic obstructive lung disease who sustains a thoracic injury. These ulcers have a tendency to hemorrhage profusely and may require operation in an already poor-risk, seriously ill patient.

Preexisting Cardiovascular Disease

Preexisting cardiovascular disease may have varying degrees of significance, depending upon the extent of the thoracic injury and its complications or upon the seriousness of the preexisting condition. The combined effects may be mild or insurmountable. The pulmonary function may be greatly compromised from extensive prior pulmonary embolization or other forms of pulmonary hypertension or congestion. Of course, poor cardiac func-

tion due to a variety of disease processes may be greatly aggravated by thoracic trauma. The combination may have overwhelming additive effects. Again, early intensive care is imperative, even though the injury may not be extensive.

The already diseased heart may tolerate poorly even minor degrees of hypovolemia, hypoxia, and hypercarbia. Arrhythmias may be a serious complication. This is another area in which much can be accomplished by a detailed history of the injured patient's prior health problems, and all can profit by early consultation and close teamwork.

Management will be facilitated by close monitoring of urinary output, blood volume, hematocrit, central venous pressure, direct arterial pressure, and determination of mean pulmonary artery pressure.

PRIOR IMPAIRMENT OF THE CENTRAL NERVOUS SYSTEM

Patients who have had a stroke or have Parkinson's disease, quadriplegia, myasthenia gravis, Guillain-Barré syndrome, or other acute or degenerative processes, already have some impairment in respiratory function as well as the inability to handle additional secretions that may result from injury to the thorax. These patients require careful attention in the matters of adequate respiratory exchange and the removal of secretions. Tracheostomy and the use of artificial respirators are often necessary for their adequate care.

REFERENCES

1. Alexander JK, Amad KH, Cole VW: Observations on some clinical features of extreme obesity, with particular reference to cardiorespiratory effects. Am J Med 32:512, 1962
2. Alexander JK, Turell DJ, Drew MJR: Mechanisms of dyspnea in obesity. Cardiovasc Res Cent Bull 2:27, 1963
3. Baker SP, Spitz WU: Age effects and autopsy evidence of disease in fatally injured divers. JAMA 214:1079, 1970
4. Bloomer WE: Respiratory function and its clinical evaluation. Edited by WL Glenn, et al. Thoracic and Cardiovascular Surgery with Related Pathology. New York, Appleton-Century-Crofts, 1975
5. Cullen JH, Formel PF: The respiratory defects in extreme obesity. Am J Med 32:525, 1962

6. Daughtry DC: Traumatic torsion of the lung. N Engl J Med 256:385, 1957

7. Murray JF: Pulmonary disability in the Hurler syndrome (lipochondrodystrophy). N Engl J Med 261:378, 1959

8. Perry JF, Galway CF: Factors influencing survival after flail chest injuries. Arch Surg 91:216, 1965

9. Renzetti AD Jr, McClement JH, Litt BD: The Veterans Administration cooperative study of pulmonary function. III. Mortality in relation to respiratory function in chronic obstructive pulmonary disease. Am J Med 41:115, 1966

10. Sankaran S, Wilson RF: Factors affecting prognosis in patients with flail chest. J Thorac Cardiovasc Surg 60:402, 1970

11. Ting EY, Lyons HA: The relation of pressure and volume of the total respiratory system and its components in kyphoscoliosis. Am Rev Resp Dis 89:379, 1964

12. Trinkle JK, Furman RW, Hinshaw MA, et al: Pulmonary contusion. Ann Thorac Surg 16:568, 1973

13. Trinkle JK, Richardson JD, Franz JL, et al: Management of flail chest without mechanical ventilation. Ann Thorac Surg 19:355, 1975

14. Yoo OH, Ting EY: The effects of pleural effusion on pulmonary function. Am Rev Resp Dis 89:55, 1964

ADDITIONAL READING

Aber CP, Campbell JA: Significance of changes in the pulmonary diffusing capacity in mitral stenosis. Thorax 20:135, 1965

Adhikari PK, et al: Pulmonary function in scleroderma. Am Rev Resp Dis 86:823, 1962

Andrial M: Influenzal pneumonia and blood gas analysis. J Thorac Cardiovasc Surg 40:79, 1960

Beaudry PH, Wise MB: Respiratory gas exchange at rest and during exercise in normal and asthmatic children. Am Rev Resp Dis 95:248, 1967

Boushy SF, Coates EO Jr: The prognostic value of pulmonary function tests in emphysema. Am Rev Resp Dis 90:553, 1964

Colp CK, Park SS, Williams MH Jr: Pulmonary function studies in pneumonia. Am Rev Resp Dis 85:799, 1962

Cudkowicz L: Cardio-respiratory studies in patients with lung tumors. Dis Chest 51:427, 1967

Emirgil C, Zsoldos S, Heinemann HO: Effect of metastatic carcinoma to the lung on pulmonary function in man. Am J Med 36:382, 1964

Filley GF, et al: Chronic obstructive bronchopulmonary disease. Am J Med 44:26, 1968

Gaensler EA, Strieder JW: Pulmonary function before and after extrapleural pneumothorax: A comparison with other forms of collapse and resection. J Thorac Surg 20:774, 1950

Germon PA, Brady LW: Physiologic changes before and after radiation treatment for carcinoma of the lung. JAMA 206:809, 1968

Green RA, Nichols NJ, King EJ: Alveolar-capillary block due to leukemic infiltration of the lung. Am Rev Resp Dis 80:895, 1959

Huang CT, Hennigar GR, Lyons HA: Pulmonary dysfunction in systemic lupus erythematosus. N Engl J Med 272:288, 1965

Linde LM, et al: Lung function in congenital heart disease. Dis Chest 46:46, 1964

Motley HL: Impairment in blood gas exchange and types of treatment in the elderly with chronic pulmonary disease. Edited by JT Freeman. Clinical Principles and Drugs in the Aging. Springfield, Ill, Thomas, 1963

Murray JF: The spirogram in regional bronchial obstruction. N Engl J Med 264:1330, 1961

Nadel JA, Gold WM, Burgess JH: Early diagnosis of chronic pulmonary vascular obstruction. Am J Med 44:16, 1968

Oka S, et al: Pulmonary diffusing capacity and its evaluation by scintillation scanning of the lungs in lung cancer. Am Rev Resp Dis 95:239, 1967

Robin ED, et al: A physiologic approach to the diagnosis of acute pulmonary embolism. N Engl J Med 260:596, 1959

Rodman T, et al: Alveolar hypoventilation due to involvement of the respiratory center by obscure disease of the central nervous system. Am J Med 32:208, 1962

Simpson DG, Kushner M, McClement J: Respiratory function in pulmonary tuberculosis. Am Rev Resp Dis 87:1, 1963

Wise AJ, et al: The importance of serial blood gas determinations in blunt chest trauma. J Thorac Cardiovasc Surg 56:520, 1968

Woolcock AJ, Read J: Lung volumes in exacerbations of asthma. Am J Med 41:259, 1966

Woolf CR: The relationships between dyspnea, pulmonary function and intracardiac pressures in adults with left heart valve lesions. Dis Chest 49:225, 1966

17. THE MANAGEMENT OF WAR WOUNDS OF THE CHEST

William A. Cox
James M. Feltis, Jr.

The United States Army Medical Corps has performed a monumental task in caring for the wounded American soldier in World War II, in Korea, and during the recent conflict in Vietnam. Techniques of forward emergency care, continuing resuscitation, evacuation of the wounded, patient sorting, determining priority of treatment, emergency surgery as a necessary part of resuscitation, and staged treatment along the evacuation chain have been developed and markedly improved.

There must be an inherent mobility, flexibility, and adaptability to any system for the care of the wounded in warfare. This flexibility is of paramount importance because of the constantly changing tactical situation, wide variations in the number of patients and the rate at which they are received, the presence or absence of air superiority, the type of terrain and climate, the characteristics of weapons used, and the availability of supplies.

Following a survey of the six U.S. Army Hospitals in Vietnam in 1968, it was concluded that the wounded American fighting man was receiving the best medical care in the history of warfare [28]. This is largely due to: relatively stable fighting lines with fixed treatment facilities; the increased use of helicopters for rapid evacuation (Fig 17-1); well-trained, dedicated allied medical personnel; the availability of type-specific blood with improved techniques for resuscitation, anesthesia, and surgery; and ready access to improved equipment, particularly blood gas and pH analyzers as well as volume respirators.

The mortality rate of the wounded admitted to medical treatment facilities during World War II was 4.5 percent. The corresponding figure for the Korean and Vietnam conflicts is 2.5 percent. If percentage ratios of the surviving wounded to the total of battle deaths plus surviving wounded are computed, it is seen that 70.7 percent survived in all of World War II, while 73.7 percent did so during the Korean war with a further increase to 81.2 percent in Vietnam [1]. The figures gleaned from the Vietnam conflict become more impressive when it is realized that the widespread use of rapid helicopter evacuation of seriously wounded patients has meant that patients whom hitherto no skill or care would have saved are now reaching hospitals alive.

The incidence of wounds of the chest in Vietnam is approximately 7 percent [18]—a similar incidence to that of World War II and Korea. Body armor was used in the Korean conflict for the first time in modern warfare; prior to its adoption the occurrence of chest wounds had been 19 percent [2]. In November, 1970, the Defense Department reported that 147,000 U.S. military patients had been hospitalized for wounds suffered in Vietnam. Approximately 10,300 of this group had sustained wounds of the chest; in many instances there was multiple system involvement. Almost 6500 patients were evacuated from Vietnam to the Surgical Services at Brooke General Hospital between 1965 and 1970. Of this group, 201 had thoracic wounds.

BASIC PRINCIPLES IN THE MANAGEMENT OF CHEST WOUNDS

The basic principles for the treatment of thoracic wounds in warfare are presented below and were formulated during World War II by Col. Edward D. Churchill and his staff of thoracic surgeons during a meeting at Marcianise, Italy, in March 1944 [7].

1. The majority of chest injuries are best managed by providing and maintaining a clear tracheobronchial tree, with endotracheal suctioning and bronchoscopy when necessary; administering oxygen; and prompt needle aspiration of collections of blood and air from the pleural space to regain complete expansion of the lung.
2. Formal thoracotomy should be performed only for: (a) continued intrathoracic bleeding; (b) continued excessive air leak from the respiratory tract; (c) thoracoabdominal wounds; (d) injury to vital structures (esophagus, heart);

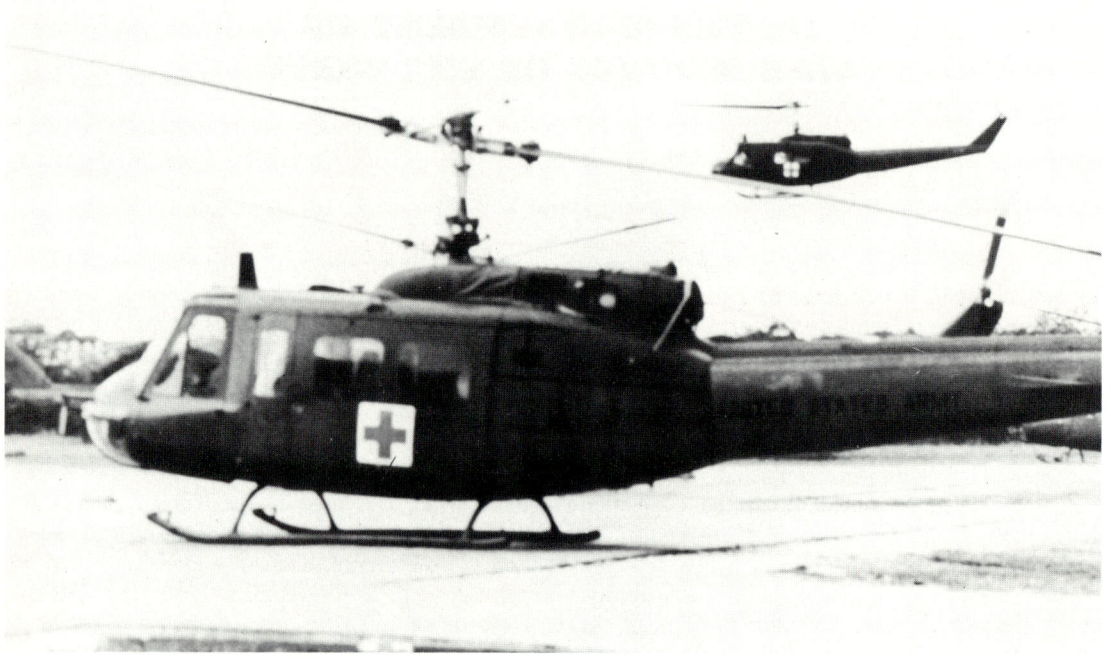

(e) large intrapleural foreign bodies readily accessible by simple extension of the wound.
3. Pulmonary resection is rarely indicated and should be conservative when done.

These principles put emphasis properly on first the restoration of altered cardiopulmonary physiology and secondly definitive treatment of the thoracic wound. Following their widespread adoption, the mortality rate in patients with chest wounds was reduced from 25 percent in World War I to approximately 9 percent in World War II. As guidelines to chest wound management they have been used successfully in Korea and Vietnam with few basic changes.

To obtain adequate pleural drainage, large-bore plastic thoracostomy tubes attached to an underwater seal or temporarily to Heimlich valves are used during evacuation rather than multiple thoracenteses. In the management of most thoracoabdominal wounds, the thoracic component is dealt with by adequate pleural drainage with large-bore thoracostomy tubes, followed by exploratory laparotomy rather than a thoracoabdominal approach. If the thoracic involvement is too extensive to be treated by closed-tube thoracostomy, then a formal thoracotomy is performed to stabilize cardiopul-

Fig 17-1. U.S. Army helicopter ambulance, UH-IH "Huey." (Courtesy Capt. Lynn W. Rasmussen, MSC, U.S. Army, 507th Medical Company Air Ambulance, Fort Sam Houston, Texas.)

monary function followed by laparotomy through a separate abdominal incision.

IMMEDIATE MEASURES

Depression of cardiopulmonary function is the common denominator in war wounds of the chest. During the initial care of these injuries, all measures should be directed toward aggressively restoring cardiopulmonary function as early as possible. This can be achieved by ensuring a clear tracheobronchial tree, an intact and stable chest wall, a well-drained pleural space with completely expanded lungs, and an adequate circulating blood volume.

The medical aidman, the most forward appendage of emergency medical care, is trained to apply occlusive dressings to all chest wounds, whether sucking or not. Large, snug, supporting dressings are applied to large defects to help stabilization of the chest wall and to control hemorrhage. The patient is encouraged to cough frequently to keep his airway clear. He is positioned with the injured side down and supported with folded blankets [18]. He is then evacuated, usually by helicopter, to the forward aid station, brigade clearing station, or forward surgical hospital, depending on the tactical situation and his condition. At the clearing station, the airway is checked, a tracheostomy is done, or an endotracheal tube is placed and respiration supported with an Ambu bag if necessary. Blood volume is restored with colloid. Pleural drainage is established by thoracentesis or by placing a large-bore (40 or 45F) plastic thoracostomy tube dependently in the midaxillary line. Pneumothorax can be vented temporarily with a needle placed in the second intercostal space midclavicular line and held by a hemostat securely taped flush to the chest wall. A flutter valve can be constructed, using a rubber glove finger split at the end and tied to the thoracentesis needle hub. This temporary measure may be lifesaving. While the patient is being evacuated, continuing decompression of a pneumothorax can also be achieved with a thoracostomy tube placed in the second intercostal space anterior axillary line and attached to a Heimlich flutter valve. Antibiotic treatment is initiated and tetanus toxoid booster given. If the patient is hypoxic and acidotic from respiratory insufficiency or hypovolemia, nasal oxygen is started and sodium bicarbonate administered. The conditions of severely injured patients, such as those with large sucking wounds of the chest, are stabilized as much as possible, and they are given priority evacuation to the nearest forward surgical hospital. Resuscitative measures are continued en route. Upon arrival, an endotracheal tube is placed immediately, if this has not already been done, and respiration is supported with an Ambu bag. Blood is given, acidosis is corrected, and the patient is operated on for debridement and necessary repair of the chest wall and associated defects.

Only a small number (approximately 10 percent) of patients with chest injuries require formal thoracotomy [19]. The majority can be managed by conservative techniques that restore depressed cardiopulmonary function. These techniques must be applied in a timely, aggressive, and continuing manner to gain a clear tracheobronchial tree, an intact stable chest wall, a well-drained pleural space with completely expanded lungs, and an adequate circulating blood volume. Autotransfusion is being used more widely when uncontaminated blood can be collected and reinfused.

HEMOTHORAX

Hemothorax is the most commonly seen lesion following chest injury. Probably every casualty with a penetrating chest wound suffers some degree of hemothorax. In the Mediterranean Theater in World War II, hemothorax comprised 80 percent of chest wounds and 752 cases were treated at the 300th General Hospital Chest Center [9]. In the Korean War, between 1950 and 1952, Valle [27] reported 952 patients with hemothorax out of 1535 patients with penetrating chest injuries. In January 1968, Patterson and associates [19] reported on 476 patients evacuated to the Clark U.S. Air Force Hospital who had sustained intrathoracic injuries in Vietnam; 331 or 69.4 percent of these patients had hemopneumothorax.

Hemothorax interferes with cardiorespiratory function by causing collapse of the lung and by producing blood loss from the circulating blood volume (Fig 17-2). Pain from the chest injury

Fig 17-2. Chest roentgenogram demonstrates a large left hemothorax.

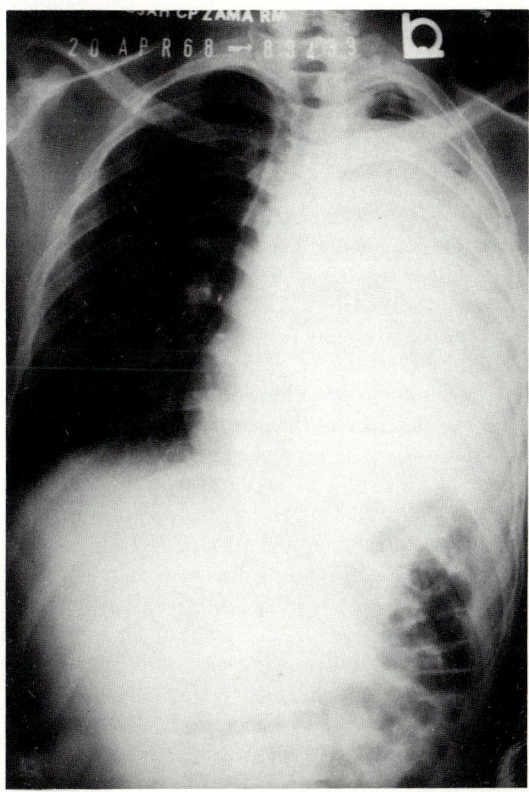

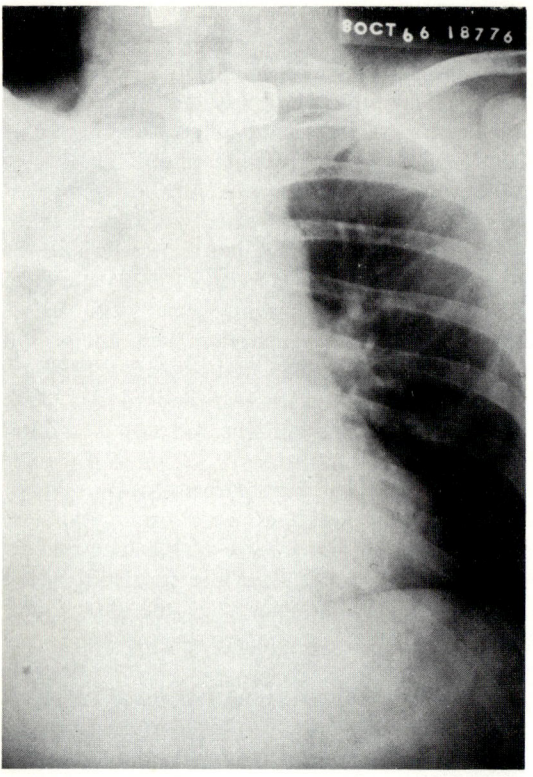

Fig 17-3. Inadequate drainage of a right hemothorax because of a small rubber catheter.

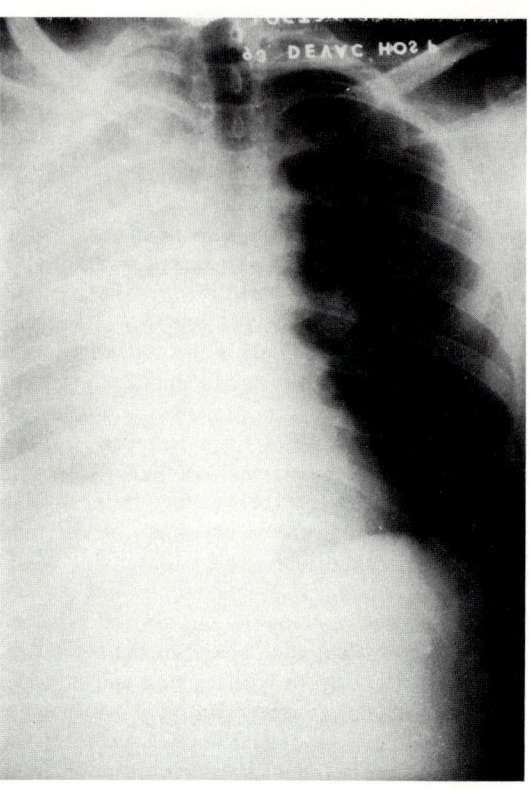

Fig 17-4. Restrictive right fibrothorax following incomplete drainage of a hemothorax.

will cause splinting and poor excursion of the chest wall. The pleural space of a 70 kg man will accommodate several liters of fluid and, depending upon the size of the hemothorax, varying degrees of hypotension, hypoxia, hypercarbia, and acidosis will be produced.

Approximately 90 percent of hemothoraces are caused by bleeding from the pulmonary circuit—a low pressure circuit of between 20 and 25 mm Hg. The vast majority of these patients will stop bleeding if the lung is promptly and completely reexpanded. This is best accomplished by adequate pleural drainage with a large-bore (40 to 45F) plastic thoracostomy tube placed dependently in the midaxillary line and attached to underwater seal drainage. Early reexpansion of the lung and complete drainage of the pleural space may be augmented by applying suction to the underwater seal. Following drainage of the hemothorax, roentgenograms should be taken periodically to demonstrate clinically unrecognizable sequestration of blood in the pleural space.

Figure 17-3 shows inadequate drainage of a hemothorax due to the use of a small rubber catheter in which clotting took place.

Approximately 10 percent of hemothoraces are caused by bleeding from a damaged intercostal or internal mammary artery. These patients will not respond to adequate pleural drainage. They are easily recognized by refractory shock, despite blood replacement, and persistent bleeding of 100 cc or more of blood per hour from the thoracostomy tube. Such patients require immediate thoracotomy and suture ligation of the bleeding artery.

Blood usually will not clot in the pleural space unless the rate of bleeding is quite rapid. It becomes defibrinated by the respiratory movements and hence remains liquid. It is most important to evacuate completely all of the blood in the pleural space to prevent fibrothorax. If a significant amount is left in the pleural space, the resulting fibrothorax will limit lung, chest wall, and diaphragmatic excursion and may require thoracotomy and decortication to relieve the restrictive defect (Fig 17-4).

In a small percentage of hemothoraces, the blood will not remain fluid but will coagulate. Closed tube thoracostomy will not provide adequate drainage in these instances. In World War II, Burford [9] pioneered the important concept that a clotted hemothorax was a clear indication for early open thoracotomy, complete removal of the clot, reexpansion of the lung, and adequate pleural drainage. Blood retained in the pleural space following chest wounds is also fertile ground for the development of empyema and its debilitating sequelae.

PNEUMOTHORAX

Pneumothorax occurs less commonly than hemothorax after war wounds of the chest. In the report from Clark Air Force Base Hospital [19] on the intermediate care of 476 patients with chest injuries from Vietnam, there were 25 patients with pneumothorax (6 percent); however, there were 331 patients with hemopneumothorax (69 percent). The pleural air in pneumothorax may come from a penetrating wound in the chest wall or from an air leak from injury to the underlying lung. If the air leak persists, the lung will collapse completely, causing moderate respiratory distress. If a one-way ball valve leak occurs from the lung or chest wall, tension pneumothorax will develop with a shift of the mediastinum to the contralateral side, compressing the contralateral lung (Figs 17-5, 17-6) and precipitating severe respiratory distress. *Tension pneumothorax is a lethal lesion unless promptly decompressed.* The temporary expedient of thoracentesis in the second intercostal space midclavicular line will relieve the tension. During evacuation of the patient prior to definitive treatment, continuing temporary decompression of the pleural space is achieved by leaving the needle in the space indicated, holding it there by a hemostat securely taped flush to the chest wall. Again, a flutter valve can be constructed with a rubber glove finger split on the end and tied to the thoracentesis needle hub. Definitive treatment is best accomplished with a large-bore (40 to 45F) thoracostomy tube placed in the second intercostal space midclavicular line and attached to underwater seal and suction. With the patient in a semi-Fowler's position, the second intercostal space is as high as the apex of the pleural space. This tube placement will achieve complete removal of air, full expansion of the lung, and abutment of the parietal and visceral pleuras, in turn causing

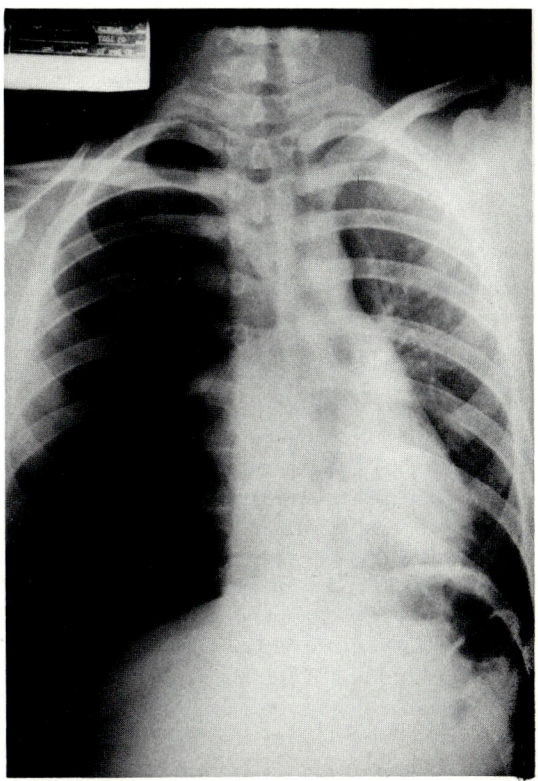

Fig 17-5. *Chest roentgenogram shows widened intercostal spaces, shift of the mediastinum to the left, and depression of the right hemidiaphragm due to tension pneumothorax.*

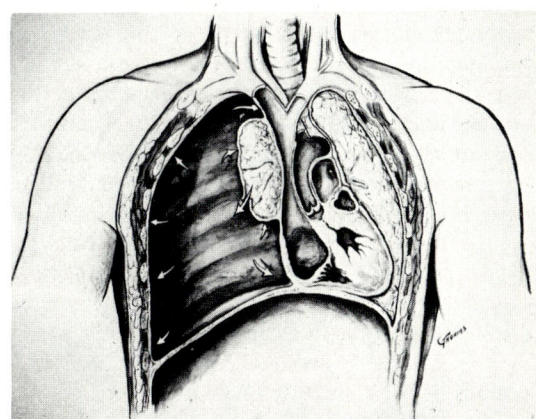

Fig 17-6. *A tension pneumothorax with a one-way ball valve leak from the injured lung. The increased intrapleural pressure has depressed the right diaphragm and displaced the mediastinum to the left, compressing the contralateral lung.*

early pleural symphysis and sealing of the air leak.

Persistent excessive air leakage, continuing pneumothorax associated with hemoptysis, respiratory distress, or significant mediastinal emphysema, signal injury to a major bronchus or to the trachea. The site of injury can be localized by bronchoscopy. A persistent excessive air leak is an indication for thoracotomy and repair of the defect, or if the injury is too extensive for repair, it may be managed by resection.

SUCKING WOUNDS OF THE CHEST

Sucking wounds of the chest, also termed *open pneumothoraces,* are caused by penetrating injuries that expose the pleural space to atmospheric pressure. All such penetrating wounds are potentially sucking wounds, particularly if they are large. Lesions located on the anterior or medial chest wall where the extracostal musculature is sparse tend to cause communication with the atmosphere, as compared to posterior wounds. This is due to the protection afforded by the thick muscle layers posteriorly. Some wounds are of the sucking variety only when the skin and muscle layers are in a certain alignment. Penetrating injuries inflicted by missiles traveling in an oblique trajectory are less likely to cause a sucking wound than those that enter at right angles to the chest wall.

Penetrating wounds of the chest cause pneumothorax, hemothorax, and paradoxical motion of the mediastinum (Fig 17-7). If the defect is larger than the glottic opening, more air will move through the site of injury, causing severe respiratory insufficiency and death. These physiological changes can be reversed by sealing the opening in the chest wall with a large occlusive dressing applied over vaseline gauze and draining the pleural space to remove the air and blood (Fig 17-8). Before sealing the wound, much of the air and blood can be drained by having the patient perform the Valsalva maneuver. Following this, the defect is sealed with hand pressure on the dressing while the patient breathes. This procedure is repeated as necessary. Since all penetrating wounds of the chest may be or may become sucking wounds, they should be treated initially with an occlusive dressing. In patients with extensive injuries, pleural drainage should be established as early as possible, and these patients should be given priority for helicopter evacuation to the most forward surgical hospital.

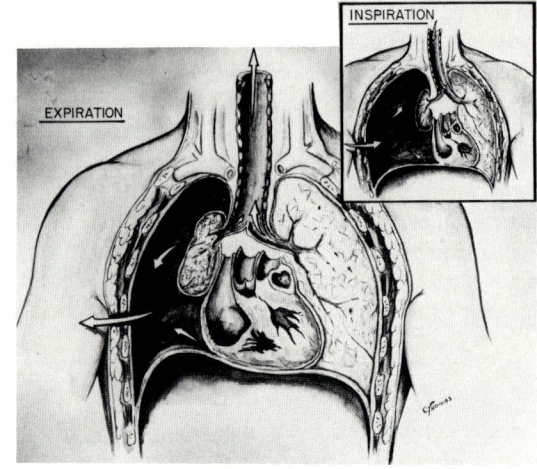

Fig 17-7. *Sucking wound of the chest with mediastinal flutter. When the patient breathes in, air is drawn through the wound into the pleural space, shifting the mediastinum to the left, and when he breathes out, air exits through the wound, shifting the mediastinum to the right, both shifts interfering with ventilation of the contralateral lung.*

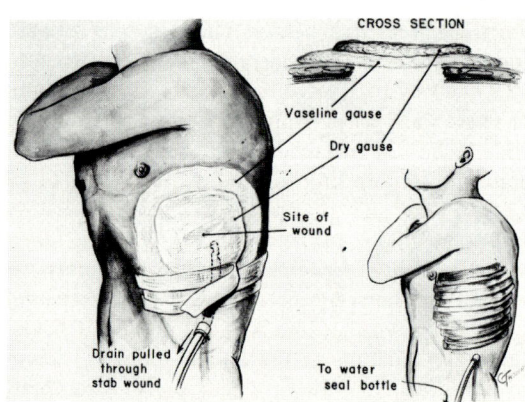

Fig 17-8. *Emergency dressing for sucking wound of the chest uses a large occlusive dressing and establishes pleural drainage with a thoracostomy tube to underwater seal.*

At operation, all nonviable tissue is debrided, rib fragments are removed, injured rib ends are smoothed, the wound is irrigated with copious quantities of saline, and the chest wall is closed. The skin is left open for delayed primary closure, unless the wound is relatively clean and the patient is seen early. The pleural space is properly drained with large-bore thoracostomy tubes attached to underwater seal and suction.

Many large defects of the chest wall can be closed by using a relaxing incision, rib shingling, or turning muscle or skin flaps. To prevent necrosis tissues must be approximated without significant tension. To stabilize respiratory function, it is imperative that adequate closure be obtained and it is far better to achieve this by using adjacent normal tissues. In massive defects with extensive tissue loss with which the above methods will not suffice, the defect should be meticulously debrided and irrigated, adequate pleural drainage established, and closure obtained by using coarse weave Marlex mesh, followed by loose suturing of the skin. We have used this technique successfully in 4 severe chest wounds that were relatively clean and seen soon after they had been inflicted. Such patients must be maintained, as indicated, with suitable broad spectrum antibiotics and appropriate pleural drainage for a longer period. When the chest wall is unstable after repair and there is significant paradoxical motion, insert an endotracheal tube or perform a tracheostomy. Then aerate the lungs by using a volume respirator with mild hyperventilation until the chest wall stabilizes.

"Traumatic thoracotomy," as advocated by Churchill [11] in World War II, may be done through a large chest wall defect or by extending the defect. Accessible foreign bodies, bone fragments, and blood clots are then removed. Damage to the underlying lung is repaired by removing detached nonviable parenchyma. Significant air leaks and bleeding points should be controlled with absorbable sutures. Because of its amazing recuperative powers *conservatism* must be the rule in excising damaged pulmonary tissue.

It was thought that chest injuries from high-velocity missiles (over 2500 ft/sec) in Vietnam might require many more pulmonary resections but, to date, this fear has not been realized [28]. Pulmonary tissue, due to its great compliance and compressibility, suffers less destruction from high-velocity missiles than the more dense organs. There have been, however, several cases of such missile injury involving a major bronchus in which lobar resection was required for a persistent excessive air leak that did not respond to pleural drainage [26].

A report on 20 patients at Letterman General Hospital and Walter Reed General Hospital described persisting traumatic cavities following wounds from high-velocity missiles in Vietnam

[22]. Ten of these patients required lobar or segmental resection for delayed hemoptysis, pneumothorax, or infection; Geiger [14] emphasizes the importance of obtaining bronchograms on patients who have had persisting traumatic cavities prior to judging these cavities as closed. Two patients with small cavities of this type but without symptoms have been followed at Brooke General Hospital and resolved without surgery.

Another unusual type of high-velocity missile injury to the chest has been described by Thomas [26] and Geiger [14]. They saw 7 patients in whom the bullet did not penetrate the pleural space. However, the force from the tangential trajectory produced massive contusion and infarction of the underlying lung, as illustrated by the patient in Figure 17-9. These patients were acutely hypoxic, had gross hemoptysis, and on roentgeno-

Fig 17-9. Tangential high-velocity bullet wound of the chest that did not penetrate the pleural space but did produce infarction of the right upper lobe. (Courtesy Brig. Gen. David E. Thomas, MC, U.S. Army.)

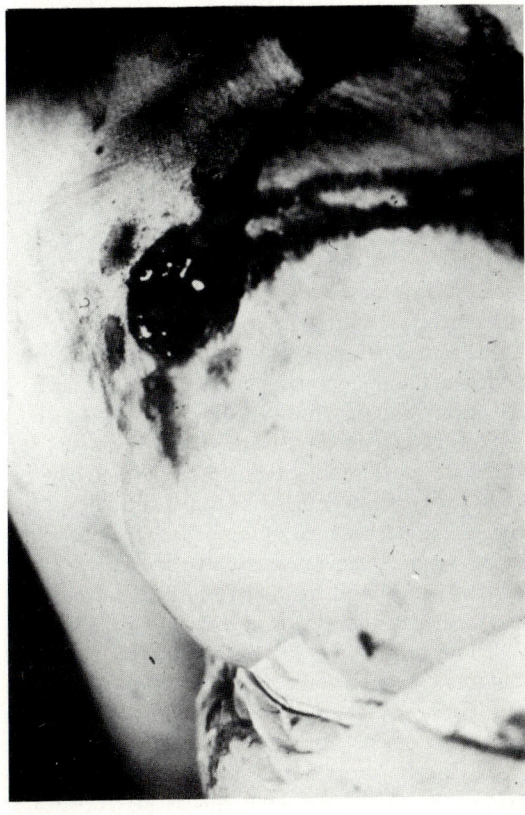

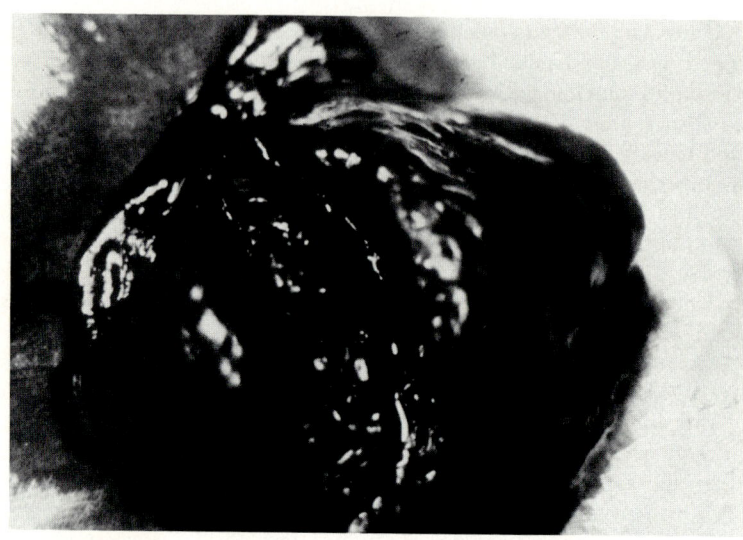

gram showed opacification of the involved lobe. In each instance, lobe resection resulted in dramatic improvement. The resected right upper lobe from one of these patients is shown in Figure 17-10.

Fig 17-10. Same patient as in Figure 17-9. Resected infarcted right upper lobe of the lung. (Courtesy Brig. Gen. David E. Thomas, MC, U.S. Army.)

THORACOABDOMINAL WOUNDS

In World War II, thoracoabdominal wounds accounted for approximately 5 percent of all wounds attributable to battle [3]. A thoracoabdominal wound is defined as one due to a single penetrating missile that causes damage to structures in both the chest and abdomen. In approximately 90 percent of cases the missile enters the chest first, penetrates the diaphragm, and enters the abdomen. With the dome configuration of the diaphragm, penetrating injuries of the lower chest, even with a straight trajectory, may easily cause concomitant abdominal penetration, and abdominal injury should always be suspected when there is lower chest involvement. Wounds of the left chest are more serious than those of the right because of possible damage to the splenic flexure of the colon, stomach, or spleen. Nonetheless, right-sided wounds can cause massive blood loss from hepatic injury and necessitate hepatic lobar resection or hepatic debridement and drainage [14].

Thoracoabdominal wounds represent some of the most severe of all battle injuries and often entail depressed cardiopulmonary function and an acute abdomen. Patients with them should be given high priority for evacuation and should be treated as early as possible and as far forward as possible. The mortality rate increases with the time lag between injury and operative treatment. During World War II, with an elapsed time of 12 hours, mortality was 24 percent; with an interval of 30 hours it increased to 39 percent [3].

In the management of thoracoabdominal wounds, the thoracic component in most instances can be treated with adequate pleural drainage by closed-tube thoracostomy, using 40 to 45F tubes attached to underwater seal and suction. Following stabilization of cardiopulmonary function, the abdominal component of the injury is managed by exploratory laparotomy. It is important that adequate pleural drainage be provided in these patients prior to the administration of closed endotracheal anesthesia for laparotomy. This prevents tension pneumothorax and occult hemothorax from occurring during the exploratory procedure.

If the thoracic component of the thoracoabdominal injury is too extensive to be managed by closed-tube thoracostomies, a formal thoracotomy is done, thereby stabilizing cardiopulmonary function. An exploratory laparotomy through a separate abdominal incision is subsequently performed.

FLAIL CHEST

Flail chest is caused by loss of the bony support of the chest wall due to multiple fractures of several ribs from compression or penetrating injuries. This loss of structural support causes paradoxical motion of the involved segment of the thoracic wall. When the patient breathes in, the increased negative intrapleural pressure pulls the flail segment in, causing interference with aeration of the lung on the injured side. Concomitantly, the mediastinum shifts toward the uninvolved side and compresses the contralateral lung. Flail chest also depresses ventilation by causing splinting due to the severe pain associated with the multiple rib fractures. The summation of these factors is respiratory insufficiency, the extent varying with the size of the flail segment.

Many techniques have been used to help stabilize flail chest. Having the patient lie on the injured side may be employed as a temporary measure and is particularly useful during evacuation. Another temporary procedure that may be applied by the forward medical aidman is fixing the flail segment in the "in position" with a bulky supportive compression dressing.

When the wounded patient reaches a permanent treatment facility, various external traction devices, using pericostal wire sutures or K wires placed under the fascia and attached to two pounds of traction, may be helpful in achieving stabilization. By far the most effective treatment of flail chest (Fig 17-11) is internal pneumatic stabilization using a tracheostomy and volume respirator. The volume respirator is adjusted to provide mild hyperventilation of the patient, the CO_2 level never rising high enough to stimulate respiratory effort. The injured chest wall passively rises and falls with the respirator and chest wall pain is markedly relieved. With this technique there is an improved alignment of the fractured ribs; the flail segment will stabilize enough in several days so that the respirator can be discontinued. If there is a possibility of damage to the underlying lung, pleural drainage to underwater seal by closed-tube thoracostomy should be done prior to placing the patient on the volume respirator. This is done to prevent a possible tension pneumothorax from developing from an air leak from the injured lung.

WOUNDS OF THE ESOPHAGUS

Wounds of the thoracic portion of the esophagus are very rare. This is probably because such injury would usually be associated with damage to the

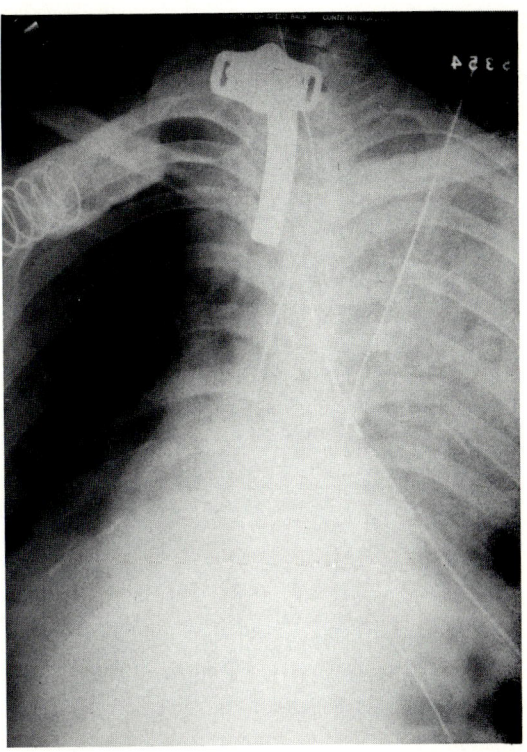

Fig 17-11. Severe flail chest due to multiple fractures of several ribs. Injury was treated with a tracheostomy and a volume respirator.

heart or thoracic aorta, or both, and prove rapidly fatal. In 2267 thoracic and thoracoabdominal wounds treated by the Second Auxiliary Surgical Group in the Mediterranean Theatre in World War II, there were 5 patients with esophageal injury [5]. All five died. Two injuries were repaired operatively and 3 were diagnosed at postmortem examination. In the past 4 years, there have been 3 patients with esophageal injury evacuated to Brooke General Hospital after successful repair of the injury in Vietnam. These patients have continued to do well.

The most common symptom of esophageal injury is substernal discomfort with acute pain in the same area on swallowing. Cervical subcutaneous and mediastinal emphysema are usually present and there is a peculiar nasal twang to the voice, originally described by Boerhaave [13] in his description of spontaneous perforation of the esophagus. As the mediastinitis progresses, clinical findings of toxicity appear and progress rapidly unless immediate thoracotomy is done with repair of the esophagus and transpleural drainage of the widely opened mediastinum by means of large-bore thoracostomy tubes attached to underwater seal drainage and suction. These patients should be given broad spectrum antibiotics and at operation the widely opened, contaminated mediastinum should be well irrigated with copious quantities of saline and, again, broad-spectrum antibiotics. Some patients are so ill they will require respiratory support with a volume respirator postoperatively. The integrity of the esophageal repair should be checked with a radiopaque "swallow" before beginning oral feedings. Removal of the thoracostomy tube is delayed until any possibility of a leak has been ruled out.

WET LUNG

Wet lung (also termed *pulmonary decompensation, shock lung,* or *acute pulmonary insufficiency*) is a multifaceted problem as regards both etiology and treatment. The process was first described in World War II by Burford [8]. It was postulated that wet lung was a specific response to trauma in the form of increased secretions and ineffectual coughing. This concept is supported by the experimental work of De Takats who demonstrated bronchospasm and increased secretions in animals subjected to trauma of the chest wall. Brewer and associates [4] expanded this original concept when they observed wet lung in casualties with severe head and abdominal injuries but without chest injury. Untreated wet lung progresses relentlessly, producing a high morbidity and mortality rate, even when the primary associated injuries are treated successfully. The chief measures employed effectively in its prevention and treatment during World War II were:

1. Stabilization of depressed cardiopulmonary function as early as possible.
2. Maintenance of a clear airway by encouraging vigorous coughing and employing endotracheal suctioning and bronchoscopy when necessary.
3. Relief of chest wall pain with intercostal nerve blocks and frequent small doses of morphine given intravenously.
4. Oxygen administration by nasal catheter or face mask with positive pressure.
5. Prevention of overhydration.

Today the concept of multiple etiology in wet lung has been augmented to include:

1. Hypovolemic shock resulting in increased capillary permeability with transudation of protein-rich fluid into the alveoli and interstitial space and surfactant depletion, which in turn cause decreased compliance and oxygen transfer [21].
2. Pulmonary microemboli due to fat, fibrin, cellular debris, and platelets from severe tissue injury or multiple blood transfusions, or both.
3. Humoral factors or toxins leading to intraalveolar hemorrhage and pulmonary congestion [23].
4. An increase in water and sodium retention due to a stress reaction following injury [17].
5. Endogenous water production following severe trauma [16].

Despite such a multifaceted etiology, the important factor in wet lung is failure of gaseous exchange at the alveolar capillary level. Unless it is anticipated and treated vigorously, the condition will usually progress with confluent areas of consolidation visible on chest roentgenogram (Fig 17-12), hypoxemia, and respiratory acidosis, and eventually death due to respiratory insufficiency.

Wet lung can be recognized early by suspecting it when treating the seriously injured and recog-

Fig 17-12. Chest roentgenogram of a patient with wet lung shows patchy areas of consolidation. (Courtesy Col. James P. Geiger, MC, U.S. Army.)

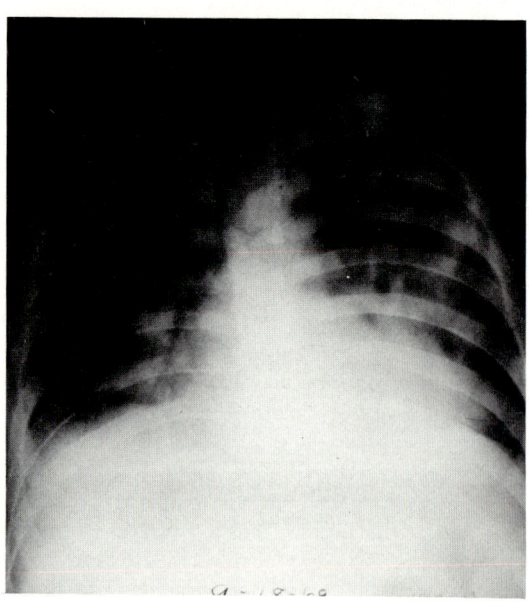

nizing the typical clinical findings of tachypnea, tachycardia, respiratory alkalosis, together with a pO_2 less than 60 mm Hg and a normal central venous pressure. Decreased pulmonary compliance may be one of the earliest findings.

The following regimen has been recommended for the treatment of wet lung [12].

1. Controlled ventilation with intubation and a volume respirator should be used. Blood gases should be closely monitored to reduce the risk of oxygen toxicity.
2. Diuresis should be induced and maintained despite a normal central venous pressure and apparently adequate urine output.
3. Fluid restriction should be instituted during the acute phase (1000 to 1500 ml/day). Administration of as little as 500 ml of saline during the recovery phase has caused a recurrence of pulmonary congestion.
4. Heparin, 3 mg per kilogram of body weight every 24 hours, in divided doses and given intravenously every 4 hours, is unlikely to provoke bleeding from the wounded area. It reduces further platelet aggregation as well as thrombus formation and has an antiserotonin effect, thereby reducing vascular damage. Heparin is also effective in treating hyperlipemia and problems related to fat embolism.
5. Dexamethasone, 12 to 16 mg given at 6-hour intervals in decreasing dosage, is also recommended. This agent appears to prevent further platelet aggregation and augments recovery of capillary and interstitial damage.
6. Pulmonary vascular spasm may be reduced by administration of chlorpromazine and oxygen. The former should be given with caution, using small but frequent doses intravenously (1 to 10 mg every 2 to 4 hours) and titrating dose to effect.
7. Appropriate antibiotic therapy, based on sputum cultures and sensitivity tests, should be given. These patients are very susceptible to pulmonary infection.
8. Sedation helps to allay anxiety and facilitates controlled respiration.

Geiger and Gielchinsky [15], in their very comprehensive report on the treatment of wet lung in Vietnam casualties, successfully treated 21 patients using combinations of the above modalities. They emphasize the importance of using a new filter for each unit of blood administered during resuscitation to reduce the number of microemboli. They also found that sodium-containing fluids and the usual volumes of intravenous or oral fluids would exacerbate wet lung for as long as several weeks following injury. These authors postulate that endogenous water production after massive body wounds may contribute to this sensitivity to fluid administration.

In patients with severe wet lung who are receiving respiratory support on the volume respirator but who have persistent hypoxia, ventilation may be augmented significantly by placing an expiratory retard valve on the expiration part of the respirator. The retard valve raises the resistance to expiration, thereby ventilating atelectatic areas of the lung that are not expanded on inspiration due to air going preferentially to the low-resistance, expanded portions of the lung.

EMPYEMA

Suppuration in the pleural cavity may occur following any penetrating wound of the chest. The incidence of this complication in World Wars I and II was approximately 30 percent [28] and 10 percent, respectively [9]. The sharp reduction was largely accomplished by adequate debridement of chest wounds, early vigorous drainage of hemothoraces by multiple thoracocenteses with prompt reexpansion of the lung, early thoracotomy for clotted hemothorax, and the widespread use of penicillin. In the Vietnam conflict, the incidence of empyema has been in the region of 6 percent [19]. This further reduction in incidence is due to:

1. Early treatment of moderate to severe wounds because of rapid helicopter evacuation (2.8 hours from wounding to the hospital) [28].
2. The use of large-bore thoracostomy tubes attached to underwater seal and suction, providing prompt, complete, and continuing drainage of the pleural space with complete reexpansion of the lung.
3. More effective broad-spectrum antibiotic therapy.
4. Prevention of recurrence of a pleural space by not evacuating a patient for at least 72 hours after removal of a chest tube and obtaining a chest roentgenogram immediately prior to evacuation.

Of the 201 patients transferred from Vietnam to Brooke General Hospital between 1965 and 1970 inclusive, 23 had empyema. A broad approach to therapy was used to achieve adequate pleural drainage and complete obliteration of any pleural space. The modalities employed have been multiple thoracenteses, closed-tube thoracostomy to underwater seal and high suction, open-tube drainage by rib resection, and formal thoracotomy.

Of the 23 patients 10 needed formal thoracotomy for adequate pleural drainage and decortication; 4 of these 10 were operated on because of an acute toxic febrile course, despite the pleural drainage by tube thoracostomy and specific systemic antibiotic therapy for gram negative organisms. Two of these four had infected clotted hemothoraces. The response of the 4 patients with the toxic febrile courses to thoracotomy, decortication, adequate pleural drainage, and reexpansion of the lung was dramatic: the toxicity and fever cleared immediately after surgery.

Two of the 23 subjects with empyema also had bronchopleural fistula. One of these was small and closed spontaneously with tube drainage. The second required thoracotomy, with decortication, suture closure of the bronchial leaks, and a tailoring thoracoplasty to obliterate the pleural space.

RETAINED METALLIC FOREIGN BODIES

The principles for the management of retained foreign bodies, developed and evolved during World War II, are still used today with little modification. Brewer and Burford [6] reported their experience with 291 cases of retained foreign bodies from the Mediterranean Theatre. There were 252 intrapulmonary and mediastinal foreign bodies and 39 intrapleural. The criteria used for removal are: an object greater than 1.5 cm in size, the presence of irregular sharp edges adjacent to a vital structure, hemorrhage (either intrapleural or hemoptysis), and infection at the site of the foreign body. Patients who required traumatic thoracotomy in forward facilities had easily accessible foreign bodies removed at that time.

These 291 cases were under observation in thoracic surgery centers for periods ranging from 2 weeks to 2 months after injury. Of the 252 with intrapulmonary and mediastinal involvement, there were 4 delayed hemoptyses, 2 secondary in-

trapulmonary hemorrhages, 18 late bronchopleural fistulas, 4 lung abscesses, 2 mediastinal abscesses, and 30 empyemas. This last number represents an incidence of 11.9 percent—an incidence very close to the overall occurrence of empyema in penetrating chest wounds in the Mediterranean Theatre. If empyema is omitted, the incidence of complications in patients with retained foreign bodies in the lung or mediastinum is 11.9 percent; if empyema is included, it is 23.8 percent. In the 39 patients with intrapleural foreign bodies 15 developed an empyema, an incidence of 38.5 percent.

Operative removal of a retained foreign body was based on the previously mentioned criteria and was carried out in approximately one-third of these 291 patients. Fifteen thoracotomies were done for the removal of intrapleural objects and 87 for intrapulmonary or mediastinal objects.

From their experience with these patients, Brewer and Burford [6] concluded that an incidence of significant complications within 60 days of wounding in 15 percent of patients with retained foreign bodies justified their removal. However, since few complications developed earlier than 10 days after wounding they found it advisable to wait until the patient could be evacuated to a permanent hospital with thoracic surgery facilities unless there was a clear indication for earlier intervention.

During the Korean conflict, Valle [27] removed 104 retained foreign bodies, basing his decision for removal on the criteria cited. Thirty-eight were from the chest wall, 35 from the lung parenchyma, and 31 from the pleural space. These patients recovered without difficulty and were returned to duty. There were 23 patients admitted to the hospital who had had thoracotomies performed in forward areas solely for the removal of a foreign body. The incidence of empyema in this group was 35 percent and further supports the conclusion that foreign bodies should be removed at a fixed installation if possible.

Of the 201 patients with chest injuries evacuated to Brooke General Hospital from Vietnam, 45 had retained metallic foreign bodies. In 11 of these patients the foreign bodies were intrapulmonary or mediastinal and met the criteria for removal. Six were removed because of size greater than 1.5 cm with irregular sharp edges and adjacent to vital structures; 3 were associated with empyema; 1 had an accompanying persistent bronchopleural fistula; and 1 had caused recurrent hemoptysis.

Multiple view roentgenograms, fluoroscopy, and arteriograms were the most useful diagnostic aids in locating the foreign bodies preoperatively. The Berman locator helped in pinpointing deeply situated objects during operation. Cultures on all of these foreign bodies were taken intraoperatively and proved uniformly negative, except those associated with empyema.

WOUNDS OF THE HEART AND GREAT VESSELS

It is rare for a patient with a major wound of the heart or great vessels to reach a medical facility alive, despite rapid transport by helicopter, although those with smaller wounds may do so [16]. Patients with penetrating wounds whose pathway might involve the heart or great vessels,

Fig 17-13. Technique of paraxyphoid pericardiocentesis for diagnosis and temporary treatment of cardiac tamponade. The treatment of choice for cardiac tamponade following a penetrating wound of the chest is thoracostomy, repair of the wound of the heart, and wide drainage of the pericardium transpleurally.

or a missile overlying the cardiac silhouette as determined by multiple view roentgenograms, should be watched closely for evidence of cardiac tamponade or refractory shock.

Cardiac tamponade results from blood accumulating in the fibrous, unyielding pericardial sac and hindering diastolic filling of the heart, particularly in the right ventricle. This results in a decreased stroke volume and decreased cardiac output. Compensatory mechanisms are increased heart rate and an elevated central venous pressure.

Pericardiocentesis (Fig 17-13) is usually diagnostic as well as being temporarily therapeutic in cardiac tamponade. Another temporary expedient in the emergency treatment of this condition is intravenous infusion of colloid to expand the plasma volume and raise the venous filling pressure, thus temporarily augmenting cardiac output.

The treatment of choice for cardiac tamponade is immediate thoracotomy and decompression of the pericardial sac by removal of blood and clot, followed by repair of the cardiac wound [24, 25]. The techniques for suturing a penetrating wound of the ventricle—a tamponading finger applying pressure, the placing of transverse mattress sutures deep to the coronary vessels for wounds adjacent to these vessels, and the use of a partial occlusion clamp for wounds of the atrium and great vessels—are illustrated in Figure 17-14. Sauerbruch's

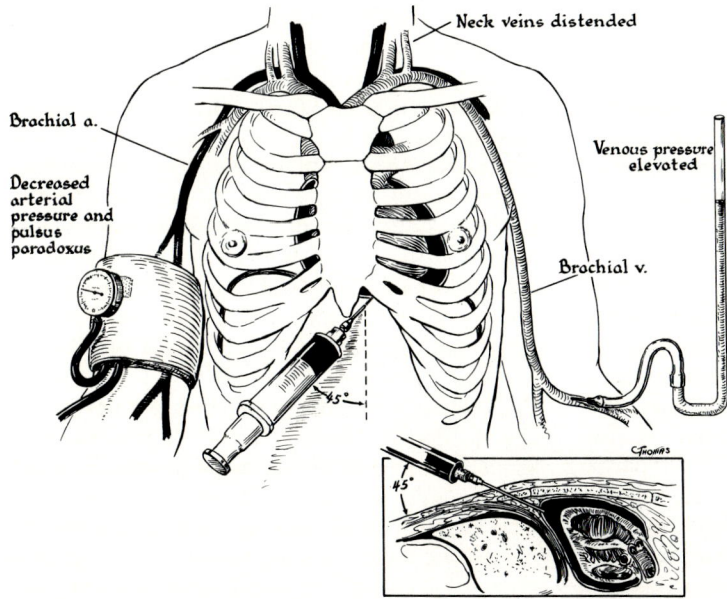

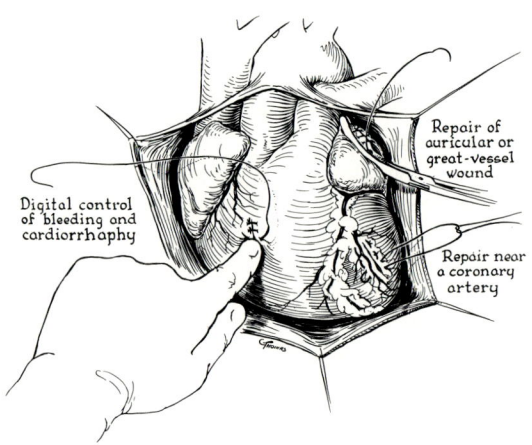

Fig 17-14. *Closed techniques for repair of penetrating wounds of the heart.*

grip for temporary occlusion of venous inflow to the heart may be useful for brief control of massive bleeding until the injury can be localized.

Wounds of the heart in which the pericardium remains open and drains freely present a different clinical picture from cardiac tamponade. Heavy blood loss dominates the clinical picture and with this type of wound there is severe refractory shock with a massive hemothorax. Blood replacement should be instituted immediately with volume expanders and low titer O blood, ventilatory support given, and the patient taken to surgery for emergency thoracostomy.

Any patient with a penetrating wound of the chest who does not respond to the usual resuscitative measures should be suspected of having injury to the heart or great vessels. In such instances appropriate therapeutic measures should be undertaken immediately.

Although contusion of the myocardium is the most common injury to the heart seen in civilian practice and is usually sustained with steering wheel compression of the chest in automobile accidents, no account of thoracic war wounds would be complete without emphasizing this subtle entity. Whenever a significant compression or deceleration injury to the chest occurs, contusion of the heart muscle should be suspected and an electrocardiogram taken.

Clinically, cardiac contusion may become apparent with a pericardial friction rub or an irregular pulse, commonly in the form of premature ventricular contractions or occasional runs of ven-

tricular tachycardia. The ECG changes most frequently seen are flattening or inversion of the T wave, decreased voltage of the QRS, and ST segment depression. These patients should be managed in the same manner as those with a myocardial infarction, and in severe contusion only the most urgent coexisting traumatic lesions should be dealt with surgically. If signs of congestive failure appear, the patient should be given digitalis. Intravenous lidocaine is the best drug for suppressing ventricular irritability, although more recently Inderal has proved to be effective in suppressing refractory ventricular irritability.

Severe compression injury may also cause tears of the heart valves and subvalvular structures, producing valvular insufficiency [10]. These injuries are rare but if the cardiac decompensation can be controlled with medical therapy during evacuation they can later be treated successfully with plastic repair or, more commonly, prosthetic valve replacement at the general hospital level.

There have been 32 asymptomatic patients with retained metallic foreign bodies in the vicinity of the heart evacuated to Brooke General Hospital from Vietnam. Based on experience gained from the implantation of myocardial pacemaker electrodes over the past 10 years, metallic foreign bodies are well tolerated in the wall of the ventricles in the absence of infection. The criteria for the removal of these fragments are: the presence of symptoms, infection, size and configuration of the fragment, proximity to vital structures, potential for embolization, and recurrent pericarditis. When there is an indication for removal, many of these fragments can be extracted using closed heart techniques; they are best treated, however, at the general hospital level where cardiopulmonary bypass facilities are available. Associated valvular injuries and intracardiac shunts can also be more successfully treated at this level [20].

ACKNOWLEDGEMENTS

The authors would like to express their appreciation to Brigadier General David E. Thomas, MC, and Colonel James P. Geiger, MC for their editorial comments.

REFERENCES

1. Allen GI: Personal communication, 1973
2. Artz CP, Bronwell AW, Sako Y: Experiences in

the management of abdominal and thoraco-abdominal injuries in Korea. Am J Surg 89:773, 1955

3. Brewer LA III: Thoraco-abdominal wounds. Thoracic Surgery. Washington, D.C., U.S. Government Printing Office, 1965, vol. II, p. 101

4. Brewer LA III, Burbank B, Samson PC, et al: The "wet lung" in war casualties. Ann Surg 123:343, 1946

5. Brewer LA III, Burford TH: Special types of thoracic wounds. Thoracic Surgery. Washington, D.C., U.S. Government Printing Office, 1965, vol. II, p. 3

6. Brewer LA III, Burford TH: Management of retained intrathoracic foreign bodies. Thoracic Surgery. Washington, D.C., U.S. Government Printing Office, 1965, vol. II, p. 325

7. Burford TH: Evolution of clinical policies in the Mediterranean Theater of Operations. Thoracic Surgery. Washington, D.C., U.S. Government Printing Office, 1963, vol. I, p. 185

8. Burford TH: Wet lung. Thoracic Surgery. Washington, D.C., U.S. Government Printing Office, 1965, vol. II, p. 207

9. Burford TH: Hemothorax and hemothoracic empyema. Thoracic Surgery. Washington, D.C., U.S. Government Printing Office, 1965, vol. II, p. 237

10. Charles KP, Davidson KG, Miller H, et al: Traumatic rupture of the ascending aorta and aortic valve following blunt chest trauma. J Thorac Cardiovasc Surg 73:728, 1977

11. Churchill ED: The surgical management of the wounded in the Mediterranean Theater at the time of the fall of Rome. Ann Surg 120:268, 1944

12. Commander-in-Chief, Pacific. Fourth Conference on War Surgery. Tokyo, Japan, 1970, p. 22

13. Editorial. The Boerhaave syndrome. JAMA 187:57, 1964

14. Geiger JP: Personal communication, 1975

15. Geiger JP, Gielchinsky I: The treatment of acute pulmonary insufficiency in Vietnam casualties. (In press)

16. Gielchinsky I, McNamara JT: Cardiac wounds at a military evacuation hospital in Vietnam. J Thorac Cardiovasc Surg 60:603, 1970

17. Gump FE, Kinney JM, Iles M, et al: Duration and significance of large fluid loads administered for circulatory support. J Trauma 10:431, 1970

18. Heaton LD, Hughes CW, Rosegay H, et al: Military surgical practices of the United States Army in Vietnam. Curr Probl Surg November 1966

19. Patterson LT, Schmitt HJ Jr, Armstrong RG: Intermediate care of war wounds of the chest. J Thorac Cardiovasc Surg 55:16, 1968

20. Rayner AVS, Fulton RL, Hess PJ, et al: Posttraumatic intracardiac shunts. J Thorac Cardiovasc Surg 73:728, 1977

21. Skilman JJ, Lawler DP, Hickler RB, et al: Hemorrhage in normal man. Ann Surg 166:865, 1967

22. Spees EK, Strevey TE, Geiger JP, et al: Persistent traumatic lung cavities resulting from medium and high velocity missiles. Ann Thorac Surg 4:133, 1967

23. Stallone RJ, Lim RC, Blaisdell FW: Pathogenesis of the pulmonary changes following ischemia of the lower extremities. Ann Thorac Surg 7:539, 1969

24. Symbas PN, Harlaftis N, Waldo WJ: Penetrating cardiac wounds: A comparison of different therapeutic methods. Ann Surg 183:377, 1976

25. Szentpetery S, Lower RR: Changing concepts in the treatment of penetrating cardiac injuries. J Trauma 17:457, 1977

26. Thomas DE: Personal communication, 1973

27. Valle AR: Management of war wounds of the chest. J Thorac Surg 24:457, 1952

28. Whelan TJ Jr, Burkhalter WE, Gomez A: Management of war wounds. Adv Surg 3:227, 1968

18. PULMONARY COMPLICATIONS OF NONTHORACIC TRAUMA, INCLUDING BURNS

Robert J. Flemma
Richard J. Thurer
Charles F. Reuben

And this is the true rule by which those who analyze natural effects must proceed; and although nature begins with the cause and ends with the experience, we must follow the opposite course, namely begin with the experience and by means of it investigate the cause.

LEONARDO DA VINCI

The effect of trauma on the lungs was first described by Burford and Burbank [17] as the "wet lung syndrome." Since then the same pathological findings have been referred to as postperfusion lung, autologous blood syndrome, respirator lung, shock lung, congestive atelectasis, Da Nang lung, adult hyaline membrane disease, and adult respiratory distress syndrome. Each of these synonyms attempts to describe what was seen in the lungs at postmortem examination following massive trauma of varying etiology. In this chapter an attempt will be made to present the relevant information currently available and thereby establish a unifying concept of the underlying pathophysiology that at present seems the most acceptable.

Pulmonary insufficiency was often recognized as the final common mechanism in patients dying after a variety of problems, including shock of all etiologies, nonthoracic trauma, burns, or some other extrapulmonary traumatic process. The fate of a patient frequently hinges on the reaction of the lung to these various insults, the degree of respiratory insufficiency tolerated, and the success of the treatment applied. With this in mind, it may be said that the lung is the "end organ of shock" in man. In an attempt to unify this heterogeneous array of seemingly unrelated topics, a pathological as well as a clinical definition of the condition is necessary. Pathological descriptions may vary but certain basic findings are the same, despite the varying preceding events. The variances are accounted for by the particular stage of the process at which the specimens are examined as well as the duration of illness, the area of lung sampled, or the study technique used.

PATHOLOGY

In patients with this syndrome the lungs are heavy, weighing between 1,000 and 2,000 grams. They are usually dark red with focal zones of collapse and parenchymal hemorrhage. At first the ecchymotic areas are often scattered throughout the lung. Later the appearance of deep congestion becomes more confluent, often with crepitations, and a definite increase in the consistency of the lung parenchyma is noted. When the lung is transected, the cut surface bulges, showing a marked discoloration consistent with "hepatization." All major vessels are found to be patent with no evidence of pulmonary emboli or thrombi. The tracheobronchial tree is also patent and, at most, contains only modest amounts of secretions.

Microscopically, this process is seen to be primarily interstitial with secondary alveolar involvement (Fig 18-1A). In the early stages there are patchy zones of hemorrhage. The extravasated blood collects around the smaller arterioles with signs of capillary congestion and increased numbers of polymorphonuclear leukocytes. The interstitial hemorrhage progresses to involve greater areas. Schramel and co-workers [78] describe larger vessels and bronchi surrounded by sheets of red blood cells, which they believed had dissected along the perivascular planes. They also attributed the source of this bleeding to the disrupted walls of medium-sized veins and arteries.

At the same time, an edematous change takes place in the alveolar walls with thickening and broadening of the intervening septae. Neville and associates [61] have described this in association with swelling of the epithelial and adjacent endothelial basement membrane, resulting in turn in a thickened blood-air barrier. In addition, they have noted a thickening of the endothelium of many of the capillaries.

Another component of this septal thickening is described by Cederberg and colleagues [19],

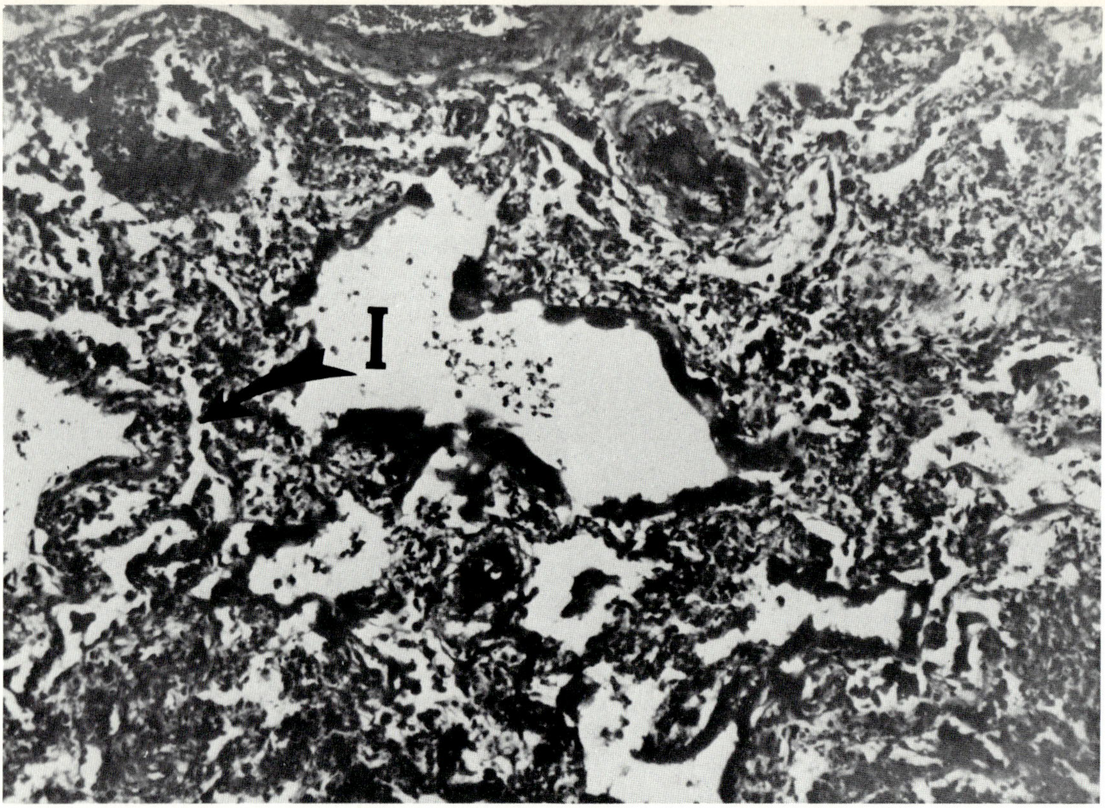

A

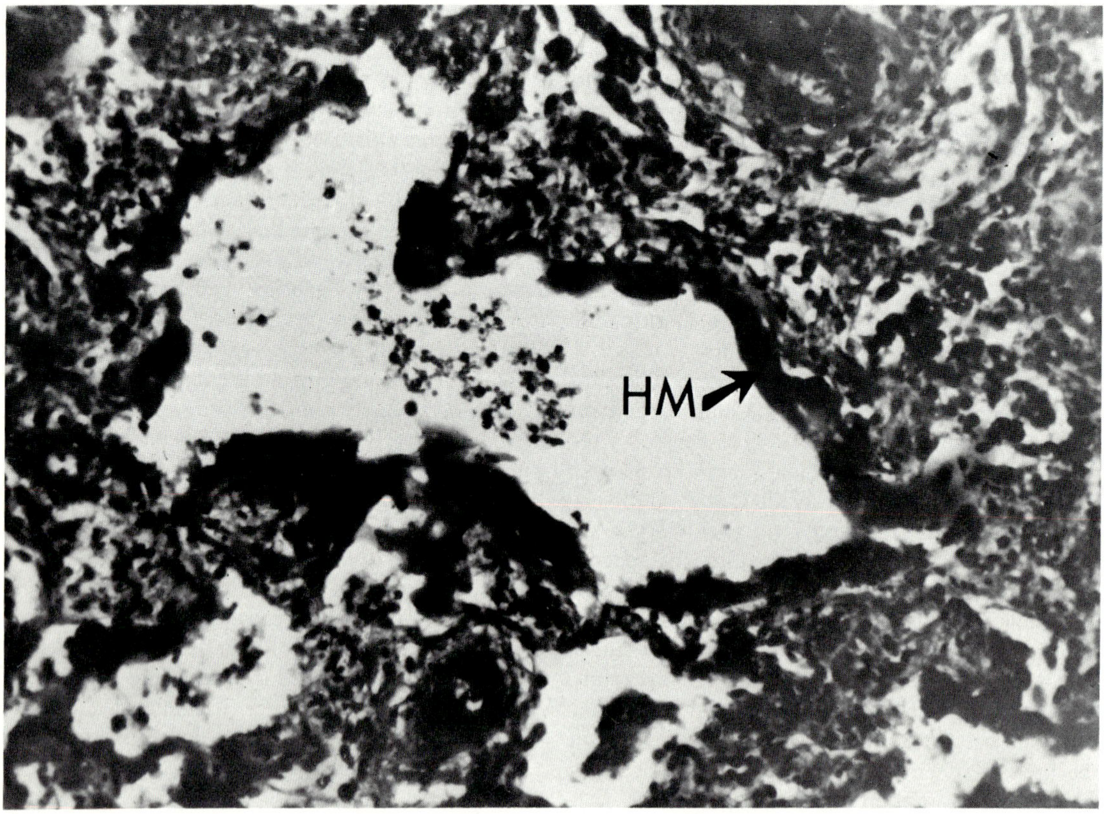

B

Nash and associates [60], Pratt [69] and others in relation to additional materials within the interstitial spaces seen particularly after excess oxygen therapy. A definite fibroblastic proliferation occurs, together with a deposition of reticulum and loose fibrillar collagenous material. This is *not* to be confused with the dense collagenous response seen in an organized pneumonia. There is often also an increase in the number of alveolar phagocytes or macrophages.

Evidence of intra-alveolar exudates is frequently present but appears to be a secondary event. A microscopic finding of interest is the characteristic and striking deposition of fibrin along the inner walls of the alveoli, alveolar ducts, and respiratory bronchioles. This layered fibrin exudate is known as a hyaline membrane (Fig 18-1B) and has been seen by many authors [11, 18, 19, 24, 36, 41, 43, 50, 77, 79, 82, 88] in a variety of conditions including uremia, rheumatic fever, radiation poisoning, and other toxic processes as well as the respiratory distress syndrome of the newborn. It comprises an eosinophilic, periodic acid-Schiff (PAS) positive-staining membrane lining the alveolar walls. Using electron microscopy, Neville and associates [61] and others have shown that this membrane corresponds to a granular, moderately dense precipitate, with the structural features of coagulated plasma proteins. Comparable studies by Van Breeman, Neustein, and Bruns [88] and the fluorescent antibody investigations of Gittin and Craig [36] have further classified the membrane as closely packed layers of fibrin. Many authors have regarded the edema and formation of the hyaline membrane as an early exudative phase in patients who subsequently died within a few days. Furthermore, they believe that this is succeeded, in those who survive longer, by fibroblastic proliferation with collagen deposition and interstitial thickening.

Electron microscopic study has revealed a fairly consistent finding in patients dying with the adult respiratory distress syndrome: alveolar lining epithelial cells are transformed into a cuboidal epithelial lining; interstitial edema and a proliferative reaction of the connective tissue elements are also described. (These are similar to the findings seen in oxygen toxicity.) The epithelial barrier is increased by a factor of 4.5. This is likely related to hypertrophy of the cuboidal Type II epithelial cells that are therefore believed to play an important role in the repair process [8].

Pulmonary Edema vs Adult Respiratory Distress Syndrome

At this point, it is important to stress a crucial aspect of the syndrome under discussion, namely, that there is a real and significant difference between this type of lung problem and the more familiar pulmonary edema. The pathological findings described above provide one way of distinguishing the two. The clinical description presented below, along with the roentgenographic aspects, are also key points in definition (Table 18-1). The differentiation between this lung picture and that of frank pulmonary edema (which may also be present to a lesser extent) is important, not only in terms of pathophysiology, but also in regard to the subsequent clinical course, mode of treatment, and ultimate prognosis.

CLINICAL FEATURES

Clinically, the syndrome usually first appears during the first few days after injury. The onset may be insidious, with restlessness and irritability. The patient exhibits progressive and severe dyspnea, tachypnea, cyanosis, and the thoracic cage retracts on inspiration. Surprisingly, there is, as a rule, no history of previous respiratory disease, and when pulmonary function studies are performed after recovery there are frequently no demonstrable residual effects [23, 53, 87].

The chest may contain coarse breath sounds. The patient becomes progressively cyanotic and does not improve with administration of pure oxy-

Fig 18-1. (A) *Photomicrographs of postmortem lung tissue from a patient with the adult respiratory distress syndrome. Low-power magnification shows interstitial exudative process within alveolar septae, with thickening of the alveolar walls and congestion of the arterioles and venules. (B) High-power magnification of the same area shows characteristic intra-* alveolar fibrinous deposition appearing as a hyaline membrane (HM). Note that the alveolus proper is relatively spared the main reaction and is only secondarily involved. (Photomicrographs courtesy of the Department of Pathology, St. Luke's Hospital, Milwaukee, Wisc.)

Table 18-1. Diagnostic Features Differentiating Adult Respiratory Distress Syndrome from Pulmonary Edema

	Pulmonary Edema	Adult Respiratory Distress Syndrome
Microscopic picture	Primarily alveolar exudate	Primarily interstitial process
Tracheal secretions	Copious amounts of frothy sputum	Little mucoid secretions
Chest roentgenogram	Hilar congestion	Peripheral fluffy infiltrates
Arterial pO$_2$	Low; due to diffusion block but increases with oxygen therapy	Low; due mainly to shunting and refractory to oxygen therapy
Treatment	Responds well to intermittent positive pressure breathing and diuretics	Requires continuous positive pressure breathing, corticosteroids and diuretics

gen or intermittent positive pressure breathing. The tracheobronchial tree produces little sputum during this process, unlike the frothy secretions seen in pulmonary edema. As the respiratory rate and minute ventilation increase, the pulmonary compliance steadily decreases. The rigid lungs need increasingly greater opening pressures and require up to 60 cm of water or more to maintain adequate tidal volume.

Arterial Blood Gases

Characteristically these patients are hypoxemic with an arterial PO$_2$ as low as 30 mm Hg. These levels continue to drop and are not corrected by the administration of oxygen. The arterial PCO$_2$ is initially low and represents hyperventilation by the patient. However, as the process reaches the terminal stages, the PCO$_2$ rises abruptly to very high levels.

Roentgenographic Findings

Initially the chest roentgenogram may appear to be normal (Fig 18-2A). The first signs appear as a patchy interstitial infiltrate with a somewhat "fluffy" or "snowball" appearance. These infiltrates can be bilateral or located predominantly in a single lobe but are more marked at the periph-

ery. There is relatively little hilar involvement (Fig 18-2B). As the process develops, the areas of infiltration may increase and coalesce, both lung fields appearing almost completely opaque (Fig 18-2C). If the patient survives, resolution takes place, and subsequent chest films appear identical to those taken before the onset of the illness (Fig 18-2D). Of special interest is the fact that while the patient is recovering, the roentgenogram picture improves at a slower rate, thus producing a discrepancy between the patient's clinical appearance and the roentgenographic findings.

Etiology

There are many conditions in which this type of pulmonary problem arises but nonthoracic trauma and shock appear to be among the most frequent. Various reports [4, 6, 16, 38, 40, 57, 69, 70, 80, 90] have related the condition to war injuries, automobile accidents, elective surgery, and so on. Different types of shock have also been implicated, including hemorrhagic, endotoxic, cardiogenic, and septic. It has been clearly shown [11, 19, 48, 60, 68] that oxygen toxicity following prolonged administration of high concentrations of oxygen has produced this syndrome.

Several other factors have been reported as causing the gross and microscopic pathological findings. However, the available data do not establish that all these processes originated in the same type of problem since the information was based on postmortem anatomical studies. Many investigators have reviewed the findings of various series of postmortem examinations and found similar pathological features, especially hyaline membrane formation, in patients suffering from viral pneumonia, rheumatic pneumonia, influenza, pneumonic plague, uremia, radiation poisoning, and miscellaneous thoracic and nonthoracic neoplastic processes [4, 6, 18, 24, 43, 50, 82].

Our own experience has involved patients who were subjected to periods of controlled shock, namely, extracorporeal circulation. There are numerous accounts devoted to "postbypass" or "postpump" lung, and many different etiological theories have been suggested [1, 9, 49, 56, 61, 63, 64, 67, 89]. Using this well-controlled setting, a large volume of information has been obtained that can provide insights into the basic mechanisms involved [66].

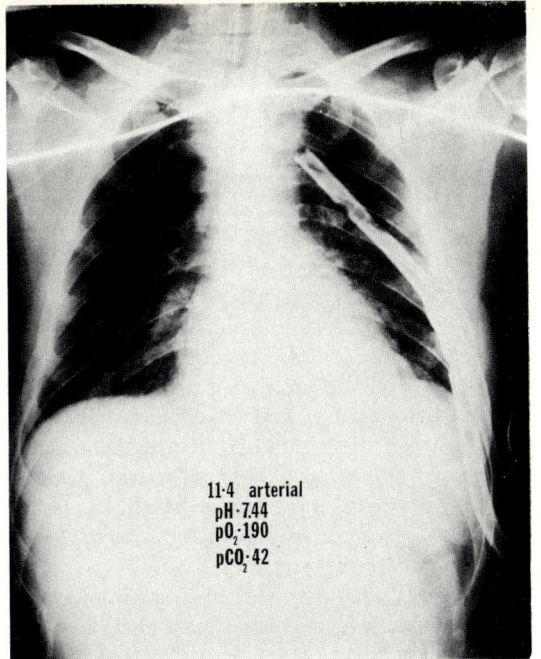

11·4 arterial
pH · 7.44
pO₂ · 190
pCO₂ · 42

A

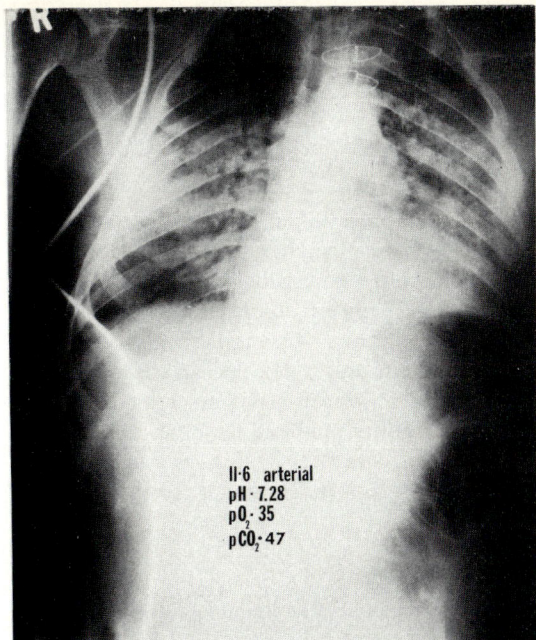

11·6 arterial
pH · 7.28
pO₂ · 35
pCO₂ · 47

B

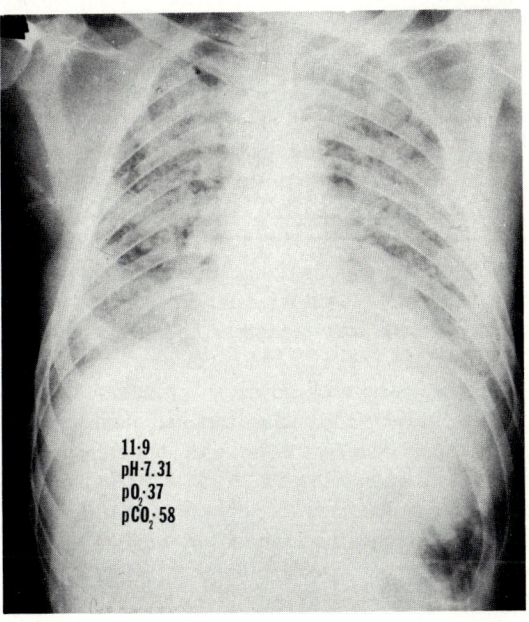

11·9
pH · 7.31
pO₂ · 37
pCO₂ · 58

C

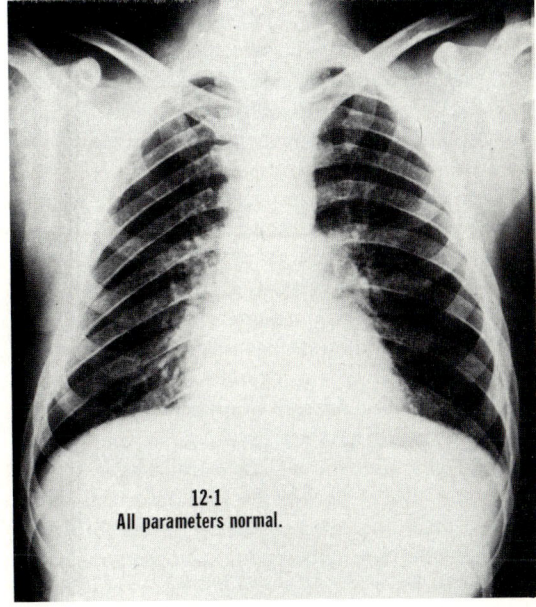

12·1
All parameters normal.

D

Fig 18-2. *Chest roentgenograms of a patient with adult respiratory distress syndrome following cardiopulmonary bypass. (A) Immediate postoperative chest roentgenogram shows the lung fields to be well expanded and within normal limits. Arterial blood gases were normal while the patient was on ventilatory support. (B) On the second postoperative day, evidence of bilateral interstitial infiltrates is seen with patchy appearance. Note fluffy peripheral infiltrates bilaterally. Blood gases revealed marked hypoxemia with minimal CO₂ retention. (C) The chest film on the fifth postoperative day shows marked worsening.*

There is now essentially total lung field involvement with coalescence of these infiltrates. Despite continuous positive pressure ventilation and steroids, blood gases at this time were still abnormal. As is usual, return of blood gas values toward normal preceded roentgenographic improvement. (D) By the twenty-seventh postoperative day, the patient had recovered. The chest film taken then shows almost complete resolution. Blood gases were normal. (Roentgenograms courtesy of the Department of Radiology, St. Luke's Hospital, Milwaukee, Wisc.)

PATHOPHYSIOLOGY

Many of the processes, e.g., shunting and hyaline membrane formation, that lead to and occur in association with the syndrome seem fairly well established. Nonetheless, there are numerous other less obvious factors. The earliest identifiable lesions are probably not the initiating factors themselves but instead represent a final common pathway of injury produced by more obscure antecedent events. These early changes may, however, furnish a direction in the search for the initiating factors.

Interstitial Changes

The earliest identifiable lesion appears as pulmonary congestion with interstitial edema and often hemorrhage. This represents a change in the vascular permeability and even disruption in the continuity of the vessel walls themselves. Henry [40] has pointed out that the end results of the shock state can affect the pulmonary vasculature in two ways: (1) by altering capillary permeability, and (2) by altering the tonicity of the vascular bed. Both of these mechanisms seem to be involved.

Teplitz [85], utilizing electron opaque tracers, has demonstrated that the site of vascular leakage in trauma victims occurs at the capillary level. This is to be distinguished from the protein exudate of inflammatory edema that occurs at the level of the venule. He has shown that "blisters" may form between the endothelium and its thin basement membrane and ultimately rupture. The damaged area may then give rise to the protein exudate characteristic of the early stages of the syndrome. Likewise, Neville and associates [61] believe that increased capillary permeability in patients who have undergone cardiopulmonary bypass precedes the other demonstrable pulmonary changes. Nash and associates [60] have shown similar findings associated with oxygen toxicity.

Veith and colleagues [89, 90] on the other hand, believe that the earliest changes consist of periarterial hemorrhage without capillary congestion. They feel that pulmonary arterial constriction of the small and medium-sized vessels is followed by a secondary vasodilatory phase. This reaction may compound tissue hypoxia or may in itself be a major cause of hypoxia in the pulmonary capillary, thus affecting the integrity of the vasculature in the lung and changing the structure and permeability of the pulmonary bed. The end result is diffuse interstitial hemorrhage and edema.

Still others, such as Berry and co-workers [13], Schramel and colleagues [78], Keller and associates [45], and Kuida and co-workers [46] believe the site of vascular tone to be at the postcapillary venule level, resulting in increased hydrostatic pressure in the capillaries with increased transudation and exudation. Shanklin [79] regarded these pressure changes as a manifestation of left heart failure. However, Jenkins and colleagues [44] have shown that the syndrome can be brought about rapidly and completely with no rise in left atrial pressure.

A review of patients with this syndrome after cardiopulmonary bypass has shown that they exhibit a low cardiac output as manifested by low blood pressure, elevated central venous pressure, lower pulse pressure, and increased arterial-venous oxygen saturation differences. These episodes usually precede roentgenographic evidence of abnormality but often occur during hypoxic periods (after the process has begun); thus left heart failure, at least in this patient population, seems to represent an effect and not a cause of the pulmonary insufficiency [87]. Similarly, the work of Henry and associates [41] has shown that lung changes following shock are due primarily to intrinsic processes within the pulmonary parenchyma and are not secondary to left ventricular failure.

Another aspect of intrinsic processes is fluid overload aggravating the vascular damage and permeability changes. After the hypovolemic period found in patients in shock, a period of hypervolemia often ensues. Significant volumes of fluid are frequently required by trauma victims due to loss of vascular integrity, sequestration, and other processes. Overly vigorous fluid therapy can be hazardous in a situation in which a vascular bed has been previously insulted by poor perfusion, hypoxia, and so on. Jenkins and colleagues [44] noted such fluid overload as a major contributing factor in the congestive atelectasis seen in posttrauma patients and felt that fluid *restriction* should be employed. Mills [57] has also stressed a more conservative approach to volume administration, especially in the resuscitation of patients in whom there has been a significant period of hypoxia.

Postperfusion hypervolemia after a cardiopulmonary bypass procedure is also a well-established phenomenon. This finding is particularly notice-able since the introduction of hemodilution for priming the pump oxygenator [62]. However, the use of such a system has certain implications as far as fluid balance is concerned. Neville and co-workers [63, 64] have shown that when hemo-dilution is utilized, the perfusate permeates many other areas of the body and sequesters in these areas. Such storage compartments (referred to as the "third space") show marked increases in vol-ume after perfusion. As soon as bypass is com-pleted, a postperfusion hypovolemia occurs with both whole blood and partial hemodilution. Gad-boys and Litwak [31] have attributed this to se-questration of fluids, the lung parenchyma being a major location of this sequestration. Reinfusion of the oxygenator contents may cause the blood volume to return to normal. Component analysis reveals, however, that there is a significant rise in plasma volume and a decrease in red cell mass, a situation analogous to the traumatized patient re-covering from hemorrhagic shock with fluid ther-apy. Later this fluid is mobilized from storage areas and returned to the circulation with a pro-found concomitant hypervolemia.

Patients can be monitored by means of such in-dicators as weight, central venous pressure, he-matocrit, and blood volume. In our experience with cardiopulmonary bypass, patients who were on it who develop this syndrome demonstrate a profound weight gain during the first 5 postop-erative days, and the above findings were encoun-tered with equal frequency whether hemodilution was utilized or homologous blood was the sole priming agent [87]. It appears that excess fluid volume is more of a compounding and aggravat-ing factor than an initiating one.

Hyaline Membrane Formation

The formation of a hyaline membrane is related to exudation. This finding of a granular, some-times layered, fibrin lining of the alveoli, alveo-lar ducts, and respiratory bronchioles is believed by Teplitz [85] to represent protein that has leaked into the alveolus proper. The protein exu-date in the alveoli is cleared slowly while serving as an osmotic force for further loss of fluid and protein from an abnormally permeable microcir-culation. As further water resorption takes place, the fibrinous protein material remains as inspis-sated and possibly air-dried denatured plasma pro-tein. This process may represent a secondary selec-

tive fluid resorption of a previous exudative process.

Capers [18] has studied the relationship be-tween blood transfusions and hyaline membrane disease in adults. He found that 47 percent of one group of patients had had transfusions at some time during the clinical course of the syndrome, usually shortly before death. One patient with aplastic anemia required 192 transfusions over an extended period of time. Special stains showed the hyaline membranes to be markedly and dif-fusely positive for iron. The latter finding was in-terpreted as proof that the material had originated from blood plasma. This may well confirm that the membrane results from a transudative process rather than one of aspiration.

It has been suggested that such a transudative process may not be abnormal in itself, but rather that the process of resorbing this material may be the main problem. Lieberman and Kellog [51] have postulated that the defect is manifested by the inability of the patient to effect lysis of the fibrin deposited on the alveolar membrane. They have demonstrated deficiencies in profibrinolysin (plasminogen) in the lungs of neonates with hya-line membrane disease. MacLeod, Stalker, and Ogston [55] performed assays of lung tissue for fibrinolytic activity in patients with renal failure who have such membranes; they found that the defect was caused by an inhibitor of the substance that activates profibrinolysin. Fleming and col-leagues [28] found similar results in patients with hyaline membranes following radiation ther-apy. Thus, the qualitative difference between pul-monary edema and hyaline membrane disease in adults may be explained on the basis of differences in the fibrinolysin activity in the lungs. The pre-cise nature of the inhibitor of fibrinolysin activa-tion is as yet undetermined.

It is difficult to assess the degree of respiratory embarrassment seen in these patients in relation to the effects of the membrane per se. The mem-brane appears to increase the size of the blood-air barrier and may represent the effects of a relative diffusion deficit. It may also add to the instability of the alveolus and promote atelectasis and resul-tant shunting. With the information presently at hand, it is believed that the formation of the membrane is probably a reversible phenomenon, at least in the early stages, as judged by complete clearing without apparent subsequent respiratory impairment. Furthermore, it appears to play a far less significant role than the shunting that seems to be the cause of the major respiratory difficulties in these patients.

Role of Atelectasis and Surfactant

The problem of alveolar instability resulting in atelectasis and right-to-left intrapulmonary shunting is believed by many to be the main manifestation that must be recognized and reversed if patients who develop this syndrome are to survive. The atelectasis may begin as a patchy process scattered in different areas of the lung. It then progresses to become a more diffuse process, resulting in profound changes in the patient's clinical, roentgenographic, and laboratory status. Among the reasons for this atelectasis may be a compressive effect on the alveoli due to interstitial edema and hemorrhage. It is this type of mechanism that seems implied in the term *congestive atelectasis* referred to by Jenkins and associates [44].

A much more prominent factor in the etiology of atelectasis is alveolar instability following an alteration or destruction of a phospholipid lining material that Lieberman [50] has referred to as the "surface-tension-lowering" substance, also known as *surfactant*. This acellular coating has been the subject of much investigation and its many properties are discussed in detail by Scarpelli [76] as well as others. It is known to be a lipoprotein complex, dipalmitoyl lecithin, and is synthesized in the Type II alveolar cells or granular pneumocytes of the lung. These alveolar cells are extremely active with a very high metabolic rate and hence are quite vulnerable to adverse changes in their milieu. They appear quite dependent upon an adequate pulmonary capillary blood flow to maintain their ability to synthesize surfactant.

The normal pathways for removal of surfactant are not well understood, but phagocytosis and ciliary elimination are two possibilities. Surfactant may also be inactivated by any number of the different materials found within the alveoli during the pathological process. Pattle and Burgess [65] have shown that some lipids such as lecithin, lysolecithin, and Tween 80 may interfere with the normal surface-tension-lowering substance in the lung. Taylor and Abrams [84] and Gardner, Finley, and Tooley [33] have described the elimination of surface activity in alveoli when contact is made with blood or plasma by surfactant. These factors may further increase the tendency toward

loss of the alveolar lining layer during the period when the cells that synthesize surfactant are unable to meet the metabolic demand.

When recovery takes place after the period of insult to the alveolar lining cells, there is another time lag. Alveolar cells are known to have a half-life of approximately 4 to 5 days under normal circumstances. In patients with the metabolic derangements under review this time may be correspondingly shortened. The cellular unit that will ultimately form the surfactant-producing cells may also have been compromised or even destroyed. If the atelectatic alveoli are to reexpand, they must have a new lining of surfactant and this also requires time.

These processes, which prevent or destroy surfactant, thus result in atelectasis due to alveolar instability secondary to surfactant loss. An increased stiffness and decreased compliance of the lung follows. Once the alveoli have collapsed, relatively high opening pressures are required to reinflate them so that ventilation can be distributed to those alveoli that remain free of atelectasis. This difficulty in reopening alveoli merely compounds existing difficulties in further promoting ventilation-perfusion inequalities. The end result of these phenomena is shunting with all its accompanying physiological abnormalities.

Right-to-Left Intrapulmonic Shunting

The shunting of deoxygenated blood across the pulmonary bed appears to have a significant role in causing the profound systemic derangements seen in this syndrome. It has been suggested that such shunting is secondary to precapillary arteriolar constriction, resulting in a divergence of pulmonary artery blood flow directly through anastomotic channels to the pulmonary veins without the benefit of a perfusing capillary system [16]. Likewise, shunting may be due to alveoli being filled with proteinaceous material, causing a relatively nondiffusable barrier.

There are various ways of measuring these shunts. The assessment of alveolar-arterial oxygen tension while the patient is inhaling 100% oxygen is a commonly used method. Dye dilution curves are also employed. Germon, Kazem, and Brady [34] have advocated as yet another means of detection the use of the cardiopulmonogram utilizing ^{131}I-labeled human serum albumin macroaggregates. When significant shunting is suspected because of hypoxemia and hypocarbia with increased alveolar ventilation, the hypoxic component is characteristically found to be refractory to the administration of 100% oxygen. Compensatory mechanisms occur secondary to these blood gas abnormalities. Cardiac output is usually increased to compensate for arterial hypoxemia, yet this may only lead to increased oxygen consumption [16]. Similarly, hyperventilation occurs, as evidenced by a low arterial PCO_2, but this also adds to oxygen consumption.

It is important that the arterial PCO_2 is normal to low until the late stages of the process while the arterial PO_2 remains consistently diminished despite the breathing of 100% oxygen. This situation is best understood in relationship to the oxyhemoglobin dissociation curve and the CO_2 blood dissociation curve. These curves demonstrate that an amount of CO_2 in excess of normal may be lost from a particular aliquot of blood traversing the pulmonary capillary bed. At the same time, a limit is set on the amount of oxygen that a similar aliquot is able to acquire in spite of high arterial partial pressures of oxygen. This is due to the leveling off of the oxyhemoglobin curve at higher PO_2 values. Thus, when shunted blood, which is essentially venous, is admixed to the pulmonary flow that has successfully undergone gaseous exchange, the limited oxygen content of the aerated blood is not sufficient to compensate for the venous oxygen content of the shunted blood. On the other hand, the successful excess desaturation of CO_2 in the blood perfusing the ventilated areas of the lung more than compensates for the hypercapnic status of the shunted blood, the result being arterial normocapnia or even hypocapnea until the late stages of the syndrome when the shunt is of such proportions that even the CO_2 relationship is not compensated for sufficiently. The shunting component of this syndrome therefore takes on great importance as arterial hypoxemia causes compensatory mechanisms to become operable, although these mechanisms are often quite inadequate. This may end in a vicious cycle as the metabolic derangements are further aggravated by inadequate oxygenation.

Final Common Pathway

Lieberman [50] states that the etiology of this syndrome may be summarized by what he calls the "unified theory" of hyaline membrane disease. He refers to three variables as an explanation of this particular spectrum of pulmonary disease in the following order: (1) pulmonary exudations; (2) deficient surface-tension-lowering substance; and (3) deficient fibrinolysis within the lungs. Ashbaugh and colleagues [4] believe that a similar pulmonary response occurs to a variety of different stimuli (such as cardiopulmonary bypass, congestive atelectasis, fat embolism, and sepsis) as a result of a common mechanism of injury. The major events appear to be decreased compliance, refractory cyanosis, and microscopic atelectasis, all of which point to alveolar instability.

Veith and co-workers [90] state that postoperative and posttraumatic factors such as hypotension and homologous blood transfusions can lead to a common vascular reactivity. Replogle, Gazzaniga, and Gross [74] have pointed to the circulatory insult resulting from cardiopulmonary bypass as being analogous in many respects to the circulatory insufficiency of hemorrhagic shock, especially in terms of tissue damage due to inadequate perfusion. Young [92] has also found some similarities between the lungs of animals subjected to hemorrhagic shock and those of human patients after cardiopulmonary bypass. Lesage and associates [49] have stated that "perfusion" lung corresponds to "shock" lung and that the shock is probably of the toxic variety. Finally, Lee and colleagues [48] have questioned whether the "pump" lung or the congestive atelectasis seen after cardiopulmonary bypass is analogous to oxygen toxicity that results in inactivation of surface active material by an unknown circulating inhibitor.

The above considerations suggest the occurrence of a final common pathway to injury of the lung. With this in mind, we must consider the actual initiating factors that begin the chain of events that lead to the syndrome under discussion.

PATHOGENESIS

In view of the complexity of the interactions following nonthoracic trauma and shock, it is doubtful that only a single factor is responsible for the manifestations noted. The numerous etiological possibilities would need a separate book for their complete discussion. Consequently, only the major categories of investigation relevant to this area will be mentioned.

Preexisting Physical Factors

Conditions present prior to injury must be kept in mind. For example, there is a decreased amount of surfactant in bronchial washings from smokers as compared to normal individuals [20]. However, preceding lung disease, as detected by pulmonary function studies, may not be a prerequisite since many patients who develop this syndrome have previously been in good physical condition.

Role of Toxins

Patients with the adult respiratory distress syndrome have sustained tissue injury with concomitant hypoxia. Hypoxia may cause various toxins to be released from tissue cells, blood cells, or other sources not yet identified. Some of the better known of these agents are free hemoglobin, serotonin, bradykinin, catecholamines, homologous blood, bacterial toxins, circulating lysosomal enzymes, surfactant and fibrinolysin inhibitors, altered blood cells or proteins, fibrin microemboli, platelet and blood emboli, and fat emboli.

Extracorporeal Circulation

Many of the elements of hypoxia or pathophysiological changes from hypoxia seem more likely to be involved than others. For example, in extracorporeal circulation, the bypass system itself is often implicated in the pathogenesis of the ULT adult respiratory distress syndrome. Direct trauma to the various blood constituents by mechanical means is one possibility. Further, the abnormal contact of blood and oxygen is another source of damage. The type of oxygenator used has been shown to affect the degree of alteration of the various blood elements, the bubble oxygenator being more traumatic in this way than the disc mechanism. The membrane oxygenator is the least offensive [49]. Veith and associates [89], utilized isolated lung perfusion, venovenous bypass, and total cardiopulmonary bypass, found that a similar pulmonary lesion occurs with all three systems and concluded that the common denominator was blood flowing through an extracorporeal pump gas exchanger system and that this effect is not altered by passage through the systemic capillaries. To a lesser degree, this problem is also encountered with transfusions of blood or plasma to trauma victims.

That damaging toxins circulate under these conditions has been demonstrated by Lesage and associates [49]. These investigators employed a standard bypass system, one in which a homologous lung was placed in series with the pump as a filter, and one system where an isolated lung was intro-

duced into the circuit after the bypass was completed. The homologous lung showed little difference from the other lung in the circuit and therefore did not act as a filter. When the isolated lung was introduced after bypass, the damage present in the lung already in the circuit was reproduced. This provided good evidence of the occurrence of a toxic shock process. Such toxins can also alter the plasma proteins that are ultimately seen in the pulmonary exudates and hyaline membranes found in patients with this syndrome.

Sepsis

Sepsis plays an important, although as yet not completely understood, role in the development of pulmonary insufficiency in a number of clinical settings. There is a direct association between sepsis and acute respiratory failure in patients who have undergone general operations without trauma. Respiratory failure also occurs when a septic focus is present secondary to any cause. The underlying mechanism of pulmonary damage remains obscure, however. Pneumonia, fluid overloading, low serum albumin, and generalized pulmonary capillary damage have been implicated.

Pulmonary capillary damage is the most attractive hypothesis for relating sepsis to respiratory insufficiency. Damage to capillaries with loss of an effective semipermeable membrane leads to protein leakage, reduction in colloid osmotic pressure, and edema formation. Various biochemical processes and functions of the lung—and the lung has many functions other than those related to gas exchange [27]—may be impaired secondary to sepsis. Surfactant production and depression of the pulmonary reticuloendothelial functions may occur, which may predispose to atelectasis and pneumonia.

Bacteria can interact with the lung, producing pulmonary damage. Direct bacterial contact with the pulmonary vasculature may occur but this is by no means necessary for the development of pulmonary damage. It has been shown experimentally that bacterial products, e.g., endotoxin, can induce pulmonary insufficiency. Plasma factors may also be involved.

Platelets play an important role in the development of pulmonary insufficiency in septic patients although their exact role is unclear [91]. Normally platelets pass through the lung with no interaction. Following endothelial damage, platelets become trapped and there is a platelet-endothelial interaction. Stiff lungs trap platelets. Aggregating platelets release serotonin and histamine. These agents initially cause bronchoconstriction in adjacent lung units [14]. Potent clotting stimuli are also present in the form of debris from injured tissue plus stasis of flow in the pulmonary capillaries. This encourages platelet aggregation and intravascular clotting. This is seen in massive tissue injury, sepsis, or atelectasis with stasis of flow in lung segments.

As has been stated, many of the pathological changes seen in the lungs are consistent with changes in vascular permeability. There is intraalveolar fibrin deposition and interstitial, periarterial, and intra-alveolar hemorrhage. Platelet masses block arterioles and hemorrhage occurs when these break up and move distally. A vascular permeability factor has been isolated from platelets. Vasoactive peptides are released when fibrinogen is converted to fibrin and these can also cause bronchoconstriction [14].

Disseminated intravascular coagulation is believed by some to be a frequent complication in patients with severe adult respiratory distress syndrome [15]. These patients have the expected clinical manifestations of disseminated intravascular coagulation with hemorrhage and ischemic necrosis of extremities. Deterioration in pulmonary function was noted with the onset of disseminated intravascular coagulation as evidenced by a fall in compliance and further impairment of gas exchange.

Many patients with pulmonary insufficiency but without disseminated intravascular coagulation had a decrease in circulating platelets during their course. When these patients were examined postmortem, a number had fibrin microthrombi in the lungs. It is felt that pulmonary capillary–endothelial-platelet interaction may be the first step in establishing disseminated intravascular coagulation. The presence of thrombocytopenia in patients without other evidence of disseminated intravascular coagulation but with the adult respiratory distress syndrome suggests that platelet aggregation occurs in these patients. The presence of microthrombi in these patients suggests that intravascular coagulation may be more frequent in these patients than the typical clinical picture of disseminated intravascular coagulation. This limited intravascular coagulation may well be initiated by capillary endothelial damage and perpetuate the syndrome. The liberation of vasoactive substances, resulting in altered capillary permeability, can, at the very least, compound the element of pulmonary edema that is commonly present.

Microemboli

The possibility of microemboli originating from an extracorporeal system seems far less likely as an etiological factor in this syndrome. Such emboli would have to first cross a systemic capillary bed before reaching the pulmonary bed. Evidence of such microemboli has not been seen at postmortem examination in the patients with adult respiratory distress syndrome.

Homologous Blood

It is of interest that the same pulmonary lesions have been demonstrated when homologous as well as autologous blood is used in perfusion, suggesting that these constitute a somewhat questionable etiological point [89]. Attempts at avoiding the homologous blood reaction by means of hemodilution have been proposed [49]. However, patients are found to be equally susceptible to this syndrome after perfusion using hemodilution as well as after perfusion in which whole blood (homologous) was the only priming agent [87].

Lung Injury Due to Hypoxia

Along with circulating toxins, a period of hypoxia and poor perfusion of the lung parenchyma itself is usually present. This aspect appears to be significant in the initiation of the syndrome. Almond and co-workers [1] have recognized three important factors in pulmonary parenchymal injury secondary to hypoxia. These are: (1) pulmonary artery flow; (2) bronchial artery oxygen saturation; and (3) bronchial artery flow. Various investigations utilizing pulmonary artery flow alterations by means of occlusive techniques have shown a delay in the development of gross changes, but following this delay, changes in compliance and pulmonary surfactant activity occur [56]. It is obvious that after pulmonary artery occlusion bronchial artery flow becomes crucial. Such studies further suggest that the origin of the pulmonary difficulties of this syndrome appear to be due at least in part to the metabolic derangements of the lung parenchyma.

As mentioned above, hypoxia of the lung parenchyma may be attributable to inadequate perfusion during periods of hypotension. Another factor may be the pattern of vascular reactivity referred to by

Veith and associates [90]. This reactivity may originate from neural reflex patterns, causing bronchoconstriction with subsequent atelectasis as well as vasoconstriction. Further, hypoxia alone is a vasoconstrictor of the pulmonary arterioles [54]. This constriction phase causes an increase in pulmonary artery pressure and this can promote the divergence of blood through anastomotic shunt channels. At the same time, poor perfusion of the capillary bed ensues with metabolic damage to the endothelium of the vessels distal to the constriction as well as to the alveolar cells. Such derangements cause a change in the permeability characteristics of the vascular bed and may account for the alterations known to occur in the syndrome.

Fat Emboli

Another factor to be considered is fat embolization. Injection of small amounts of oleic acid into the pulmonary artery has resulted in a condition very much like the adult respiratory distress syndrome [7]. A subclinical process of fat embolization may play a definite role in the lung parenchymal damage noted previously. Small emboli may lodge in pulmonary arterioles and capillaries as triglycerides. This aggravates the decreased blood flow, hypoxia, tissue acidosis, and edema in the lung. The particles are then broken down to free fatty acids by the local tissue acidosis and lipases. The consequent irritation causes a local inflammatory reaction with further hypoxia, acidosis, and stasis [5]. The fatty acids may directly affect the phospholipid lining layer of the alveolus and promote further atelectasis.

Oxygen Toxicity

The role played by high oxygen tensions in causing or aggravating the processes under discussion are in question. Their presence during extracorporeal circulation or a similar state may produce inactivation of the surfactant material in the lungs by disorganizing the oxidative enzyme systems of the epithelial cells that may be involved in fatty acid synthesis. Oxygen therapy has been discussed as an added factor in the process of nonthoracic pulmonary insufficiency. Investigations by Morgan and co-workers [58] have shown a significant reduction in surfactant in dog lungs after exposure to pure oxygen for more than 48 hours. In other studies Singer and colleagues [81] and Barber, Lee, and Hamilton [10] have investigated the effects of this type of therapy on patients after open-

heart surgery and on patients with irreversible brain damage. The former study—on patients after open-heart surgery—showed little change after a mean exposure to pure oxygen lasting 24 hours. In Barber's group, however—the patients with brain damage—there was a definite rapid increase in the amount of intrapulmonary shunting after 40 hours. It would seem that more information is necessary for accurate analysis.

The Role of Lysosomes

Perhaps a key component of this syndrome may reside in a subcellular structure known as a *lysosome*. This cytoplasmic structure contains acid phosphatases, esterases, and other enzymes, including acid ribonuclease, acid deoxyribonuclease, cathepsin, and betaglucuronidase, this last having a lipoprotein membrane that protects the cell proper from autodigestion. The lysosomal membrane has been studied by de Duve [21] and found to be susceptible to hypoxia, hemorrhagic shock, endotoxic shock, and various proteolytic agents in that these factors may cause damage to the integrity of the membrane. Replogle, Gazzaniga, and Gross [74] have noted the similarity between the circulatory insult of cardiopulmonary bypass and the poor perfusion of hemorrhagic hypotension and have stated that the ischemia of the pulmonary bed in both instances may result in damage to the lysosomal membane. The acid phosphatases and esterases may then act on various substrates, particularly dipalmitoyl lecithin (surfactant).

An interesting corollary related to lysosomal damage may involve the polymorphonuclear leukocytes. These cells have been observed to be sequestered in the pulmonary vasculature as a result of hemorrhagic shock [73]. The capillaries are particularly affected. This sequestration has also been found after cardiopulmonary bypass, with many of the white blood cells showing close apposition between their plasma membrane and that of the adjacent endothelial cell, a situation common to hemorrhagic shock [92]. The polymorphonuclear leukocytes are known to contain significant numbers of lysosomes in their cytoplasm, presumably related to their inflammatory and phagocytic function. It seems that one mechanism for the development of pulmonary injury secondary to hemorrhagic shock, cardiopulmonary bypass, and so on, may be an inflammatory reaction mediated by the polymorphonuclear leukocytes, although this has as yet to be substantiated.

Pancreatitis

Pulmonary complications of pancreatitis have long been recognized, particularly pleural effusion. Recently the adult respiratory distress syndrome has also been reported in association with pancreatitis. The mechanism of its development is not completely understood but the subject is mentioned here since pancreatitis can be associated with nonthoracic trauma and because the mechanism may be similar to those seen in other clinical settings. Blood enzyme activity, particularly lecithinase, may be increased in pancreatitis. Since a major component of surfactant is lecithin, surfactant activity may be reduced. This can then result in atelectasis. Direct pulmonary damage by enzymes does not seem likely [39].

TREATMENT

The pioneer work of such investigators as Ashbaugh and co-workers [4–6], Pontoppidan [68], and the more recent work of Gallagher and colleagues [32] has enabled us to devise effective treatment in this area without a thorough understanding of the underlying pathophysiology. Therapy is directed toward the congested, collapsed alveoli; loss of surfactant; and the exudation of fluid, albumin, and perhaps destructive enzymes. These defects together lead to respiratory distress because of stiff or resistant lungs and poor oxygen transfer at the alveolar level. Therapy is aimed at maintaining ventilation, oxygenation, and cardiac output to provide time for healing and to marshal therapeutic maneuvers. By aggressive early management of injured patients, it may also be possible to prevent development of respiratory insufficiency [32].

Continuous positive pressure ventilation in the expiratory phase of respiration prevents alveolar collapse and maintains alveolar stability. Adequate oxygenation is assured by utilizing whatever concentration of oxygen in the inspired air is necessary regardless of how high this might be. Increased oxygen does not harm the lung as long as the arterial pO_2 is not increased. The administration of corticosteroids combats alveolar edema by preserving capillary membrane permeability and lysosomal integrity. Infection is counteracted with antibiotics appropriate to the infectious agent indicated by culture studies.

Assisted Ventilation

The major problem in therapy is adequate ventilation. Pressure-regulated ventilators are unsuitable since they do not deliver an adequate volume at the increased intratracheal pressures encountered and they have no therapeutic effect on pulmonary shunting secondary to atelectasis. Volume-cycled respirators are needed to insure that the proper tidal volume is delivered to meet demands. It has been found, however, that intermittent positive pressure ventilation in this syndrome is inadequate for altering the effects of interstitial edema, congestion, and alveolar instability. This is unlike the beneficial effect seen with this mode of ventilation in patients with acute pulmonary edema resulting from left heart failure. The term *intermittent positive pressure breathing* (IPPB) refers to the fact that during inspiration, a positive airway pressure is applied. During expiration, however, the pressure in the airway (transtracheal pressure) falls to atmospheric levels. When this happens, as occurs during the expiratory phase with IPPB, alveolar collapse is permitted and a decreased functional residual capacity occurs. The pressure required to reinflate these alveoli is quite high.

It is for these reasons that continuous positive pressure breathing (CPPB) or positive end-expiratory pressure (PEEP) has been advocated [4, 6, 7, 32]. Both of these procedures comprise the application of positive airway pressure during the expiratory as well as the inspiratory phase of respiration. The theoretical basis for its advantage in situations of loss of surfactant and alveolar instability is that the positive end-expiratory pressure prevents the complete collapse of alveoli and thus improves the functional residual capacity [4, 6]. This then will establish a better ventilation-perfusion relationship and a decrease in shunting. At the same time CPPB promotes a return of the various fluids and exudates in the interstitium of the lung back to the vascular space.

Another advantage of CPPB is that it allows adequate oxygenation with lower oxygen concentrations than would be necessary with other methods. Pressures from 5 to 10 cm of water during expiration have been used with success and, when necessary, end-expiratory pressures of up to 15 to 20 cm of water or higher have been used. The pressures used are individualized for each patient and limitations are established according to blood gas requirements as well as to the degree of impairment of cardiac output. CPPB has been shown to affect the latter [6, 47], and this may be a limiting factor in rare instances. When it has been determined that the blood volume is adequate and yet significant difficulties arise with cardiac output and end-expiratory pressure is required to maintain a minimal arterial oxygen tension, a compromise may be found in the institution of end-expiratory *resistance* instead. This allows a positive pressure to exist during most of the expiratory phase, producing atmospheric levels only at the very end of expiration.

Corticosteroids

The use of steroids in the treatment of shock has long been advocated [52]. As adrenergic blocking agents they improve tissue perfusion, thus reversing some of the vasoconstriction accompanying shock. They also have been shown to increase cardiac output during experimental hemorrhagic shock [59], further improving tissue perfusion.

Steroids, in particular methylprednisolone, have been shown to have a beneficial effect in direct pulmonary trauma when administered shortly after the event [30]. This was shown with experimental pulmonary contusion. The beneficial effect was believed to be due to decreased capillary permeability, stabilization of the cell wall and perhaps lysosome stabilization. A beneficial effect has been claimed for steroids in pulmonary insufficiency associated with other predisposing factors, particularly sepsis [2]. Increased capillary permeability in sepsis was demonstrated and it is suggested that methylprednisolone reduces the transcapillary plasma leak.

Clinical experience has suggested a beneficial effect of corticosteroids in patients with the adult respiratory distress syndrome [25]. Benefit has been seen in patients following massive trauma and more particularly in those with fat embolism. In hemorrhagic shock it has been shown that steroids inhibit the adherence of leukocytes to the pulmonary vascular bed. Surfactant secretion may also be enhanced. In pancreatitis steroids may reduce the circulatory levels of myocardial depressant factor [37].

Extracorporeal Oxygenation

An attractive method for treating patients with pulmonary insufficiency would seem to be prolonged extracorporeal oxygenation. It was hoped that this might be accomplished best by means of extracorporeal membrane oxygenation (ECMO) [35]. Successful use of this method has been reported in a number of clinical situations, including posttraumatic pulmonary insufficiency [42]. Although it is clear that oxygenation can be improved and survival prolonged in certain patients in whom this method is used, it is questionable whether long-term survival rates are improved. Its real usefulness has not as yet been documented, although the recent experience with its use in infants has been encouraging [12]. The proper role, if any, of this modality should be forthcoming in the near future.

PREVENTION

The most desirable way of handling the problems resulting from nonthoracic trauma and shock is prevention. Various investigators, e.g., Sugg, Webb, and Ecker [83], have tried unsuccessfully a number of drugs and experimental procedures in attempts to prevent the adult respiratory distress syndrome. Aside from the proper treatment and monitoring of the patient, the most promising method of prevention appears to be the prophylactic use of corticosteroids as well as enthusiastic use of continuous positive pressure ventilation. Recently an experience has been reported in which aggressive monitoring and treatment with PEEP and intermittent manadatory ventilation (IMV) were applied when the intrapulmonary shunt exceeded 15 percent and before the development of hypoxemia [32]. The result seemed satisfactory. Much has been written about the use of corticosteroids in shock, trauma, extracorporeal circulation, and other similar areas.

One of the mechanisms mentioned earlier in relationship to the etiology of this syndrome is a pattern of vascular reactivity. The initiating factor appears to be a vasocontriction in the precapillary pulmonary arterioles, due either to a neural or hormonal effect or maybe both. Veith and associates [90] have speculated that the pharmacological interruption of this vasoconstriction might prevent the secondary dilatory phase that follows, thus avoiding the diffuse interstitial hemorrhage and edema. This reasoning is supported by the experiences of Lillehei and his colleagues [52].

Steroids have other effects on the cardiovascular system, particularly at the level of the small arterioles, venules, and capillaries. They have a definite beneficial action on the integrity of the small vessels in that in their absence an increase in capillary permeability is noted, as well as an inadequate vasomotor response and a decrease in the cardiac output [86], all of which effects form a prominent part of this syndrome. One of the theoretical bases for the use of steroids is the maintenance of the pulmonary microcirculation.

Another component of the problem is the inflammatory response in the pulmonary bed. It is thought that the early and late manifestations of inflammation are inhibited by steroids. This anti-inflammatory property may be related to a decrease in the permeability of the cell membrane to toxic products, which thus prevents interstitial edema with its resultant changes. These have been stressed by Ashbaugh and Petty [5] in the treatment of respiratory failure associated with fat embolism. In that syndrome steroids can obviate the action of free fatty acids in causing the inflammatory response.

The lysosome and how it functions have already been mentioned as one of the possible initiating factors in this syndrome. It is well known that corticosteroids exert a stabilizing influence on the lysosomal membrane. Since the enzymes contained within this structure interfere with lung surfactant, the use of steroids is again warranted. Replogle, Gazzaniga, and Gross [74] have used assays of beta-glucuronidase to demonstrate this in patients undergoing cardiopulmonary bypass and suggest that improvement with steroids following bypass may be related to stabilization of the lysosomal membrane.

Table 18-2 is a summation of this discussion with a proposed sequence of events that leads to the adult respiratory distress syndrome. Clinical and pathological findings are well documented and lead one back to a factor X that acts via subcellular biochemical alterations. This factor may be single or multiple, and future investigations should be most fruitful if directed to the biochemical alterations that occur in association with the clinically observed manifestations of the syndrome.

PULMONARY COMPLICATIONS OF BURNS

Twenty-five to 30 percent of all patients suffering thermal burns develop some pulmonary complication [71]. Since the treatment of such cases is usually carried out by practitioners other than thoracic surgeons, these complications might be recognized and treated more effectively if a closer rapport

Table 18-2. Pathophysiological Basis for the Adult Respiratory Distress Syndrome in Trauma Patients

Common Factor X	Hypoxia
	Humoral toxin
	Neurovascular reactivity
Subcellular damage	Mitochondria
	Lysosomes
Pathological manifestation	↑ Capillary permeability
	↑ Vascular reactivity
	Inflammation
	↓ Surfactant production and regeneration
Clinical manifestation	Interstitial edema and congestion
	Alveolar hyaline deposits
	↓ Surfactant
	↑ Atelectasis
	↑ Shunting
	↑ Hypoxemia

existed between these physicians. The remarkable reduction of mortality from burn-wound infections has caused pulmonary complications to become among the most prominent etiological factors in death from burns [71, 72]. Those commonly encountered are (1) inhalation injury, (2) pulmonary edema, (3) pneumonia, and (4) thromboembolism.

Inhalation Injury

It has been shown that direct thermal injury to the trancheobronchial tree is a rare phenomenon except when steam has been inhaled. It is also recognized that few of these people survive to reach a treatment center. The more common form of inhalation injury is that due to the products of combustion or toxic fumes. Although many refer to these as pulmonary burns, a large postmortem series has shown that these "burns" are not attributable to direct thermal injury, but rather to the reaction of the tracheobronchial tree to specific chemical components of smoke [29].

One can suspect inhalation injury simply on the basis of the history. It is not an infrequent finding in patients who sustain burns in confined spaces or who inhale large amounts of smoke. Most of these individuals have suffered burns about the face, although there is little correlation between this and injury to the tracheobronchial tree.

The critical diagnostic manifestation of this type of injury is the expectoration of carbonaceous sputum in the presence of oropharyngeal or facial burns. It should be remembered that the patient's original chest roentgenogram can be completely normal. The symptoms of wheezing, hoarseness, or dyspnea reflect a spastic reaction by the bronchi to the toxic products. Clinically, the onset of symptoms may not occur until the second day after injury when excessive cough and secretions are noted. The carbonaceous material is usually completely expelled within a few days. The earliest pathological lesion of smoke inhalation is a severe tracheobronchitis that results from the irritant effect of the products of incomplete combustion. This can lead to ulceration or even total sloughing of the mucosa with superinfection and, in severe cases, pneumonia. The organisms most likely to be found are staphylococcus, *Klebsiella,* pseudomonas and *Escherichia coli.*

Blood gas studies reveal an initial profound hypoxemia that may persist for a considerable period. Studies in patients who have been treated successfully show that pulmonary function may remain impaired for weeks and months. There have been reports of bronchiectasis developing as a result of damage to the bronchi [22].

Treatment in these patients should be aggressive. Aerosolization with mucolytic agents together with inhalation therapy, frequent nasotracheal suction, and bronchoscopy in response to any evidence of atelectasis are routine measures. Also helpful are intravenous bronchodilators for the control of the severe bronchospasm that is a manifestation of the inflammatory response to smoke. Steroids may be considered but have a limited role and have only been used in large doses on a short-term basis. They should only be used to control severe, progressive bronchospasm and in conjunction with appropriate antibiotics when the patient is exhibiting a severe metabolic deficit as a result of the increased work of breathing and in the presence of hypoxemia.

The timing of a tracheostomy in patients suffering from smoke inhalation is critical. There are no safe guidelines since the procedure has been shown to carry its own high rate of complications. While tracheostomies should definitely not be used prophylactically, the inability to control a patient in whom blood gas studies indicate a respiratory acidosis, increased work of breathing, and tremendous amounts of secretions may prompt one to take that course. The primary indication usually is difficulty in controlling secretions.

It has been shown that in patients with inhalation injury tracheostomies have been a source of increased pulmonary infections and that they cause a desquamative laryngotracheobronchitis, which may be converted to a severe airborne type of pneumonia [29]. Therefore, care has to be exerted in the evaluation of blood gas studies and the clinical picture. It is obvious that patients who require tracheostomy usually also need the benefits of artificial ventilation and this should be employed, observing the accepted criteria for removing ventilatory support in any patient.

Facial burns do not necessarily require tracheostomy. However, if severe oropharyngeal burns are present, the associated edema may well lead to a supraglottic occlusion of the airway, an indication for tracheostomy.

Pulmonary Edema

A recent extensive review of pulmonary edema discusses the various etiologies, including burns and posttraumatic pulmonary insufficiency [75]. The pulmonary edema seen in patients with burns is frequently similar to etiology to that seen in patients with other forms of trauma. The use of massive amounts of resuscitative fluids during the first 48 to 72 hours of treatment is well known. Such an aggressive approach to intravascular hypovolemia has led to a tremendous decrease in the incidence of renal failure but does introduce the problem of pulmonary edema. This occurs most commonly between the fourth and sixth day after injury when massive amounts of fluid are mobilized back into the intravascular space. For this reason, patients with burns involving over 35 percent of their body surface should undergo prophylactic digitalization for its anticipated effect on the myocardium. Most of the deaths secondary to pulmonary edema occur in patients at the extremes of age but may also occur in young, previously healthy individuals with no previous evidence of myocardial damage. The treatment of this form of pulmonary edema is similar to that used for any other type of pulmonary edema and utilizes respirators, diuretics, and digitalis. Close monitoring of blood gases allows for the appropriate cessation of respiratory support. Fatal pulmonary edema may occur with large burns, particularly in infants, young children, and elderly patients. In an elderly patient the presence of a smaller burn with its increased metabolic demands may precipitate cardiac failure despite the small size; prophylactic digitalization is recommended in such instances.

Blood gas studies in burn patients, regardless of pulmonary complications, have revealed arterial hypoxemia that may persist for up to 2 weeks [26]. It is interesting that these patients often have an accompanying respiratory alkalosis that is not only due to the hypoxic drive but tends to remain present through the period when the pO_2 returns to normal. It is believed by some that the different forms of treatment for burns may play a role in causing alkalosis, but as is evident with other trauma patients, respiratory alkalosis is common, and in burns it is safe to say that the adequately resuscitated patient shows acidosis rather than alkalosis [3]. The early shock in burns may lead to the same adult respiratory distress syndrome described earlier in this chapter and is found at postmortem examination in its advanced stages, complete with hyaline membranes, interstitial edema, and so on.

Pneumonia

Pneumonia in burn patients is usually either airborne or hematogenous. Airborne pneumonia tends to occur earlier during the postburn course and histologically can be seen to start with deposition of organisms in the bronchioles due to spread of exudate and bacteria down the respiratory ducts. It can be distinguished grossly by large confluent lesions involving lobar segments or entire lobes of the lung. These lesions are also commonly seen as a complication of tracheostomy and in patients with pneumonia following smoke inhalation.

The latter occurs late in the postburn course and represents spread of infection from a distant source to the lungs [71]. The earliest identifiable septic changes occur in the alveolar capillaries. The gross pulmonary picture reveals hemorrhagic subpleural nodules distributed in all segments of the lung. In the past, the hematogenous pneumonias were caused by metastatic emboli from invasive burn wound sepsis. At the present time, with better control of infection, this type of pneumonia is more likely to be due to spread from areas of suppurative thrombophlebitis.

A rare and unusual pneumonia secondary to hematogenous spread from the burn wound is that caused by *Pseudomonas pseudomallei*. Pulmonary meliodosis, the resulting infection, is lethal if untreated. The organism is endemic in Southeast Asia and may become evident as long as 10 years after exposure in any exposed patient suffering trauma. The infecting agent may lie dormant but with decreased systemic resistance after burns or other trauma, there is spread to the lungs, causing a hematogenous pneumonia. A rapidly fatal septicemia is manifested by an abrupt, strikingly elevated temperature (105°F to 106°F), mild abdominal distress, and a flush originating on the face and neck that spreads caudally. These signs and symptoms in any patient who has returned from Southeast Asia should prompt massive antibotic therapy with tetracycline. Many of those properly treated will survive.

Thromboembolism

It is interesting that thromboembolism is a relatively rare entity in burn patients, even those who have been in bed for considerable portions of their convalescence. In a postmortem series in which 96 percent of all patient deaths involving burns were examined, thromboembolism was found in only 5 of 700 patients. The reason for this in a group thought to be highly susceptible can be attributed in part to the stress now placed on ambulating patients soon after sustaining a burn. The use of open treatment without immobilization may also play a part in the low incidence of thromboembolism.

The burned patient has long been an ideal subject in any study of the effects of massive trauma. Improved treatment of burn complications has led to an increased appreciation of the attendant pulmonary problems. While these problems are not confined to burns, the usual principles of thoracic surgery are sometimes not as easily applicable to burn patients as in other trauma patients. Nonetheless the use of respirators, blood gas studies, careful pulmonary toilet, and the support of the cardiovascular system in the early postburn period are all in the area of thoracic surgery and contribute to the care of patients with thermal injuries. It has been observed that the burned patient and his cardiovascular responses can resemble the patient who develops pulmonary complications after extracorporeal circulation, the same principles of cardiovascular and pulmonary physiology being applicable in both situations.

An understanding of lung responses to major trauma is now recognized as essential to a more complete understanding of human reaction to injury. As we move toward a better comprehension at the biochemical and molecular level, we once again underscore the "unity" of medicine.

REFERENCES

1. Almond CH, Jones JC, Snyder HM, et al: Hypoxin of the lung parenchyma during cardiopulmonary bypass. Arch Surg 93:986, 1966
2. Anderson RR, Sibbald WJ, Holliday RL, et al: Increased pulmonary capillary permeability in human sepsis—reduction with steroid therapy. Presented at the Annual Meeting of the Association for Academic Surgery, Seattle, November 1977
3. Asch MJ, White MG, Pruitt BA Jr: Acid base changes associated with topical sulfamylon therapy: Retrospective study of 100 burn patients. Ann Surg 172:946, 1970
4. Ashbaugh DG, Bigelow DB, Petty TL, et al: Acute respiratory distress in adults. Lancet 2:319, 1967
5. Ashbaugh DG, Petty TL: The use of corticosteroids in the treatment of respiratory failure associated with massive fat embolism. Surg Gynecol Obstet 123:493, 1966
6. Ashbaugh DG, Petty TL, Bigelow DG, et al: Continuous positive pressure breathing (CPPB) in adult respiratory distress syndrome. J Thorac Cardiovasc Surg 57:31, 1969
7. Ashbaugh DG, Uzawa T: Effect of continuous and intermittent positive pressure breathing on experimental respiratory distress. Surg Forum 19:268, 1968
8. Bachofen M, Weibel ER: Basic pattern of tissue repair in human lungs following unspecific injury. Chest 65:14S, 1974
9. Baer DM, Osborn JJ: The postperfusion pulmonary congestion syndrome. Am J Clin Pathol 34:442, 1960
10. Barber RE, Lee J, Hamilton WK: Oxygen toxicity in man—a prospective study in patients with irreversible brain damage. N Engl J Med 283:1478, 1970
11. Barter RA, Finlay-Jones LR, Walter MN: Pulmonary hyaline membrane: Sites of formation in adult lungs after assisted respiration and inhalation of oxygen. J Pathol Bacteriol 95:481, 1968
12. Bartlett RH, Gazzaniga AB, Jefferies MR, et al: Extracorporeal membrane oxygenation (ECMO) cardiopulmonary support in infancy. Trans Am Soc Artif Intern Organs 22:80, 1976
13. Berry WB, McLaughlin JS, Clark WD, et al: The effects of acute hypoxia on pressure, flow and resistance in the pulmonary vascular bed. Surgery 58:404, 1965
14. Blaisdell WF: Pathophysiology of the respiratory distress syndrome. Arch Surg 108:44, 1974
15. Bone RC, Frances PB, Pierce AK: Intravascular coagulation associated with the adult respiratory distress syndrome. Am J Med 61:585, 1976
16. Border JR, Tibbetts JC, Schenk WG: Hypoxic hyperventilation and acute respiratory failure in the severely stressed patient: Massive pulmonary arteriovenous shunts? Surgery 64:710, 1968
17. Burford TH, Burbank B: Traumatic wet lung; observations on certain physiological fundamentals of thoracic trauma. J Thorac Cardiovasc Surg 14:415, 1945
18. Capers TH: Pulmonary hyaline membrane formation in the adult. Am J Med 31:701, 1961
19. Cederberg A, Hellsten S, Miorner G: Oxygen treatment and hyaline pulmonary membranes in adults. Acta Pathol Microbiol Scand Sect B 64:450, 1965
20. Cook WA, Webb WR: Surfactant in chronic smokers. Ann Thorac Surg 2:327, 1966
21. de Duve C: Lysosome Concept in Lysosomes. Edited by AVS de Reuck, MP Cameron. London, J&A Churchill, 1963, p. 362
22. Di Vincenti FD, Pruitt BA Jr, Reckler JM: Inhalation injuries. J Trauma 11:109, 1971
23. Downs JB, Olsen GN: Pulmonary function following adult respiratory distress syndrome. Chest 65:92, 1974
24. Editorial: Hyaline membrane formation in the adult lung. Lancet 1:362, 1962
25. Eiseman B, Ashbaugh DG: Pulmonary effects of non-thoracic trauma. J Trauma 8:624, 1968
26. Epstein BS, Hardy DL, Harrison HN, et al: Hypoxemia in the burned patient: A clinical pathologic study. Ann Surg 158:924, 1963
27. Fishman AP, Pietra GG: Handling of bioactive materials by the lung. N Engl J Med 291:884, 1974
28. Fleming WH, Szakacs JE, Hartney TC, et al: Hyaline membrane following total body irradiation—relation to lung plasminogen activator. Lancet 2:1010, 1960
29. Foley FD, Moncrief JA, Jason AD: Pathology of the lung in fatally burned patients. Ann Surg 167:251, 1968
30. Franz JL, Richardson JD, Grover FL, et al: Effects of methylprednisolone sodium succinate on experimental pulmonary contusion. J Thorac Cardiovasc Surg 68:842, 1974
31. Gadboys H, Litwak R: The postperfusion hematocrit. J Thorac Cardiovasc Surg 46:772, 1963
32. Gallagher TJ, Civetta JM, Kirby RR, et al: Post-traumatic pulmonary insufficiency: A treatable disease. South Med J 70:1308, 1977

33. Gardner RE, Finley TN, Tooley WH: The effect of cardiopulmonary bypass on surface activity of lung extracts. Bull Soc Int Chir 21:542, 1962

34. Germon PA, Kazem I, Brady LW: Shunting following trauma. J Trauma 8:724, 1968

35. Gille JP, Bagniewski A: Ten years of use of extracorporeal membrane oxygenation (ECMO) in the treatment of acute respiratory insufficiency (ARI). Trans Am Soc Artif Intern Organs 22:102, 1976

36. Gittin D, Craig JM: Morphological studies of hyaline membranes in the newborn infant. Arch Pathol 59:207, 1955

37. Gleen TM, Lefer AM: Autitoric action of methylprednisolone in hemorrhagic shock. Am J Pharmacol 13:230, 1971

38. Gomez AC: Pulmonary insufficiency in nonthoracic trauma. J Trauma 8:656, 1968

39. Hayes MF, Rosenbaum RW, Zibelman M, et al: Adult respiratory distress syndrome in association with acute pancreatitis. Am J Surg 127:314, 1974

40. Henry JN: The effect of shock on pulmonary alveolar surfactant, its role in refractory respiratory insufficiency of the critically ill or severely injured patient. J Trauma 8:756, 1968

41. Henry JN, McArdle AH, Scott HJ, et al: A study of the acute and chronic respiratory pathophysiology of hemorrhagic shock. J Thorac Cardiovasc Surg 54:666, 1967

42. Hill JD, O'Brien TG, Murray JJ, et al: Prolonged extracorporeal oxygenation for acute post-traumatic respiratory failure (shock-lung syndrome). N Engl J Med 286:629, 1972

43. Holland RH, Capers TH: Pulmonary hyaline membrane disease in adults—A cause of postthoracotomy mortality. Am Rev Res Dis 84:719, 1961

44. Jenkins MT, Jones RF, Wilson B, et al: Congestive atelectasis; a complication of the intravenous infusion of fluids. Ann Surg 132:327, 1950

45. Keller CA, Schramel RJ, Hyman AC, et al: The cause of acute congestive lesions of the lung. J Thorac Cardiovasc Surg 53:743, 1967

46. Kuida H, Hinshaw CB, Gilbert RP, et al: Effect of gram-negative endotoxin on pulmonary circulation. Am J Physiol 192:335, 1958

47. Kumor A, Falke KJ, Geffin B, et al: Continuous positive pressure ventilation in acute respiratory failure—effects on hemodynamics and lung function. N Engl J Med 283:1430, 1970

48. Lee CJ, Lyons JH, Konisberg S, et al: The effects of spontaneous and positive pressure breathing of ambient air and pure oxygen at one atmosphere pressure on pulmonary surfactant characteristics. J Thorac Cardiovasc Surg 53:759, 1967

49. Lesage AM, Tsuchioka H, Young WG, et al: Pathogenesis of pulmonary damage during extracorporeal perfusion. Arch Surg 93:1002, 1966

50. Lieberman JA: A unified concept and critical review of pulmonary hyaline membrane formation. Am J Med 35:443, 1963

51. Lieberman J, Kellog F: A deficiency of pulmonary fibrinolysin in hyaline membrane disease. N Engl J Med 262:999, 1960

52. Lillehei RC, Longerbeam JK, Block JH, et al: Nature of irreversible shock: Experimental and clinical observations. Ann Surg 160:682, 1964

53. Llamas R: Adult respiratory distress syndrome. Chest 65:468, 1974

54. Lloyd TC Jr: Effect of alveolar hypoxia on pulmonary vascular resistance. J Appl Physiol 19:1086, 1964

55. MacLeod M, Stalker AL, Ogston D: Fibrinolytic activity of lung tissue in renal failure. Lancet 1:191, 1962

56. Mandelbaum I, Giammona ST, Shumacker HB: Extracorporeal circulation, pulmonary compliance and pulmonary surfactant. J Thorac Surg 48:881, 1964

57. Mills M: The clinical syndrome. J Trauma 8:651, 1968

58. Morgan TE, Finley TN, Huber GL, et al: Alterations in pulmonary surface active lipids during exposure to increased oxygen tension. J Clin Invest 44:1737, 1965

59. Nagy S, Tarnoky K, Petri G: Cardiac output of bled dogs after intravenous administration of corticosteroids. Acta Physiol Scand 27:257, 1965

60. Nash G, Blennerhassett JB, Pontoppidan H: Pulmonary lesions associated with oxygen therapy and artificial ventilation. N Engl J Med 276:368, 1967

61. Neville WE, Balis JV, Talso PJ, et al: Postbypass histochemical alterations following overinfusion of noncolloids. J Trauma 8:827, 1968

62. Neville WE, Colby C, Peacock H, et al: Superiority of buffered Ringer's lactate to heparinized blood as total prime of the large volume disc oxygenator. Ann Surg 165:206, 1967

63. Neville WE, Talso PJ: Postperfusion compartmental fluid alterations. Surgery 63:220, 1968

64. Neville WE, Thomason RD, Hirsch DM: Postperfusion hypervolemia after hemodilution cardiopulmonary bypass. Arch Surg 93:715, 1966

65. Pattle RE, Burgess F: The lung lining film in some pathological conditions. J Pathol Bacteriol 82:315, 1961

66. Pennock JL, Pierce WS, Waldhausen JA: The management of the lungs during cardiopulmonary bypass. Surg Gynecol Obstet 145:917, 1977

67. Philbin DM, Sullivan SF, Bowman FO, et al: Low cardiac output and postcardiotomy hypoxia. Circulation 6:156, 1968

68. Pontoppidan H: Treatment of respiratory failure in non-thoracic trauma. J Trauma 8:938, 1968

69. Pratt PC: Oxygen toxicity as a factor. J Trauma 8:854, 1968

70. Proctor HJ, Ballantine TVN, Broussard ND: An analysis of pulmonary function following non-thoracic trauma, with recommendations for therapy. Ann Surg 172:180, 1970

71. Pruitt BA, Di Vincenti F, Mason A, et al: The occurrence and significance of pneumonia and other pulmonary complications in burned patients: Comparison of conventional and topical treatments. J Trauma 10:519, 1970

72. Pruitt BA, Flemma RJ, Di Vincenti F, et al: Pulmonary complications in burn patients: A comparative study of 697 patients. J Thorac Cardiovasc Surg 59:7, 1970

73. Rattliff NB, Wilson JW, Mikat E, et al: Altered leukocytes in pulmonary vessels of dogs in hemorrhagic shock. Microvasc Res 2:7, 1970

74. Replogle RL, Gazzaniga AB, Gross RE: Use of corticosteroids during cardiopulmonary bypass: Possible lysosome stabilization. Circulation 33:86, 1966

75. Robin ED, Cross CE, Zelis R: Pulmonary edema. N Engl J Med 288:239, 1973

76. Scarpelli EM: The surfactant system of the Lung. Philadelphia, Lea & Febiger, 1968

77. Schaefer KE, Avery ME, Benoch K: Time course of changes in surface tension and morphology of alveolar epithelial cells in CO_2-induced hyaline membrane disease. J Clin Invest 43:2080, 1964

78. Schramel R, Hyman A, Keller CA, et al: Congestive atelectasis. J Trauma 8:821, 1968

79. Shanklin DR: Cardiovascular factors in development of pulmonary hyaline membrane. Arch Pathol 68:49, 1959

80. Simeone FA: Pulmonary complications of non-thoracic wounds: A historical perspective. J Trauma 8:625, 1968

81. Singer MM, Wright F, Stanley LK, et al: Oxygen toxicity in man—A prospective study in patients after open-heart surgery. N Engl J Med 283:1473, 1970

82. Stowens D: Hyaline membrane disease—morbid anatomy, hypothesis of its pathogenesis and suggested method of treatment. Am J Clin Pathol 44:259, 1965

83. Sugg WL, Webb WR, Ecker RR: Prevention of lesions of the lung secondary to hemorrhagic shock. Surg Gynecol Obstet 127:1005, 1968

84. Taylor FB, Abrams ME: Effects of surface active lipoprotein on clotting and fibrinolysis, and of fibrinogen on surfactant tension of surface active lipoprotein; with a hypothesis on the pathogenesis of pulmonary atelectasis and hyaline membrane in respiratory distress syndrome of the newborn. Am J Med 40:346, 1966

85. Teplitz C: The ultrastructural basis for pulmonary pathophysiology following trauma—pathogenesis of pulmonary edema. J Trauma 8:700, 1968

86. Travis RH, Sayers G: Adrenocorticotrophic hormone: adrenocortical steroids and their synthetic analogs. Edited by LS Goodman and A Gilman. The Pharmacological Basis of Therapeutics. New York, Macmillan, 1967, p. 1624

87. Unpublished data by Flemma et al. (1971) on the adult respiratory distress syndrome in postoperative cardiac surgery patients.

88. Van Breeman VL, Neustein HB, Bruns PD: Pulmonary hyaline membrane studied with the electron microscope. Am J Pathol 33:769, 1957

89. Veith FJ, Deysine M, Nehlsen SL, et al: Pulmonary changes common to isolated lung perfusion, venovenous bypass and total cardiopulmonary bypass. Surg Gynecol Obstet 125:1047, 1967

90. Veith FJ, Panossion A, Nehlsen SL, et al: A pattern of pulmonary vascular reactivity and its importance in the pathogenesis of postoperative and post-traumatic pulmonary insufficiency. J Trauma 8:788, 1968

91. Vito L, Dennis RC, Weisel RD, et al: Sepsis presenting as acute respiratory insufficiency. Surg Gynecol Obstet 138:896, 1974

92. Young WG: Personal communication on the inflammatory response in the lung's reaction to acute hemodynamic injury, 1971

19. MANAGEMENT OF PROBLEMS RELATED TO DIVING

Ronald Samson
Eugene L. Nagel

The incidence of accidents related to underwater diving is difficult to ascertain. This is especially true when the activity is recreational since systematic reporting of such accidents does not exist. Instances of chest trauma in this context are even more difficult to identify. One study in 1963 [14] stated that the U.S. Navy had reported only 7 fatal accidents attributable to skin and scuba diving during the preceding 16 years. A comparative survey by the same authors failed to define the incidence of such accidents in the civilian population of the United States. The same study did reveal, however, that in Florida there was an increasing number of accidents and fatalities associated with pleasure diving each year [15]. Another study, by the Department of Engineering of the University of Rhode Island [12], showed that there were 124 fatal diving accidents in the United States in 1970. Of these 124 21 occurred while the person was skin diving and 103 while he or she was using some form of compressed gas. Just as the incidence of these accidents is difficult to ascertain, it is equally difficult to evaluate their etiology.

This chapter will discuss certain clinical conditions found in trauma associated with diving in terms of pathophysiology, signs and symptoms, treatment, and preventive measures. Our discussion will deal primarily with chest trauma related to the direct and indirect effects of pressure, as well as some miscellaneous problems that may be encountered.

The term *scuba* is an acronym for "self-contained underwater apparatus." Typically when diving for sport, the participant maintains himself submerged and air is delivered from a compressed air supply. This is generally contained in cylinders at initial pressures approximating 3000 pounds per cubic inch. The compressed air flows to the diver via a demand-regulated system. On demand (inhalation) air at the diver's ambient pressure is made available; on exhalation, the air flow is terminated. Of necessity, a pressure-reducing apparatus is incorporated to reduce high tank pressure to that at which the diver is breathing (ambient pressure).

THE PROBLEM

Chest trauma resulting from pressure may be due to decreasing or increasing ambient pressure. By far the most significant problems are those associated with decreasing ambient pressure, which falls as a diver at depth (high ambient pressure) ascends toward the surface. It is a common misconception that the danger exists when a person is diving rather than coming to the surface. Problems associated with ascent include air embolism, pneumothorax, mediastinal emphysema, pericardial emphysema, and pulmonary interstitial emphysema. Recently all of these entities have been included under the heading of extra-alveolar air syndrome [10]. The pathophysiology is essentially the same for all of these entities. An excessive intrapulmonary gas pressure relative to surrounding tissue results in the disruption of lung integrity and the escape of gas from the lung to other areas of the body. The intrapulmonary pressure necessary to cause rupture of the lung (80 mm Hg) was determined in 1933 in dogs by Adams and Polak [1]. In 1958 Schaefer and co-workers [11] (also working with dogs) showed that the production of gas emboli from the lung was not related to absolute pressure but was due to differences between intrapulmonary and intrapleural pressures (transpulmonic pressure). It has also been shown that a transpulmonic pressure of 50 to 70 mm Hg can cause rupture of lung tissue [3]. If the pressure difference is calculated in terms of alteration of depth, then a change in depth of approximately 2 to 3 feet could, theoretically, cause an increase in transpulmonic pressure sufficient to rupture the lung, provided the lungs are initially fully expanded, more specifically:

$$\frac{55 \text{ mm Hg}}{760 \text{ mm Hg}} = \frac{x}{33 \text{ ft}}$$

where $x = 2.39$ ft

Air embolization has been reported at depths of only 6 to 10 feet [5]. The physical changes producing lung rupture upon ascent are defined by Boyle's law, i.e., if the temperature of a gas is kept constant, then the volume will vary inversely with absolute pressure $(P_1V_1 = P_2V_2)$. Thus an initial volume of gas contained in the lungs will increase as the pressure upon it decreases during ascent. If the increasing volume is not allowed to escape, as when the breath is held or in respiratory obstruction, then a rise in intrapulmonary pressure sufficient to disrupt the pulmonary tissue may be reached. Ultimately, it is the inability of expanding gas to escape that causes lung rupture. As is frequently the case, a diver may panic at a given depth, holding his breath and rising rapidly, with the subsequent occurrence of lung rupture. The same occurrence can be seen in various disease states—e.g., as with bronchiolitis, pulmonary cysts, severe generalized obstructive lung disease, and even in patients in whom calcified hilar lymph nodes (Ghon complex) have impinged on a bronchus—when air becomes trapped. These conditions are obviously significant when the physical status of a potential diver is being evaluated, and anyone who wishes to undertake diving should first check with his physician as to his physical status.

CLINICAL MANIFESTATIONS AND TREATMENT

Air embolism resulting from pulmonary rupture resulting from diving accidents is associated with a high mortality [16]. Gas is released directly into the pulmonary circulation from the alveolus via the lung capillaries, and thence to the pulmonary vein, left heart, aorta, and carotid arteries. Due to the effect of gravity and the commonly adopted perpendicular position of a diver, the gas is trapped selectively in the cerebral circulation (cerebral air embolism). Less frequently, it may return to the pulmonary circulation and cause air embolism. It may also pass into the coronary circulation and produce myocardial ischemia.

With the introduction of gas bubbles into the cerebral circulation, acute occlusion of the involved vessels occurs. As shown by Waite and associates [16] the occluding air lodges in vessels from 2 to 30μ in diameter. As a result, there is ischemia, hypoxemia, and often acute pulmonary edema, the last occurring within 1 hour. Clinical signs and symptoms are directly related to the pathological

process taking place in the lung or central nervous system or both. The onset is sudden, usually within 1 minute of surfacing, and this is important in the differential diagnosis [3]. If more than 5 minutes elapse before the onset of tangible signs, other causes should be considered.

Symptoms can be nonspecific and often comprise a rapid onset of weakness, disorientation, and vascular collapse. Chest pain is more frequent if there has been associated pulmonary embolization. When coupled to a pulmonary episode, cough, nausea, and a "millwheel" cardiac murmur may all be significant. The ECG may show a pattern suggestive of ischemia or acute right heart strain. A frothy, bloody sputum may result from tearing of lung tissue. Symptoms of pneumothorax also may be present. Central nervous system involvement as evidenced by headache, vertigo, auditory disturbance, speech and visual defects, paralysis, paresthesia, and convulsions may manifest itself, together with apnea or Cheyne-Stokes breathing. Other signs include bubbles in the retina that can be easily seen by ophthalmoscopy, and Liebmeister's sign, which consists of sharply defined areas of pallor on the tongue and a marbling of the skin, a condition sometimes confused with skin bends.

The only effective treatment for air embolization is immediate recompression. The rationale, in general, is to reduce bubble size and permit normal circulation to resume. Treatment necessitates a recompression chamber. During the time necessary to transport the victim to a chamber, certain supportive therapy should be instituted. A head-down position may be beneficial in reducing the amount of air reaching the cerebral circulation by causing gravity displacement. Keeping the feet up will also improve the cardiovascular status if shock is present. Placing the victim in a position somewhere between the left lateral decubitus and the prone positions so as to prevent further embolization is also advocated [9]. It should be pointed out, however, that these maneuvers will have no effect on bubbles already in vital organs; these require recompression. If no chamber is available and a life-threatening situation exists, the patient may be recompressed while still in the water although this is obviously an effort almost certainly doomed to failure from the start; recompression by redescent can be carried out successfully only if an experienced team is available with a virtually unlimited supply of air. Such facilities permit a proper schedule to be maintained. Administration of 100% oxygen will also help reduce bubble size slightly by decreasing the partial pressure of nitrogen. Fluids may be necessary to support circulation, and steroids are frequently used to reduce cerebral edema. If cardiovascular collapse ensues, cardiopulmonary resuscitative measures may be necessary in order to support a failing circulation.

No detailed discussion of recompression treatment in a chamber will be presented here, although certain comments are appropriate. The treatment tables most widely accepted are those distributed by the U.S. Navy [15]. In general, they consist of specific depths of staged decompression for varying amounts of time. The rationale is a reduction in bubble size by redissolving the gases into solution, followed by slower elimination of these gases from the circulation. Other methods of recompression treatment have been advanced by organizations interested in diving, but the reasoning behind these is essentially the same. One interesting study by Waite and associates [16] suggests that "bounce" dives (rapid descent to 165 ft) may be just as effective as prolonged treatment. He also claims that 4 atmospheres (approximately 130 ft) may be the greatest depth necessary in such a situation.

Mediastinal emphysema is another manifestation of lung tissue rupture, this time with release of gas to a different body space. The etiology is the same as for vascular air embolism except that the air does not enter the circulation to any marked degree; instead, it moves into the mediastinum and compresses the structures contained therein. The signs and symptoms may include cyanosis, dyspnea, and occasionally a generalized circulatory collapse. Another finding that may be diagnostic is mediastinal "crunch." This sign, however, can be confused with the "millwheel" murmur heard in pulmonary embolization. If symptoms of mediastinal emphysema are not severe, no treatment is necessary. On the other hand, if there is any doubt, or if the patient's distress is more marked, then the condition should be treated by recompression.

Under these circumstances pneumothorax has the same etiology, except that air escapes into and accumulates in the pleural space. It is often associated with vascular air embolism and may complicate its treatment. Such an occurrence may become evident after recompression for air embolism, at which time reascent dyspnea presents itself again due to the pneumothorax. The relevant signs and symptoms are cyanosis, chest pain, splinting, tachypnea, mediastinal shift, absent or decreased breath sounds, and an alteration of the percussion note. If the pneumothorax is not associated with air embolism, treatment consists of removal of trapped air via chest tubes or needle aspiration; if there is associated air embolism, recompression becomes a necessary additional measure.

Pulmonary interstitial emphysema is another sign of lung rupture wherein air escapes into the lung tissue [6]. Therapy should be essentially supportive until the air is reabsorbed and eliminated, unless distress becomes marked at which time recompression is indicated.

Chest trauma directly related to increasing ambient pressure is exemplified by lung "squeeze"—an entity that applies to breathholding or "free" diving. The diver takes in a certain volume of air, holds his breath, and descends to a maximum depth. As he descends, the ambient pressure increases, and by Boyle's law, the gas in his lungs decreases in volume proportionate to the increased pressure. When the lung volume diminishes to a value below or near residual volume, the pulmonary vessels rupture and blood is released into the alveoli. Should this occur at the residual volume, then a diver whose vital capacity is 5 liters should increase the pressure and decrease the lung volume to this critical residual volume at a depth of 4 to 5 atmospheres (approximately 120 to 150 ft). Calculations based on vital capacity, residual volume, and the theoretical squeeze level do not always apply in actual situations. Examples of squeeze have been found at depths much less than theoretical predictions, while in other instances there has been no squeeze at depths greatly in excess of those calculated [13]. Obviously, there are undelineated factors involved. The most common symptom associated with the condition is hemoptysis and perhaps mild chest pain. The clinical signs are considered benign, and no definitive treatment is recommended other than observation and supportive therapy.

Decompression sickness, most frequently called "the bends," does not come under the category of direct chest trauma. It is nonetheless important in that it may first appear like air embolism and in many instances the resultant process and associated symptoms are similar. However, the pathophysiology is quite different. Since detailed coverage of decompression sickness could in itself be the subject of a book, only a brief description will be attempted here.

The so-called bends were probably first noted by Boyle as early as 1670, the first clinical case being reported by Trigor in 1841, with the etiology and incidence reported by Burt in 1880. The disease process has a number of manifestations and synonyms and is also called caisson disease, compressed air illness, divers' problem or itch, aeroemphysema, and "the staggers." The most commonly accepted term today is *decompression sickness,* sometimes abbreviated to DCS.

To understand the etiology of this disease, we must again consider the general gas laws, and additionally, the concept of partial pressure plus the theory of bubble formation. According to Dalton's law, the total pressure of a mixture of gases is equal to the sum of the partial pressures of each gas in the mixture, while Henry's law states that the amount of gas dissolved in a liquid is proportional to the partial pressure of that gas at a fixed temperature.

As a gas, nitrogen obeys the above laws so that when a diver descends there is a tendency for more nitrogen to dissolve in the blood and tissues. Complete tissue saturation at any given depth occurs in about 12 hours. Nitrogen is eliminated over the same time lapse, being less diffusable than the oxygen and carbon dioxide normally found in compressed air. As a diver ascends, the dissolved nitrogen is in disequilibrium with the air mixture being breathed and has a tendency to leave the tissues, enter the blood, and ultimately be passed out through the alveoli. The rate of elimination depends on its diffusion rate into the blood, which is relatively slow. If the rate of pressure change on ascent is rapid enough, the tissues become relatively supersaturated with nitrogen, which bubbles out into the vascular space. Formation of bubbles thus depends on a driving force, defined as $\Delta P = T\text{-}P$, where ΔP is the driving force for the total pressure of dissolved gases and P is the ambient pressure [7]. There are modifying factors involved in bubble formation, i.e., cavitation, Bournoulli's effect, turbulence, vortex, positional negative pressure pulses, as well as tearing and shearing forces within the blood vessel. When a bubble nucleus of nitrogen is formed, aggregation to a larger bubble is fostered by the remaining gases because nitrogen is five times more soluble in lipid compared to aqueous tissues, and, because perfusion of fatty tissue is less, bub-

bles are more commonly formed in adipose tissue or tissues with a high lipid content, e.g., the central nervous system. Most significant effects occur in areas where terminal arteries are found—generally in the brain and spinal cord. It is the bubble, like the air of air embolism, that causes vascular occlusion. However, the bubble itself does not seem to explain the whole picture and a number of factors can modify the pathological course. Temperature causes vasoconstriction as it is decreased; fright may do the same as a result of catecholamine release. Tissue injury, either acute or chronic, causes an alteration in blood flow. Exercise causes an increased production of carbon dioxide, which in turn increases the driving forces required for bubble formation. Obesity and alcohol ingestion also favor the production of bends.

Signs and symptoms of decompression sickness depend upon the organ system or tissue involved. Incidence is greatest in the musculoskeletal system compared to the central nervous system, skin, and respiratory systems. The speed of onset is variable. Usually half of the victims experience symptoms within 1 hour of ascent and at least 97 to 99 percent feel the effects within 12 hours. In most instances, onset of symptoms is less rapid than those of air embolism, although symptoms can have their onset even while the person is still in the water.

The bends are now generally regarded as purely musculoskeletal manifestations of decompression sickness. Localized pain is usually felt and there may be an associated weakness or swelling at the site of injury. The pain is often described as deep, severe, and boring in nature. Frequently the patient experiences a generalized malaise, fatigue, fever, and chills. The occurrence of vascular occlusion by bubbles is aided by exertion or prior injury, or both. Immersion in hot water tends to increase the pain of bends and may be of assistance in the differential diagnosis, the pain of purely mechanical injury usually being decreased by such treatment. Dermal manifestations of bends are of less importance but are often associated with decompression sickness in other systems. They may include itching, pain, cyanosis, increased temperature, urticaria, and blebs. The lesions occur most often on the shoulders, abdomen, forearms, and thighs and tend to remain for several days after the initial incident.

Although the nervous system is affected less often, when it does become involved, there is a greater potential for lethal damage. Decompression sickness in the central nervous system may mimic air embolism and it becomes very difficult to determine which particular disease entity has produced the clinical picture. In general, air embolism causes purely cerebral symptoms while decompression sickness shows signs of spinal cord involvement, either alone or in association with cerebral injury [8]. The more rapid onset of air embolism may also serve as a rough guide to differential diagnosis. Signs of spinal cord injury may include paraplegia, monoplegia, paralysis, spasticity, loss of bladder and bowel control, and paresthesia. Cerebral signs include convulsions, unconsciousness, stupor, collapse, nausea, vomiting, visual disturbance, vertigo, headache, nystagmus, speech defects, restlessness, agitation, confusion, and personality changes. When the more severe of these indications are present, it may be difficult or impossible to differentiate between decompression sickness and air embolism.

Respiratory pathology related to decompression sickness is usually referred to as "the chokes," although they are considered relatively uncommon in comparison to other signs of decompression sickness. The etiology is thought to be formation of bubbles in the venous system that are carried to the right heart and then to the pulmonary arterial tree. The occlusion at this level is held responsible for the clinical picture. The symptoms and signs consist of substernal distress, cough, a burning sensation in the laryngotracheobronchial tree, hyperpnea, dyspnea, cyanosis, and shock. A mill-wheel murmur is frequently heard on examination. The physical picture is otherwise nonspecific and may be difficult to differentiate from that of the burst lung syndrome. If untreated, this type of decompression problem is associated with the highest mortality.

The only definitive treatment of the various manifestations of decompression sickness is recompression. Again, a detailed discussion of the exact therapy schedule will not be undertaken here. The standard U.S. Navy decompression tables 1–4, and more recently 5–6, should be consulted [15]. The trend recently is to use tables 5–6, which involve recompression with periods of oxygen breathing at depths equal to or lesser than 60 feet; tables 1 to 4 have been all but abandoned. The rationale for using oxygen with pressure is to provide a higher PO_2 to ischemic tissues; it also increases the gradient for movement of other gases from the air

bubbles by reducing the pressures of these other gases in the blood by having the patient breathe 100% oxygen for various intervals [15].

Treatment other than this definitive treatment of recompression may also be of value. Such measures may be undertaken both before and after recompression and include the use of intravenous fluids. Low molecular weight dextran is often advocated to increase blood flow and decrease the occurrence of hypercoagulability and sludging, phenomena that occur in association with bubble formation. Heparin is also used. Some investigators claim that fat embolization may take place with decompression sickness. Aspiration of gas from the heart may be necessary [4]. Cardiovascular support with cardiac stimulation and either vasoconstrictors or vasodilators may be necessary. Steroids are advocated to reduce an inflammatory reaction and central nervous tissue edema. Hypothermia may be required to diminish metabolic requirements.

It should be mentioned that when moving the patient to an area where recompression treatment is to take place, the transportation, if it is by air, should be at as low an altitude as possible.

In summary, it is evident that the syndrome of decompression sickness, although not directly related to thoracic trauma (except in the case of the chokes), presents problems of differential diagnosis and may furnish other pathology besides that of the specific chest injury.

REFERENCES

1. Adams BH, Polak IB: Traumatic lung lesions produced in dogs by simulating submarine escape. USN Med Bull 31:18, 1933
2. Behnke MB: Decompression sickness: Advances and interpretations. Aerospace Med. 42:255, 1971
3. Gillen HW: Symptomatology of cerebral gas embolism. Neurology 18:507, 1968
4. Hoff EC: A bibliographical sourcebook of compressed air. Diving and submarine medicine. Bureau of Medicine and Surgery, Navy Med 2:1191, 1954
5. Lanphier EH: Diving medicine. N Engl J Med 256:120, 1957
6. Macklin MT, Macklin CC: Malignant interstitial emphysema as an important occult complication in many respiratory diseases and other conditions. Medicine 23:281, 1944

7. Merrill RH: Diving physiology and decompression illness. Milit Med 135:464, 1970

8. Miles S: Underwater Medicine. London, Staples Press, 1962

9. Musgrove JE, MacQuigg RE: Successful treatment of air embolism. JAMA 150:28, 1952

10. Samson RL: Diving accidents and near drowning. Emergency Med Care 2:151, 1975

11. Schaefer KE, et al: Mechanisms in development of interstitial emphysema and air embolism on decompression from depth. J Appl Physiol 13:15, 1958

12. Schenk H, et al: Skin and scuba diving fatalities involving U.S. citizens. Scuba Safety Report Series, No. 2, University of Rhode Island, 1970

13. Strauss MB: Mammalian adaptations to diving. US Navy Submarine Medical Center Rep No. 562, Groton, Conn., 1969

14. Taylor GD, et al: Skin and scuba diving fatalities. J Fla Med Assoc 49:808, 1963

15. US Department of the Navy: U.S. Navy Diving Manual. (NAVSHIPS 250–538.) Washington, DC, US Government Printing Office, 1958

16. Waite CL, et al: Dysbaric cerebral air embolism. Proceedings of the Third Symposium on Underwater Physiology. Natl Acad Sci Natl Res Counc: 205, 1967

20. LATE RESULTS IN WAR WOUNDS OF THE CHEST

Lyman A. Brewer III

The chapter entitled "Management of War Wounds of the Chest," Chapter 17, outlines the fundamental principles of treatment of wounds of the thorax worked out in the Mediterranean Theater of Operations in World War II and presents the basis for current therapy of thoracic trauma. Employment of these principles, together with the many technological advances of the past 25 years, has reduced the immediate mortality following today's treatment [1, 5, 6, 11, 15, 18]. However, there are no up-to-date statistics on the late results of chest injury, military or civilian.

In 1965, while compiling the history of thoracic surgery during World War II, I had the opportunity to review a group of men with chest wounds whom I had treated at the front lines [4]. Since their treatment had involved the same basic principles as those currently employed in civilian and military practice, it should be possible to gain an insight into the long-term results that can be anticipated from today's regimens of therapy. Some of the significant findings of this study are reported here with the permission of the Surgeon General, United States Army Medical Corps.* Of approximately 1000 wounded men treated by the author, only 167 found it necessary to report at a later date to the Veteran's Administration, where their records became available for scrutiny. It would thus appear that more than 833 individuals did not consider themselves in need of further treatment. It may be assumed that the late results in this group were as good and probably much better than in the first group.

The ages of the wounded referred to ranged from 18 to 39 years at the time of wounding. Shell fragments caused 77 percent of the wounds and small arms fire the remainder. In roughly one-half (86 cases) wound debridement was carried out, while in the other half (81 cases) a thoracotomy was performed; the latter includes 25 who underwent a thoracoabdominal operation. The high percentage of thoracotomies was due to the fact that the majority of these patients who underwent them were critically wounded and nontransportable and so were treated at field hospitals set up next to the clearing station.

Supported by the Brewer Medical Foundation, Suite One, 225 Grand Avenue, South Pasadena, California 91030.

* Hal B. Jennings, Jr., M.D., Lieutenant General, The Surgeon General, Department of the Army, Washington, D.C.

BLAST INJURIES

In 21 patients in this series of 167, generalized blast injury presented a serious problem of management. Severe dyspnea, wet lung syndrome, transient cardiac irregularities, and signs of cerebral anoxia were the initial findings. In 4 instances, perforation of the ear drums indicated a very severe blast effect. Localized blast injury, due to the impact force of a high explosive shell fragment on the thoracic cage and its contents, was present in practically every patient with a major chest wall or intrathoracic wound. In these patients, because the management of the wound itself dominated the clinical scene, it was very difficult to evaluate precisely how much the localized blast added to the severity of the injury (see Figs 20-1, 20-2).

All these patients were evacuated. Two of them later succumbed to wounds other than the blast injury. Among the remainder, 6 were able to return to limited duty while the rest were subsequently given a disability discharge. It is of interest that 2 individuals received their discharge because of psychoneuroses; they were followed for periods up to 17 years and showed an excellent complete recovery. In the group as a whole, dyspnea was minimal and the roentgenograms revealed only slight pulmonary emphysema. It would appear, therefore, that even with a severe blast injury, if the patient recovers from the initial thrust of the positive and negative pressure waves, his outlook, physically speaking, for the future is excellent.

SEVERE CHEST WALL WOUNDS

Extensive trauma to the thoracic musculature and bony cage created challenging clinical problems in 145 cases. There were 88 sucking and 4 thoraco-

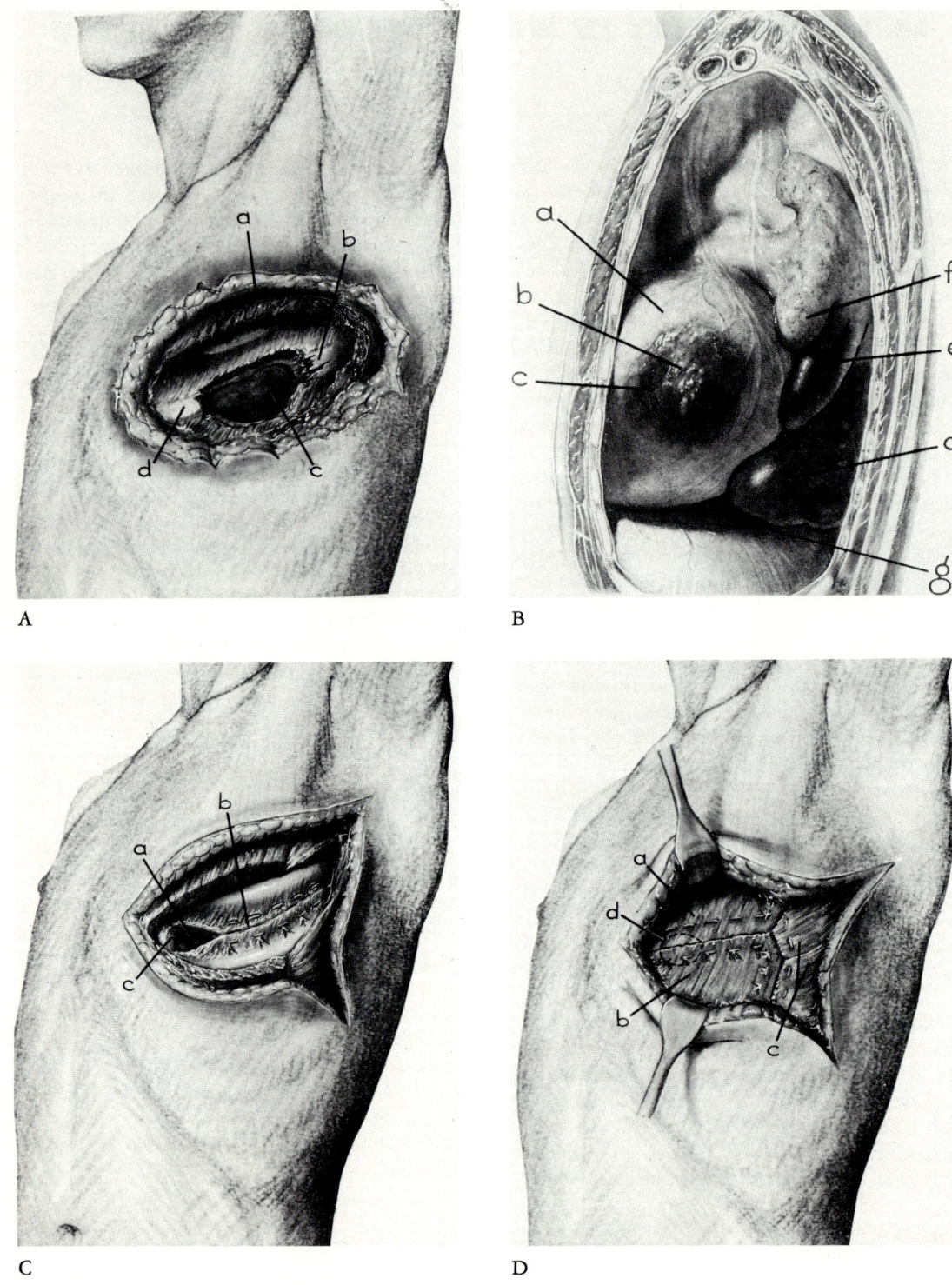

A

B

C

D

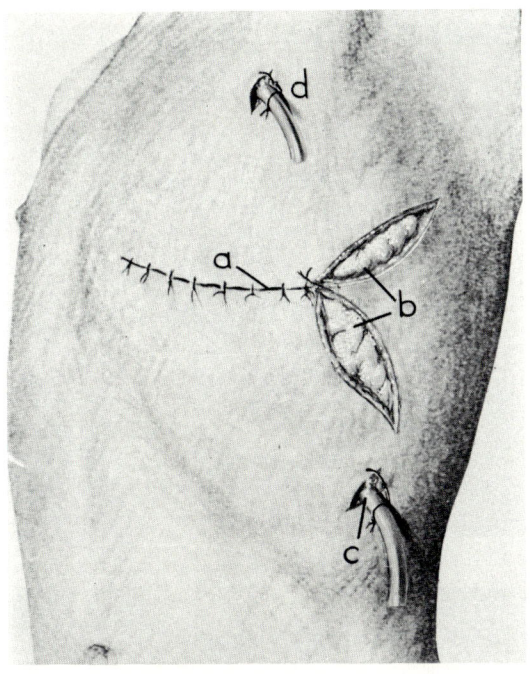

E

Fig 20-1. Case 1. *Anterolateral sucking wound of left chest. (A) Anterolateral aspect of left chest after removal of petrolatum-impregnated gauze pack: (a) large, dirty wound, 5" × 8", involving pectoralis major and serratus magnus muscles; (b) stump of fifth rib; (c) defect in pleura 2.5" × 3"; and (d) stump of fifth costal cartilage. (B) Findings at thoracotomy: (a) tense hemopericardium; (b) nonopaque foreign bodies (dirt, bone, cloth) in pericardium; (c) hematoma of pericardium; (d) hematoma of entire left lower lobe; (e) laceration and hematoma of lingula of left upper lobe; (f) accessory lobe; and (g) hemothorax (3000 cc). (C) First step in wound closure: (a) residual defect in pleura, 1" × 1.5", impossible to close; (b) closure of intercostal muscles, and (c) anterior stump of fifth cartilage. (D) Closure of muscles of anterior chest wall over pleural defect: (a) upper portion of pectoralis major muscle; (b) lower portion of pectoralis major; (c) serratus magnus muscle; and (d) pleural defect. (E) Wound closure: (a) anterior reinforcement of closure by skin suture; (b) skin wound left open posteriorly; (c) posteroinferior closed intercostal drainage tube; and (d) anterior intercostal closed drainage tube. (Illustrations from LA Brewer III, Wounds of the chest in war and peace, 1943–1948. Ann Thorac Surg 7:387, 1969. By permission.)*

abdominal wounds. With careful excision and cleaning only 10 patients needed additional drainage of the wound and in these initial surgery had been delayed up to 72 hours. The emphasis was placed on careful, thorough debridement rather than antibiotics (see Figs 20-1, 20-2). Penicillin was valuable, however, in the presence of massive soft tissue destruction or when surgery had been postponed.

HEMOTHORAX

Hemothorax was a clinical challenge in 91 cases. Prompt removal of the blood from the pleural cavity was carried out in all of these patients. In only 14 instances was there a persistent or clotted hemothorax; decortication was carried out in 9 of these, 7 for organizing hemothorax and 2 for hemothoracic empyema. This represents an incidence of 5.3 percent in the entire series and 10 percent of those with severe hemothorax. Two patients who developed late empyema responded to drainage. Thus, the aggressive management of hemothorax and prompt open evacuation of the pleural cavity as a part of the initial treatment was highly successful (see Figs 20-1, 20-2). These results are in sharp contrast to the results obtained in World War I during which, because early open evacuation of the hemothorax was not uniformly performed, empyema and draining sinuses were the rule.

TRAUMA TO THE LUNG

Laceration of the lungs was present in 61 of the patients in the series. Thirteen were managed conservatively by pleural decompression while open repair was necessary in 48. In only 1 was pulmonary resection employed and this was segmental in type. Recently in Vietnam, a much larger percentage of resections were performed.

Intrapulmonary hematomas were found in 89 persons. Diagnosis was made by direct inspection of the lung or by roentgenographic findings when pneumonitis and atelectasis could be ruled out. In patients undergoing thoracotomy, the entire lobe appeared on occasion to be boggy and hemorrhagic. Since the lung has great recuperative powers because of its dual blood supply from the pulmonary and bronchial arteries, great restraint must be exercised by the surgeon to overcome the temp-

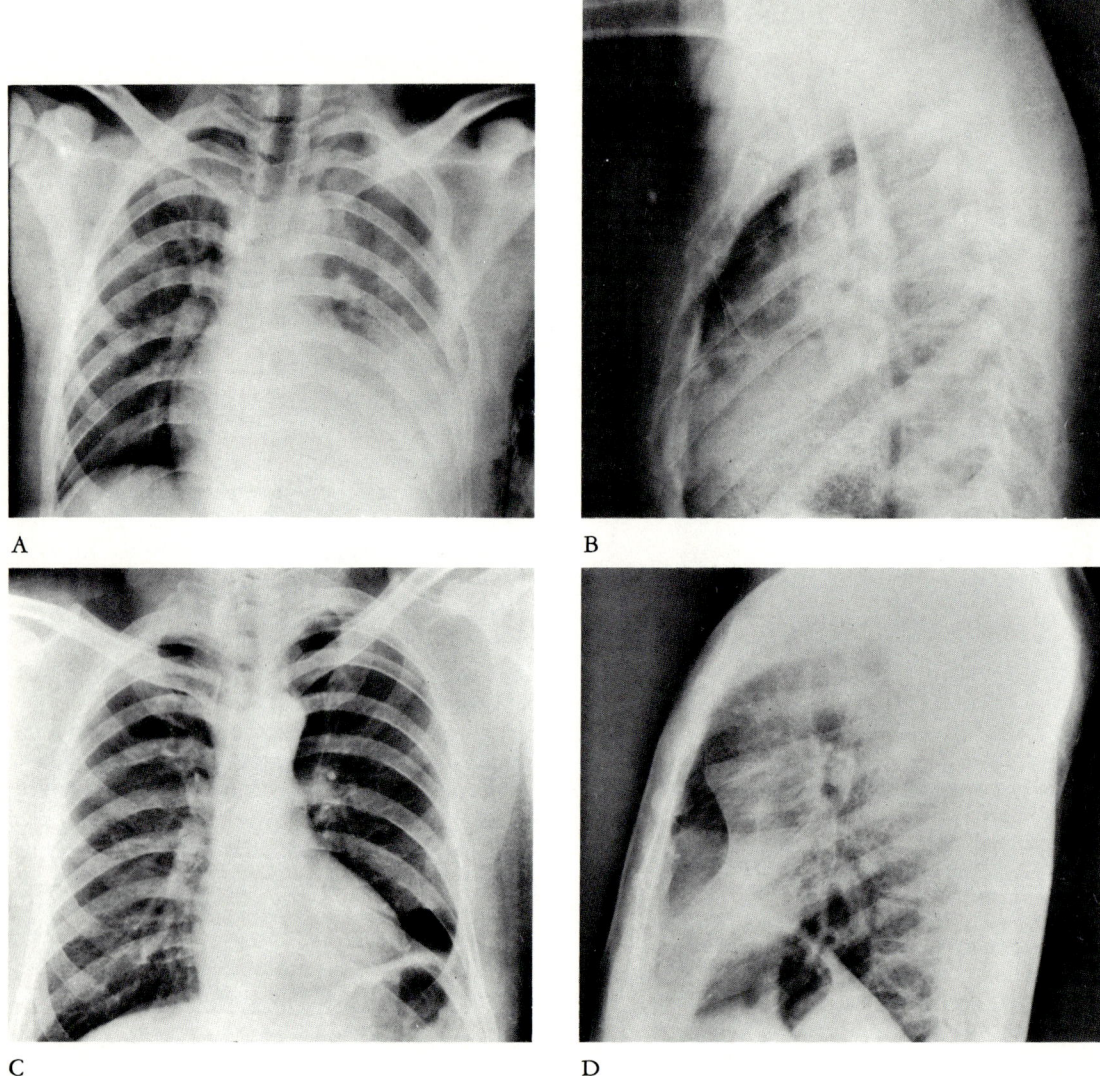

A

B

C

D

Fig 20-2. Serial roentgenograms in mediastinal injury with intrapericardial foreign bodies and hematoma. (A) Posteroanterior roentgenogram, November 8, 1944, taken immediately after wounding, shows massive left hemothorax with a slight shift of mediastinum to the right and extensive emphysema of left chest wall. Right lung is clear. (B) Lateral roentgenogram taken on same date shows diffuse haziness. No radiopaque foreign body is seen. (C) Posteroanterior roentgenogram, November 22, 1960, taken 16 years after wounding, shows clear lung fields and normal heart shadow. Note muscular defect of left anterior chest wall, with resection of anterior portion of fifth rib and tenting of left diaphragm. (D) Lateral roentgenogram taken on same date shows defect of left anterior chest wall with pleural reaction posterior to it and high anterior tenting of left diaphragm. Otherwise, the findings are within the normal range. (Illustrations from LA Brewer III, Wounds of the chest in war and peace, 1943–1948. Ann Thorac Surg 7:387, 1969. By permission.)

tation to remove extensively involved lobes. In each of these 89 cases, however, the hematoma resolved spontaneously, usually in 4 to 6 weeks. The important lesson to be learned from this experience is that pulmonary hematoma following trauma does not provide an indication for pulmonary resection (see Figs 20-1, 20-2). On the other hand, if a hematoma should become infected or form a persistent cavity, then resection should be performed.

The "Wet Lung of Trauma," a condition characterized by the persistence of fluid in the lung in the bronchial tree, was a major problem in 65 of the group studied. This syndrome was first described by our group in the Mediterranean Theater in World War II [3, 7]. The recognition for the first time that the lung reflected severe trauma not only to the chest, but to the abdomen and brain has led to extensive investigation of this condition [3]. This syndrome is now known as respiratory distress syndrome or RDS. It soon became evident that such patients did not tolerate surgery, nor did they tolerate travel well. Consequently no attempt at transfer was made, regardless of the type of wound, until the lungs were comparatively dry. Our management of wet lung included intercostal nerve block, catheter bronchial suction, and intermittent positive pressure breathing that I introduced for the treatment of pulmonary edema, the advanced state of "Wet Lung of Trauma" in 1944. Follow up studies show that if the wet lung received early and careful treatment there were few, if any, pulmonary problems to be dealt with at the base installations (see Figs 20-1, 20-2). However, pulmonary complications were the rule in untreated cases of the syndrome and mortality and morbidity were high.

Only 2 of the 65 patients with severe wet lung syndrome later developed a pneumonitis. Bronchiectasis and chronic abscess, the hallmark of similar wounds in World War I, were not a late feature. None developed the massive atelectasis reported after that conflict. If the patient received proper and early treatment for the wet lung, his chances for complete recovery were excellent.

Case 1

A 19-year-old infantryman sustained a massive sucking wound of the left anterior chest due to a high-explosive shell fragment in France during World War II. Airtight packing was applied as a first aid measure and he received two units of plasma. Almost 3 hours later, he was admitted to the hospital in deep shock. Blood pressure was 80/70; pulse 128; and respirations 40.

Roentgenograms showed obscuration of the left lung (see Fig 20-2A, B). Pulmonary edema occurred after the administration of plasma and intravenous fluids. Large amounts of a thin, pinkish material were aspirated repeatedly by transnasal bronchial suction. Pulmonary edema was again precipitated by an attempt at blood transfusion, which had to be discontinued. Over a period of *8 hours, intermittent positive pressure oxygen therapy was administered.* This consisted of employing a portable anesthetic machine and squeezing the inflation bag with each respiration of the patient. Pressures from 6 to 12 cm of water were generated [3]. The packing was adjusted to allow blood to escape from the chest periodically.

Approximately 10 hours after admission to the hospital his condition was judged to be satisfactory enough to allow him to undergo thoracotomy. This procedure was indicated because of continued intrathoracic hemorrhage, the possibility of diaphragmatic and cardiac injury, and the need for closure of the very large wound.

Surgery consisted of debridement of the chest wall where the pectoralis and serratus muscles were extensively destroyed (Fig 20-1A–E). A long segment of the shattered fifth rib had to be removed down to the cartilage, leaving an opening 2½″ × 3″. By extending the incision in the fifth intercostal space posteriorly, the left thoracic cavity was well exposed. The left lower lobe and the lingula of the left upper lobe were involved in an extensive hematoma. One liter of blood was removed from the pleural space and 90 ml of blood from the tense pericardium. Pericardial bleeding was controlled, and dirt, cloth, and rib fragments were removed. A window was made to drain the pericardium and the pleural cavity. Closure of the chest wall was carried out as shown in Figure 20-1C, D, and E. The left arm was then cleansed and the brachial artery was repaired after milking a clot out of the vessel and restoring proximal and distal flow. The ulnar nerve was traumatized but not completely severed.

The patient made a satisfactory recovery. The extensive hematomas of the left lung absorbed completely and no further chest surgery was needed. Following his return to the United States, the ulnar nerve was repaired and the patient was discharged from the Army.

The late results were excellent. Six years after sustaining his injuries, the serviceman reported that he was working 40 hours a week as a building materials salesman. Chest roentgenograms, made 16 years after wounding, demonstrated clear lung fields and a normal heart shadow. There was, however, a residual muscular defect evident on this film (Fig 20-2C).

RETAINED FOREIGN BODIES

Shell fragments and other retained metallic foreign bodies also presented a challenging problem. There were 102 instances of retained thoracic foreign bodies—35 in the chest wall, 35 in the lung, 22 in the pleura, and 11 in the mediastinum. These objects were removed as soon as possible if they measured over 1 to 2 cm in diameter or were positioned where a major vessel, the heart (Case 1), a bronchus, the trachea, or the esophagus might become involved. Forty-one patients were ultimately discharged with retained foreign bodies, but only 1 had symptoms necessitating subsequent removal. The conservative approach to intrathoracic foreign bodies adopted in these cases still appears to be sound.

THORACOABDOMINAL WOUNDS

Twenty-five thoracoabdominal wounds caused serious problems involving both body cavities. Wounds of the upper abdomen were repaired through a thoracoabdominal incision, which offered superb exposure through the widely opened diaphragm (Fig 20-3A–H). This is in contrast to practice in Vietnam and at the Los Angeles County/USC Medical Center where both wounds are handled separately. Each method has certain advantages. In this series, prompt repair of gastrointestinal perforations and exteriorization of the wounded colon were employed in all patients. The subsequent surgery included five drainage procedures (for three empyemas and two subphrenic abscesses), as well as the removal of a foreign body. No patient with a thoracoabdominal wound returned to active duty and all were evacuated to the continental United States. Three died at the base hospitals of complications. At the time of late follow-up it was shown that the remaining patients who returned to this country were well and working. These excellent late results indicate

a complete return to health in those surviving the early surgery.

Case 2

While serving in France during World War II, a 21-year-old infantryman received wounds of the lower chest, shoulder, upper arm, and scalp. On admission to hospital he complained of severe chest and abdominal pain. His blood pressure was 130/80, pulse 80, and respirations 36. Breath sounds were diminished on the left but an improvement took place after an intercostal nerve block. The persistence of deep and rebound tenderness together with absent bowel sounds in the left upper quadrant indicated peritoneal contamination. Roentgenograms of the chest showed minimal pleural involvement on the left while abdominal films revealed a shell fragment in the left upper quadrant of the abdomen (Fig 20-3D–H). A 500 cc blood transfusion was administered slowly and the stomach emptied with a Levin tube.

Four hours after wounding his condition had improved enough to perform emergency surgery. A left thoracolaparotomy was performed (Fig 20-3A–C). Physical findings and the position of the foreign body in the left upper quadrant influenced us to use this approach, although it certainly could have been handled from below. After debriding the chest wall, the incision was extended along the eighth intercostal space, opening the pleural cavity. A moderate amount of bloody fluid was aspirated. A laceration of the left lower lobe was repaired and, after opening widely the wound of the diaphragm, an excellent exposure of the left upper quadrant was obtained. The lacerated colon was also repaired and brought out through a left upper quadrant incision, the loop being held in place by a glass rod. The diaphragm and chest wall were then closed with appropriate drainage. The wounds of the shoulder, upper arms, and scalp were cleaned and excised. The postoperative course was uneventful. The colostomy was closed at a later date and no further surgery was needed. After a period of service on limited duty he was discharged.

About 7½ years after receiving his wounds, the patient reported that he had worked as a truck driver since the war. Although he had no shortness of breath nor digestive symptoms, he did complain of an occasional twinge of pain in the left chest. The follow-up roentgenogram 16½ years after wounding showed clear lung fields (Fig 20-3G, H).

MEDIASTINUM

Since the mediastinum houses the great vessels, heart, esophagus, trachea, and bronchi, major wounds in this area are often rapidly fatal. In the series under review there were only 13 patients in whom such injuries were treated. It seems likely that these wounds may have been tangential or the result of spent missiles. Hemomediastinum was demonstrated on the chest roentgenogram in 5 patients but blood was absorbed without surgery in all of these. Foreign bodies were removed from 4 individuals. In the late follow-up, bronchial and esophageal obstruction were not encountered and neither was other symptomatology present.

FOLLOW-UP STUDIES

Subsequent surgery performed in 127 patients at a base hospital is presented in Table 20-1. Primary closure of the wound was carried out in 59 patients and removal of foreign bodies in 13. Drainage of the chest wall, including empyema, was performed on 14 individuals. In the continental United States 3 patients underwent removal of foreign bodies; 2 had drainage of an empyema; and in 1 patient there was excision of an arteriovenous fistula involving the internal mammary vessels. All were discharged with their lungs expanded and chest walls healed.

Subsequent roentgenograms (taken 3 to 17 years after wounding) showed substantially similar findings to those found on the predischarge films. Healed scars or tenting of the diaphragm were seen in 57 patients, and "thickening" of the pleura in 27. Only 5 had pulmonary emphysema.

This group of 167 patients was predominantly asymptomatic. The records show that only 3 complained of symptoms of moderate chest pain and dyspnea. Practically all were working. Eighteen had a psychoneurosis, probably related to the total war experience and the fact that they had been wounded, rather than the chest wound per se.

Thoracic disease following discharge from the Army was not a significant problem. Two patients contracted pulmonary tuberculosis and recovered with treatment, while another developed bronchogenic carcinoma on the same side as the penetrating chest wound. Some were hospitalized at various times for pneumonia and other acute respiratory infections. It should be emphasized, however, that this incidence of pulmonary infection was no greater than that in the general population.

CONCLUSIONS

This follow-up study offers strong support for a physiologically oriented treatment regimen, and one that provides rapid restoration of the function of the lungs and heart. In most instances, minor procedures were found to be effective. These included closed thoracostomy, catheter bronchial suction or tracheostomy, packing of a sucking wound, and stabilization of the chest wall. In some cases, thoracotomy was necessary to reestablish the cardiopulmonary function. This was most

Table 20-1. Surgery Required in Fixed Hospitals in Patients Who Underwent Surgery in Forward Hospitals

| Surgery in Fixed Hospitals | Previous Surgery in Forward Hospitals | | | |
| | Thoracotomy | | Thoraco-laparotomy | Total |
	Yes	No		
Drainage of chest wall	2	3	2	7
Drainage for empyema	5	1	1	7
Removal of foreign body	5	7	1	13
Decortication	4	4	1	9
Abdominal surgery	2	—	4	6
Delayed primary wound closure	26	31	2	59
Other	8	12	6	26

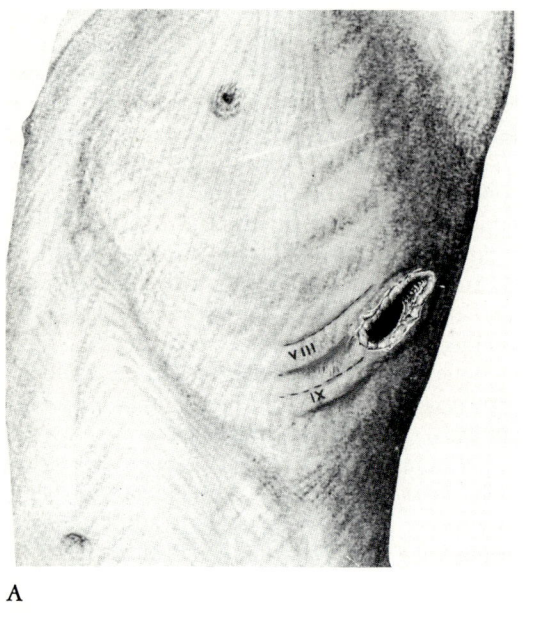

A

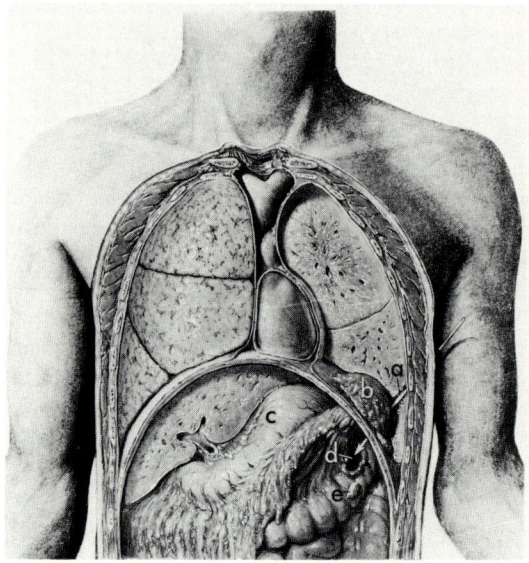

B

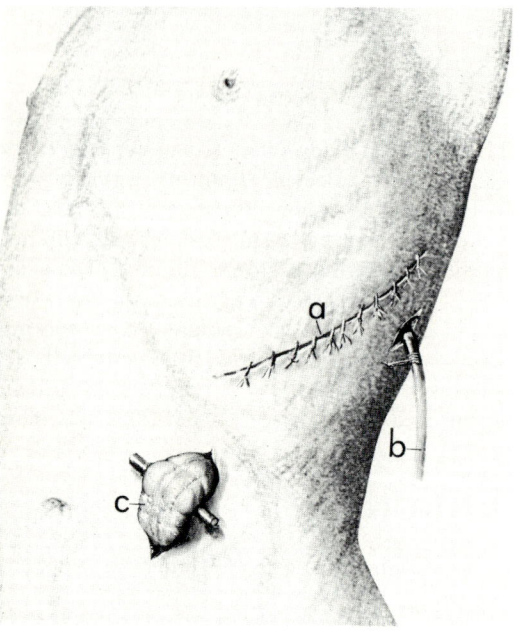

C

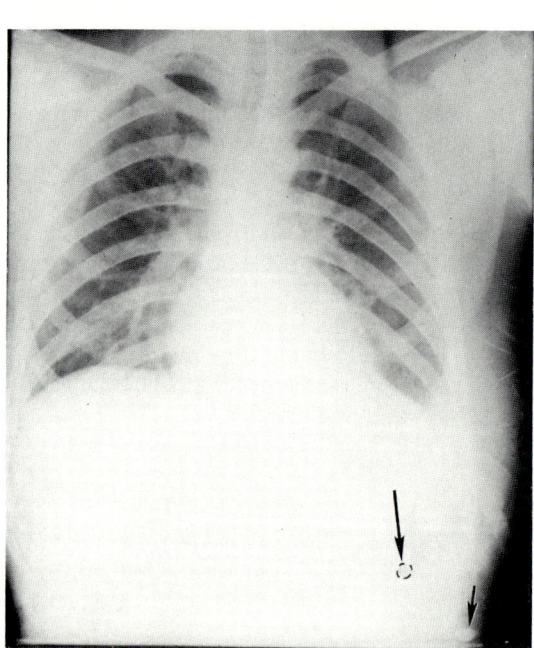

D

Fig 20-3. **Case 2.** *Schematic showing of thoraco-abdominal wound with serial roentgenograms. (A) Small penetrating wound in left eighth intercostal space in midaxillary line. (B) Pathological findings: (a) laceration of lung; (b) omentum plugging laceration of diaphragm; (c) intact stomach; (d) laceration of splenic flexure of colon; and (e) foreign body. (C) Anterolateral chest wall at conclusion of* operation: (a) closed thoracotomy incision; (b) closed pleural drainage tube; and (c) exteriorized loop of colon over glass rod. (D) Posteroanterior roentgenogram of chest, September 22, 1944, taken shortly after wounding, shows relatively clear lung fields, small amount of fluid in left pleural cavity, and small metallic foreign body in left upper quadrant of abdomen. Levin tube is in the esophagus.

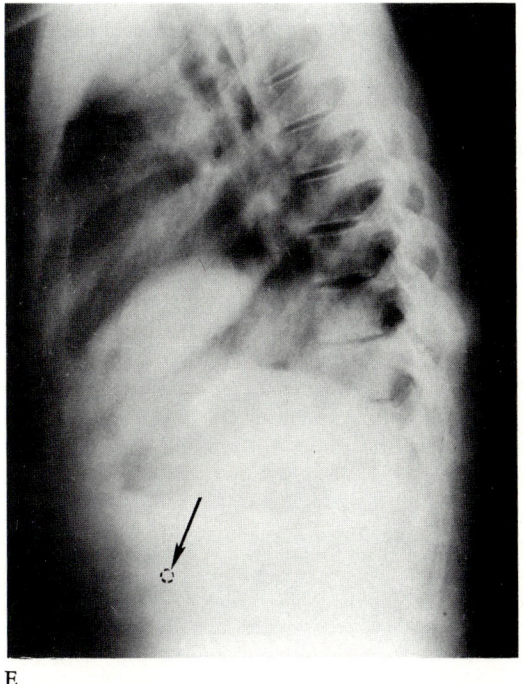

E

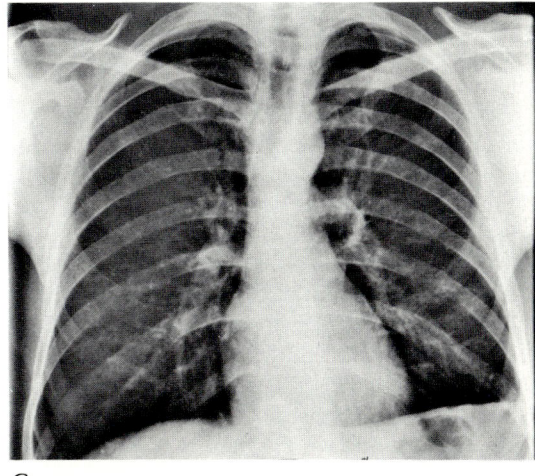

G

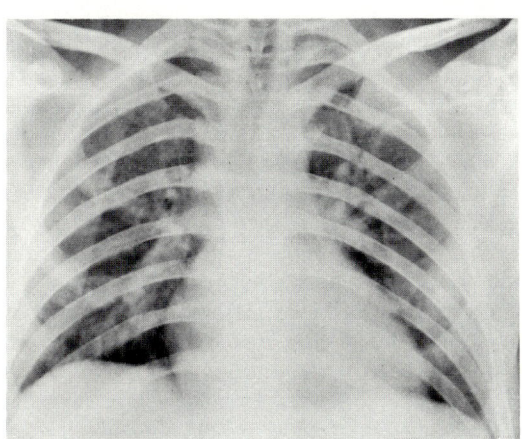

F

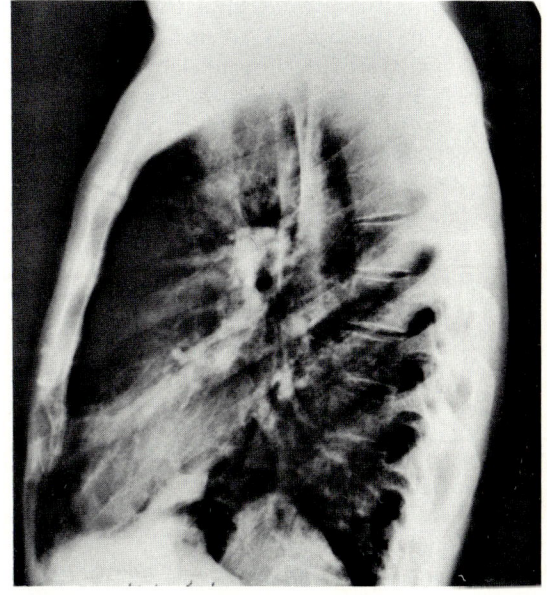

H

(E) *Lateral roentgenogram taken on same date shows small metallic foreign body in left upper quadrant of abdomen and haziness of lungs.*
(F) *Posteroanterior roentgenogram shows expansion of left lung on sixth postoperative day. (G) Postero-anterior roentgenogram of chest, February 14, 1961, taken 16½ years after wounding, shows clear lung fields. Left diaphragm is flat, and costophrenic sinus*

is blunted laterally. (H) Lateral roentgenogram taken on same date shows prominent bronchovascular markings, tenting of diaphragm anteriorly, and sharp posterior diaphragmatic sulcus. (Illustrations from Medical Department, United States Army, Surgery in World War II—Thoracic Surgery, *Vol. II, p. 487, 1965. By permission.)*

often for massive hemorrhage, air leak, or thoracoabdominal wounds. Following the careful stabilization of cardiorespiratory physiology and debridement of the wound, thoracotomy could be performed safely. Indications for the latter included sucking wounds, thoracoabdominal wounds, continued intrathoracic hemorrhage, air leak, and injury to vital mediastinal structures (esophagus, trachea, heart, great vessels, and thoracic duct). There seems no valid reason to revise these indications, the more so since they have been retested carefully in Korea and Vietnam and in civilian practice.

Certain other lessons should be underlined. The vigorous treatment of "traumatic wet lung" by clearing the airway and using intercostal nerve block and intermittent positive pressure breathing will not only save life but will also prevent late pulmonary infections and invalidism. Hemothorax must be promptly evacuated and effective pleural drainage must be maintained. As a rule, pulmonary laceration responds to closed thoracostomy but at times does need direct suture. Hematomas of the lung are usually absorbed. If patients with blast injury to the heart and lungs survive the initial trauma they have an excellent prognosis. Asymptomatic small intrathoracic foreign bodies (1 cm or less) may be left undisturbed. Patients with mediastinal wounds who survive the initial wounding do well. Prompt closure of gastrointestinal wounds and exteriorization of the traumatized colon were found to be justified. Patients with thoracoabdominal wounds recovered completely if they survived the initial operation and the postoperative complications.

The excellent late results reported here provide solid support for the principles of treatment of chest wounds which we developed in the Mediterranean Theater of Operations during World War II. The same principles have been employed successfully in Korea, Vietnam, and civilian life.

RECENT PROGRESS

To put these follow-up studies in perspective, it is important that a brief review of current practices in the management of trauma be presented. During the past 14 years (1965 to 1979), there have been no revolutionary advances in the management of thoracic wounds per se. This period of time has seen, however, the perfection of established methods of handling patients with trauma, which has resulted in the improvement of the treatment of patients with thoracic injuries.

The institution of the paramedic ground and air ambulance system by the police and fire departments in major cities has been a definite step forward. This system, patterned after programs perfected in the Vietnam War, has resulted in the rapid transport of the patient wounded in a traffic accident (the greatest source of civilian trauma) to the hospital [8, 9]. Equipped with special two-way radio communication and ECG transmission, well-trained paramedics are able to resuscitate the critically injured patient at the scene of the accident, under the radio direction of an emergency room physician who remains at the medical center. Once the patient has had the initial resuscitation, he is speedily transported to the hospital for definitive treatment. Thus, with the prompt action of the paramedic team usually called promptly through the police and fire departments, precious time that may be lifesaving in patients with cardiac or aortic wounds is not lost. The patient is saved from the hazard of lying unattended on the highway waiting for an ambulance which might not have trained paramedics and in deep shock from hemorrhage or another potentially lethal cause.

When he or she arrives at the hospital, rapid restoration of cardiopulmonary function of the patient with the severe chest wound is mandatory, as cited previously. This is effected by the identification and treatment of the cause of the shock with correction of blood loss and improvement of tissue perfusion in the hypoxic patient. Hypoxia, readily detected by monitoring the arterial blood gases, may be corrected by the prompt insertion of an intratracheal tube, which not only insures the airway for the administration of positive pressure oxygen but also permits a constant toilet for the tracheobronchial tree. Central venous pressure and, in certain cases, pulmonary artery wedge pressures will detect overloading of the right and left ventricles. Because patients who have sustained major injuries are very susceptible to infection, scrupulous aseptic techniques must be employed on all minor surgical procedures performed on the patient: intravenous cannulation, intratracheal intubation and suction, bladder catheterization, and so on [16]. The sooner a prophylactic intravenous injection of a broad spectrum antibiotic, such as cephalothin for thoracic wounds or gentamicin for thoracoabdominal wounds, is given, the better the chance to control potential infection.

The introduction of computerized axial tomography (CAT), isotope scans, and regional angiography has led to a more precise diagnosis, making decisions for or against surgery more certain. As emphasized by several authors in this book, minor surgical methods (closed thoracostomy, wound debridement and closure, airway establishment, and chest wall stabilization, and so on) are sufficient for the majority of patients. Continuing massive pneumothorax and hemothorax, as well as thoracoabdominal, esophageal, cardiac, and great vessel wounds, still remain sound indications for emergency thoracotomy. The techniques for these major procedures have been refined, but the principles remain the same. Certain newer operative techniques are discussed later. Intraoperative filtering, heparinizing and returning to the patient the blood lost in the pleural cavity in severe hemorrhage has resulted in a great saving in the number of units of banked blood that were formerly necessary to restore blood volume [2]. This method conserves a vital public resource.

Current operative techniques, based on more precise diagnosis, can be more accurately planned and expeditiously executed. However, the general approach to treatment is still the same as those presented earlier in this chapter. Current procedures are mainly refinements in anesthesia and operative procedures, with two exceptions: (1) intra-aortic balloon pumping and (2) extracorporeal circulation. The former is a product of the past decade and the latter of over the past two decades. Intra-aortic balloon pumping has been proved to be of value in combatting hypotension secondary to a failing myocardium. This technique has had its greatest value, however, in maintaining blood pressure and lessening cardiac strain in acute myocardial infarction and following cardiac operations. Although it is infrequently employed in acute trauma, it perhaps should be used more often.

Extracorporeal circulation (discussed in Chapter 12) is now available in many centers treating victims of trauma. This technique for the management of massive intrathoracic bleeding in the acute stage and later for the repair of subacute or chronic posttraumatic conditions, is a great addition to the surgeon's armamentarium. Although

the heparinization, which is mandatory for the above procedures, is a disadvantage in the trauma patient with severe hemorrhage, otherwise uncontrollable bleeding may be managed by this technique [17].

Postoperative treatment in the intensive care wards has improved by: (1) better monitoring of the patient's cardiac and respiratory functions and (2) the use of more highly trained physicians, nurses, and ancillary personnel who treat the patient on an around-the-clock basis [16]. The teaching of registered nurses the rudiments of electrocardiography has given more meaning to the use of the electrocardiographic oscilloscopes that are now found in all intensive care wards.

Respiratory care, so important to the patient with a severe thoracic wound, has improved with the development in many hospitals of departments specializing in this form of treatment. The more frequent monitoring of arterial blood gases, the development of more efficient respirators, and the early employment of intratracheal tubes instead of tracheostomy have been important advances [19].

The perfection of the use of positive end-expiratory pressure (PEEP) has made it possible to maintain a satisfactory PO_2 with a FIO_2 of 40 percent [13]. It has its greatest use in patients who needed from 60 to 100 percent FIO_2 to maintain proper oxygenation of the blood. With the employment of PEEP, the omnipresent danger of oxygen toxicity and hyaline membrane disease, which occurs in 24 hours with the administration of high oxygen concentrations, may be avoided. Sometimes it may be necessary to gradually raise the pressure with PEEP to levels as high as 20 to 40 cm of water. Great care must be taken with this technique to avoid impairment of left heart function or the development of pulmonary edema. This may be done by means of measuring the peripheral or wedge pulmonary artery pressure, which reflects left atrial and ventricular diastolic pressure, and by calculation of the cardiac output [13]. Although the management of these patients is difficult, at times these patients—who would otherwise die—will be saved.

Membrane oxygenators have been employed for days or a week or more to oxygenate the blood in trauma patients who were in respiratory failure and all other methods had failed [10, 12]. Although a few successes have been reported, there have been more failures, so that this form of treatment should still be considered as experimental. This technique demands elaborate equipment and a large, highly trained staff that, because of the enormous expenses involved, is beyond the reach of most hospitals. Open-lung biopsy should be performed prior to the use of this technique to make sure that fibrosis of the lung has not developed, which would doom this form of treatment to failure [12].

To be sure, with the arrival of more of the critically injured persons to the emergency rooms of hospitals, the overall mortality for trauma patients has only slightly improved. The death rate for these patients who have lived to reach the hospital is inevitably higher [14, 15, 17], which in turn effects the overall mortality figures. Yet fewer "dead-on-arrival" casualties means that more patients will be saved who otherwise would not have survived to receive hospital care. This is particularly true of patients with injuries to the heart and major vessels.

With a society in America that is extremely mobile, follow-up studies of patients who have had chest wounds has been extremely difficult, and there have been no long-term reports available. Those included in this chapter were made through a study of Veterans Administration Hospital records. Since identical principles of treatment are being used at this time for the management of thoracic trauma, it seems reasonable to assume that the excellent 16-year results herein reported could currently be a bit better due to the advances in treatment that have been cited. Sufficient time has not elapsed to develop such statistics on patients who have been managed by the improved methods discussed earlier in this section. Nevertheless, if the current mobility trends of the American public persist, even with the passage of sufficient time it will be difficult to assemble similar, comparable, and meaningful long-term follow-up studies.

REFERENCES

1. Aaby GV: Personal communication, 1968
2. Bregman D, Parodi EN, Hutchinson JE III, et al: Intraoperative autotransfusion during emergency thoracic and elective open-heart surgery. Ann Thorac Surg 18:590, 1974
3. Brewer LA III, et al: The wet lung in war casualties. Ann Surg 123:343, 1961
4. Brewer LA III: Long-term (1943–1961) follow-up studies in combat-incurred thoracic wounds. Edited by AL Ahnfeldt. Surgery in World War II, Thoracic Surgery. Vol. II. Washington, DC, Office of the Surgeon General, Department of the Army, 1965, p. 441
5. Brewer LA III, Steiner LE: The management of crushing injuries of the chest. Surg Clin North Am 48:1279, 1968
6. Brewer LA III: Wounds of the chest in war and peace, 1943–1948. Ann Thorac Surg 7:387, 1969
7. Burford TH, Burbank B: Traumatic wet lung: Observations on certain physiologic fundamentals of thoracic trauma. J Thorac Surg 14:415, 1945
8. Cleveland HC, Bigelow DB, Dracon D, et al: A civilian air emergency service: a report of its development, technical aspects, and experience. J Trauma 16:452, 1976
9. Felix WR: Metropolitan aeromedical service: State of the art. J Trauma 16:873, 1976
10. Geelhoed GW, Adkins PC, Corso PJ, et al: Clinical effects of membrane lung support for acute respiratory failure. Ann Thorac Surg 20:177, 1975
11. Heaton LD, Hughes CW, Rosegay H, et al: Military surgical practices of the US army in Vietnam. In Current Problems in Surgery. Chicago: Year Book, 1966
12. Hill JD, Ratliff JL, Fallat RJ, et al: Prognostic factors in the treatment of acute respiratory insufficiency with long-term extracorporeal oxygenation. J Thorac Cardiovasc Surg 68:905, 1974
13. Kirby RR, Downs JB, Civetta JM, et al: High level positive end expiratory pressure (PEEP) in acute respiratory insufficiency. Chest 67:156, 1975
14. Kish G, Kozloff L, Joseph WL, et al: Indication for early thoracotomy in management of chest trauma. Ann Thorac Surg 22:23, 1976
15. McNamara JJ, Messersmith JK, Dunn RA, et al: Thoracic injuries in combat casualties in Vietnam. Ann Thorac Surg 10:389, 1970
16. Moore FD: Post Traumatic Pulmonary Insufficiency. Philadelphia, Saunders, 1969
17. Reul GJ, Mattox KL, Beall AC Jr, et al: Recent advances in operative management of massive chest trauma. Ann Thorac Surg 16:52, 1973
18. Valle AR: Management of war wounds of the chest. J Thorac Surg 24:457, 1952
19. Yorra FH: Shock lung. Current Concepts in Chest Disease, Tuberculosis and Respiratory Disease Association of Los Angeles County, No. 3, Vol. II, 1972

21. THORACIC TRAUMA AS
SEEN BY THE MEDICAL EXAMINER

Joseph H. Davis

A medical examiner is a pathologist who has the responsibility and authority to investigate all violent, sudden, unexpected, and suspicious deaths as well as those involving workmen's compensation. The agency in which he works should amass a wealth of data pertaining to the antecedent causes and fatal end results of trauma, poisoning, and natural disease. During a 10-year period Dade County, Florida, with a population of approximately 1.3 million, had numerous fatalities; these included 1,598 homicides, 2,130 suicides, 2,341 motor vehicle deaths, and 3,154 miscellaneous accidental deaths. Postmortem examinations were performed in all and records were completed to the best possible extent. Within these case records may be found examples of practically every form of blunt and penetrating physical trauma, asphyxia, chemical, and thermal injury.

MODES OF INJURY

Each investigated death becomes an individual lesson in the study of injury causation and prevention. The circumstances of injury may be approached from three separate standpoints, each interwoven and overlapping with the others. These are the human factors, the environmental factors, and the agents that inflict the injuries. The last can include motor vehicles, weapons, machinery, poisons, and so on.

Human factors contributing to injury may be thought of as physical, meaning the presence or absence of disease states; chemical, such as the effects of alcohol or drugs; and psychological. Each of these factors can be further considered from the viewpoint of why an individual got into a hazardous situation and why he subsequently could not successfully extricate himself without injury or death. Of all the human factors that lead to injury, none is so ubiquitous as the abuse of alcohol. It may be stated without reservation that the average medical examiner facility derives its main trauma case load from such abuse. Approximately 70 percent of those drivers fatally involved in single vehicle accidents wherein no

other surviving driver can be blamed have been drinking; and in multivehicle crashes about half the dead drivers were under the influence of alcohol. In 4 out of 5 of these, blood alcohol concentration exceeded 0.10 percent and within this group, in over half it exceeded 0.20 percent. These Dade County percentages reflect the national fatality by automobile experience [11].

Two-thirds of all homicides involve drunken brawls. Alcohol also plays a role in other fatal accidents. Each year we see 6 to 8 fatal cases of asphyxia due to the impaction of a bolus of meat in the hypopharynx or larynx. These usually occur in middle-aged individuals who are wearing dentures and have a very high blood alcohol content. This provokes a lethal combination of difficulty in chewing meat, the anesthetic effect of alcohol, and carelessness. This Dade County experience with alcohol is not unique. In Finland, where the motor vehicle laws are stricter and genuinely enforced, only 22 to 27 percent of fatal vehicle crashes involve alcohol. Greater frequencies of alcohol involvement are encountered with surviving victims of injury: 36 percent in home accidents, 45 percent in other free-time accidents, and 69 percent in victims of fights, assaults, and suicide attempts [25]. Finnish studies have revealed that 30 to 35 percent of acutely injured patients treated in an emergency facility were under the influence of alcohol [24]. The thoracic surgeon should bear in mind that the acutely injured patient may well be under such influence. Blood concentration determinations of alcohol should be considered as part of the diagnostic study in order to help differentiate between the effects of injury and those of intoxication as well as to assist in making a choice of anesthetic agents. A mistaken diagnosis of intoxication, in the absence of a confirmatory blood test, has resulted in liability claims when undiagnosed injury was severe.

The role of physical, rather than chemical, impairment in accident causation is an important consideration, since such physical illness may determine the outcome of a subsequent clinical course. In a careful analysis of 1,171 dead drivers over a 12-year period, we encountered 237 individuals who died because of the careless actions of other drivers. The remainder, those who initiated the fatal crash or event, fell into two categories. In the first group were 305 drivers who collapsed at the wheel due to causes other than trauma, usually cardiac disease. However, 112 of these dying drivers caused injury and even death to others. The remaining 629 drivers who initiated or caused a crash died with severe injuries of all types: cranial, thoracic, and abdominal. Because of the fatal nature of these injuries, the pre-existing cardiovascular disease discovered postmortem could not be said to have caused death prior to the trauma. A careful analysis of the circumstances surrounding these 629 automobile crashes with fatal sequelae revealed that 5.9 percent (37) had the lethal crash sequence set into motion by preexisting disease. Of these 37 people, 7 were epileptics, 1 was a youth with a bleeding congenital cerebral vascular malformation, and the remaining 29 were individuals with severe coronary artery disease. Injured victims of automobile crashes may have underlying natural disease that may be expected to complicate treatment of the injuries.

Emphasis upon automobile-associated trauma is well justified. The first fatality occurred in New York City in 1899 and we achieved the one millionth fatality in the United States by 1954 [31] with subsequent yearly totals of 50,000 to 55,000. These are but the tip of the iceberg, the injured remainder coming under the care of the surgeon. In a 1-year period, 1966 to 1967, there were 3.5 million persons injured in motor vehicle accidents [28], an expected ratio of about 1 fatality per 60 injured patients. Motor vehicle crash injury universally accounts for a major source of multiple trauma victims encountered in surgical practice. In one French study [59] 87 percent of 168 consecutive surgical clinic multiple trauma cases were associated with automobile accidents; only 10 percent were associated with knives and bullets.

In a 16-year Denver, Colorado, study [4], confined to patients admitted with chest injuries, 73 percent of 685 patients had injuries received in automobile accidents and 13 percent had injuries associated with criminal attacks. The mortality in these patients was 8.75 percent. Within these fatalities there were 22 patients with chest injury complications, 21 with cerebral injuries, and 17 associated with other body regions and complica-

tions. With only automobile-occupant injury trauma, 70 percent of patients have involvement of more than one area, with 38.6 percent involving the thorax and only 3.35 percent involving *only* the thorax [28]. The surgeon should bear in mind that the spectrum of automobile-occupant injuries is huge. In a collective review by Sims and colleagues [51], the spectrum is reviewed, along with mechanisms whereby injury patterns arise from secondary collisions within the vehicle. Only head injuries exceed thoracic and upper abdominal injuries as causes of death in motor vehicle accidents [44].

POSTMORTEM EXAMINATION EXPERIENCE

In order to determine fatal thoracic injury frequencies, with or without other area injury, we reviewed a 3-year experience with Dade County motor vehicle fatalities. There were a total of 648 deaths of drivers, passengers, pedestrians, and cyclists. All were subject to postmortem examination. Major thoracic injury was noted in 465 (72 percent) of these vehicular deaths and was defined as intrathoracic visceral injury, bilateral rib or sternal fractures, or more than four ribs fractured unilaterally. A comparison of those who died immediately with those whose death was delayed revealed 20 percent of the former had severe aortic trauma whereas only 1.7 percent of the latter had serious aortic injury. There was thoracic aortic involvement in 36 of 94 drivers killed instantly: 6 in the ascending portion, 10 in the arch, and 20 in the descending part; whereas in 15 of the 101 passengers who died extremely quickly after the accident there were 7 who had sustained trauma to the ascending part, 3 to the arch, and 5 to the descending portion. It should be interesting to compare similar samples in the future when vehicles with obsolete non-energy-absorbing steering columns no longer remain in operation.

Only 6 persons with vertebral fractures were encountered in a total of 228 dead vehicular occupants. On the other hand, in a group of 198 pedestrians struck by cars, there were 19 associated vertebral fractures, a point of concern for the attending physician searching for hidden injury. Of the 88 pedestrians killed at the time of impact, 4 had ruptures of the ascending aortic arch and 21 of the descending aorta. Only 1 descending aortic rupture was found in the group of 110 pedestrians whose deaths were delayed. With 5 additional cases of aortic rupture in cyclists, a total of 91 such ruptures occurred in 648 vehicular fatalities in Dade County. This corresponds to the one out of six ratio reported by Greendyke [19] who studied motor vehicle deaths in Rochester, New York, from 1961 to 1965. Sevitt [47] in Birmingham, England, reported aortic rupture in 10 percent of 254 fatal road casualties: 21 percent in car occupants, 16 percent in motorcyclists, and 5.6 percent within the pedestrian group. In an excellent clinicopathological study of personally performed postmortem examinations of 37 persons with aortic rupture, his distribution was: ascending aorta, 7 cases; proximal descending aorta, 25 cases; and distal descending aorta, 5 cases [48]. The distal cases were found in pedestrians and motorcyclists with local hyperextension spinal dislocations, a point of diagnostic consideration. The frequently seen transverse intimal tear configuration of aortic ruptures indicates longitudinal stretching, e.g., localized traction injury mechanism.

The complexity of aortic injury circumstance and mechanisms are well summarized and discussed by Sevitt [49]. Recognition of surgically treatable lesions [62] may be enhanced by consideration of the potential mechanisms of injury force. Information sufficient to reveal such possible mechanisms may be gleaned from the emergency personnel or police investigators on the scene as well as by recognition of significant external abrasions, contusions, or lacerations. Recognition of injury patterns and their subsequent correlation with the circumstances of injury are also important in anticipation of questions that may be raised within courts of law, by research facilities, or by educational institutions. When a moving vehicle strikes an object, for example, the occupants are thrown toward the point of impact. In a head-on collision, the driver is thrown violently forward and upward against the steering assembly. A left front impact will throw him forward and to the left into the A pillar, the roof supports being designated A, B, and C from front to rear. A side impact results in his being propelled toward the corresponding side. Often there are multiple impacts by the vehicle as it careens off objects with corresponding interior impacts by the occupants unless they are securely restrained. The surgeon should assist in the reconstruction of the accident sequence by observing and documenting the major patterns of injury distribution, particularly skin abrasions, lacerations, or contusions. Multiple unilateral fractures indicate force from that side, although this may not necessarily be true in every case. The sum total of the apparent injuries will serve to indicate the pattern of application of force. Consideration by the physician of these forces may suggest the possibility of additional unsuspected internal injuries.

When circumstantial and clinical evidence indicates a concentration of force from nonpenetrating blunt injury, appraisal for critical injury of underlying viscera becomes obvious. In one of our cases the passenger in the right front seat of a small European automobile was thrown forward and slightly to the left as the result of a frontal impact at a speed of only 15 miles per hour. A radio knob came in contact with the left breast of the victim, producing two simple fractures. Two weeks later she suddenly complained of feeling faint and collapsed. A cardiac tamponade was found secondary to rupture of a contused left ventricle. The pericardium was intact. A similar case but with less decelerative force involved two young male baseball players who collided while trying to catch a fly ball. The elbow of one struck the other high on the anterior chest with resulting rib fractures and immediate rupture of the left ventricle.

Successful surgical repair of cardiac rupture, usually atrial, is attributed to early recognition and surgical intervention [36]. The opportunity for this is enhanced when there is an efficient paramedical emergency care and transport system [52], a service now rapidly expanding in the United States. This points out the need to recognize, too, that initial diagnosis by the surgeon is through communication with the emergency personnel. Ignorance of injury circumstances and dependence only upon an initial clinical observation can easily lead to errors or lack of recognition of critical injury, as exemplified by the case report of Bloch and Meir [7]. In their case a 20-month-old child was found under an overturned television set that rested upon his right face and hemithorax. One hour later, awake, active, and crying, and vital signs and roentgenograms considered normal, he was judged to be not seriously hurt. Six hours after discharge he was dead from an intracardiac transverse tear of the interventricular septum. More critical appreciation of the circumstance of injury should have alerted the physicians to the possibility of much more severe injury than was clinically evident.

Myocardial contusion from localized blunt trauma is less well appreciated and probably more difficult to diagnose even if thought of. Differentiation from coronary atherosclerosis and its effects may be impossible under certain circumstances. Burchell's couplet—quoted by Saunders and Doty [46], ". . . and always with a heart contusion arise both doubt and much confusion"— exemplifies the difficulty of such diagnosis. The wide spectrum of adverse cardiac effects from nonpenetrating trauma varies from disruption of the structures of the heart, at one end of the spectrum, to only demonstrable dysrhythmias without anatomical structure change at the other end. Where posttraumatic coronary occlusion has been demonstrable by angiography, one would indict trauma, especially in the absence of evidence of multiple sites of narrowing. Oren and co-workers [42] report such a case; chest pain commenced 30 minutes after a midchest fist blow with subsequent electrocardiographic and enzyme changes diagnostic of infarction. Later angiography revealed an occlusion of only the left circumflex artery. They speculate that the blow may have torn the intima or resulted in a subintimal hemorrhage, or both. I would add another hypothesis, that the blow ruptured a soft, nonoccluding, nonadvanced lipid plaque, such plaques being subject to spontaneous disruption when they are advanced [17].

The musculoskeletal wall of the thorax may be subject to great distortion from blunt trauma, especially in motor vehicle crashes. In traumatic studies of the live primate chest, up to 60 percent compression distortion is compatible with life, although cardiothoracic injuries and transient bradyarrhythmias do occur [50]. Pulmonary contusions and injuries can be expected with such compressions. Tensile stress upon the bronchi may be expected with the lateral widening associated with a shortening of the anteroposterior dimension. Bronchial disruption from nonpenetrating trauma is less common in our experience, in keeping with the reports of others [29]. The most common site of rupture is a main bronchus within 2.5 cm of the carina. In a recent fatal case that I examined postmortem the victim was a 49-year-old, moderately obese female pedestrian who was carried by an out-of-control light truck into a chain link fence. Despite an intact rib cage there was an almost complete avulsion of the left lung at the hilus with only one branch of a pulmonary vein still adherent. Left hemopneumothorax and interstitial emphysema were prominent.

Mediastinal interstitial emphysema is most commonly seen arising from the lung. This follows any episode during which hyperdistention of alveoli occur. The mechanism is dependent upon the relative distensibility of the alveoli adjacent to the nondistendible arteries and veins. The classic review of Macklin and Macklin [33] should be studied when considering this problem in its broadest sense. The complications of extra-alveolar air include not only interstitial emphysema but pneumothorax and air embolism. In our experience the most frequent complication of scuba sport diving necessitating medical treatment is such an extra-alveolar air syndrome.

It is apparent that major occupant injury occurs from secondary impact with the interior of the motor vehicle [51] or when the occupant is ejected. All clinical and pathological discussions are for naught without consideration of prevention. Human behavior modification is most difficult. Road environment modifications are less expensive and are cost-effective, especially in limited access highway design. Most effective, and least in cost, is improved use of occupant restraint devices associated with better safety design of the vehicle. In a study of 300 fatally injured vehicle occupants, Griffiths et al [20] estimate that the use of front lap belts with shoulder belts would have saved 40.6 percent of front compartment occupants and 23.7 percent of rear compartment occupants.

A clinical study by Whelan and Ackroyd [65] of patients injured in motor vehicle accidents revealed a significant reduction in the likelihood of being admitted as an inpatient if restraints were used. The problem is to persuade occupants to "buckle up," an admonition that physicians might utilize in patient dealings. Additionally there must be constant pressure upon the automobile industry to include air bag devices as standard for motor vehicles, because their worth is without question [71].

Most penetrating thoracic wounds are from bullets or similar high-velocity fragments or stab wounds during assaults. Low-energy penetration from falls onto sharp objects are infrequent. We have also investigated three motor vehicle deaths where the top rail of a roadside chain link fence penetrated the vehicle and transfixed an occupant.

Although bullet projectiles are most frequently seen, industrial stud gun injuries may occur. These are industrial instruments in which a blank pistol charge is used to drive a nail, the stud, into concrete, steel, or wood. The wounds may be quite bizarre in appearance [55].

Wounding characteristics of bullets are usually a matter of energy of motion transfer to tissues. Bullet size, caliber usually being expressed as the diameter, and weight are less significant than velocity because energy of motion is related to velocity squared. The retardant force on the projectile, e.g., that which results in energy of motion transfer to the tissue, is also proportional to the tissue density, the projected transverse area of the projectile, and the drag coefficient of the projectile at the current yaw angle. Yaw is the angle between the long axis of the projectile and its trajectory. "Tumbling" is an increase in the yaw angle. As a result of intermittent energy of motion transfers to tissue, variable-sized temporary cavities are formed in tissue with resulting serious injury to tissues and organs adjacent to but not within the pathway of the bullet [3, 10]. For further detailed discussions of the involved physics with clinical applicability, the reader is referred to the review by Rybeck [45] in conjunction with the practical clinical report by DeMuth [12]. Water, being incompressible, is quite dense, so blood-filled or moist parenchymal organs sustain explosive disruption from bullet energy. The air-containing lung, although less dense, may still have considerable cavity formation when military or hunting bullets of high velocity strike. Persistent lung cavities can complicate such wounds and require subsequent treatment [53]. Associated nervous system involvement should likewise be considered [15].

Bullet patterns are important to recognize. Entry is usually characterized by a circular abrasion with inverted margins, although some deeper strands of tissue may be everted due to blood flow. An exit wound often has slightly torn stellate margins, but in the case of an attenuated bullet it may only be represented by a tiny slit along the skin cleavage line. In this instance the bullet is usually found between the skin and the clothing. Sometimes clothing or furniture pressure over an exit wound will cause a ring-like abrasion similar to that found with an entrance wound. As a general rule bullets pursue a reasonably straight course through the body. In many cases in which the bullet does not exit, it may be palpated beneath the skin of the opposite side of the thorax. This simple maneuver enables the emergency room surgeon to establish an approximate pathway and estimate which viscera may have become involved. On the other hand, bullets entering the chest may occasionally penetrate the cardiovascular system and eventually reach an extremity, with resulting circulatory embarrassment distal to the point of occlusion. Less common is bullet embolism to the pulmonary artery [58].

Contact gunshot wounds often have a pattern of powder debris on clothing and skin [1]. This should be carefully described, as it may be a crucial point should there be an allegation of homicide when, in fact, the wound was self-inflicted. All clothing should be retained for subsequent investigation and should be held even in the absence of police investigators, who are often busy elsewhere. One need only recall the confusion and unfortunate allegations that arose in the wake of the assassination of President John F. Kennedy. This was caused by lack of communication between rescue, surgical, and investigative teams during and after the tragedy. As a result, a not unexpected flood of malicious and ridiculous speculations arose that markedly obscured the issues. All of this is directly attributable to the lack of an initial coordinated investigation in which the surgeon and medical attendants should have played a key role.

The lethality of penetrating cardiac wounds depends upon location—left ventricle injury being worse than right—and to some extent upon the instrument that caused the injury. Sugg and associates [60] note that 80 percent of the 373 persons dead on arrival at Parkland Hospital, Dallas, had gunshot wounds, whereas 56 percent of the 86 patients who survived long enough to achieve some emergency room care had stab wounds. An aggressive, open thoracotomy approach has significantly reduced mortality, particularly with regard to cardiovascular stab wounds. Treatment of thoracic stab wounds in general must be individualized although it is apparent that tube thoracostomy may be adequate for uncomplicated lung wounds [41].

Stab wounds of the thorax may be inflicted by a variety of instruments, but the vast majority involve a single-edged kitchen knife and frequently follow a domestic drunken brawl between men and women, the latter often wielding the instrument. Depending on the thrust angle, depth, and number of wounds, the injuries can be quite variable. Bear in mind that a short-bladed knife is capable of a thrust deeper than the blade length if the thrust is made with vigor against a resilient body part. Occasionally an apparently superficial stab in the shoulder will partially sever the subclavian artery with resulting subtle hemothorax. An extremely rare complication is arterial air embolism occurring when a small amount of air from the penetrating injury of a lung enters the systemic circulation to pass through the left ventricle and thence to the brain. More frequently significant air embolisms are secondary to knife wounds of the neck with venous involvement.

The courtroom question may arise as to the degree of force necessary to inflict a stab wound by a knife. Actual tests indicate a wide variation in force, depending mainly on the cutting *point* of the weapon. In general a sharply pointed knife requires between 0.5 and 3.0 kilograms pressure to penetrate abdominal skin and underlying subcutaneous tissue [30].

The infrequency of esophageal injuries in the experience of medical examiners is in keeping with the rarity of perforations due to blunt trauma and penetrating wounds noted clinically [8]. Iatrogenic perforations can result in the clinical picture of fever, mediastinal emphysema, and pain. Occasionally a perforation exists in which contrast media may not reveal the defect. Spenler and Benfield [54] include in a series of esophageal perforations a patient with nonpenetrating trauma in whom cervical esophageal perforation followed a flexion-hyperextension injury received when his vehicle was struck from the rear. They postulate that demonstrable osteoarthritic bone spurs lacerated the esophagus during the collision incident. This is feasible, since we have seen such spurs fragment, leaving cutting edges, in similar vehicle crashes.

Air under pressure can enter the esophagus and constitute an expanding foreign body with dire results. In one of our cases a man was attempting to slash the tires of a large truck during a labor dispute. The resulting blast of air dislodged his dentures and tore a vertical rent 10 cm long in the lower third of the esophagus along the left anterolateral aspect. Gastric contents entered the left pleural cavity and left pneumothorax and subcutaneous emphysema followed. Despite surgical repair of the injury he developed mediastinitis and died 2 days later.

BLAST INJURY

Thoracoabdominal blast injury with limited survival time and subsequent investigation by the medical examiner is extremely rare. Most blast injuries we investigate involve only severed limbs or victims who have been killed immediately by the blast. On rare occasion we encounter delayed death from sepsis following multiple extremity injuries. In our jurisdiction the fatal blasts are approximately equally divided between industrial premature explosive detonation and criminal bombings. Underwater detonations with injuries to swimmers are more often a wartime phenomenon, such as the sinking of the Israeli destroyer Eilat in 1967 [26]. Twenty-eight of the 32 survivors were interrogated regarding symptoms and 24 were found to have felt the blast. The most common symptom was abdominal pain in 19 of the victims, transient lower limb paralysis in 11, and nausea or vomiting in 11. Although only 6 noted sudden chest pain, 27 of the total of 32 survivors had abnormal chest roentgenograms—which varied from small to diffuse opacities—on hospital admission. Pneumothorax, pneumomediastinum, and hemothorax were frequent. The main pathological lesion of thoracic blast injury is exudation of edema fluid and blood into alveoli and interstitial spaces along with pleural tears, bullae, and arteriovenous fistulas in some instances. In those who survive hypoxemia may persist for months [9].

PULMONARY INJURY AND OTHER SUPERIMPOSED PROCESSES

Many adverse pulmonary structural and functional alterations have long been recognized in trauma and disease. Unfortunately it has been difficult for pathologists, on morphological grounds, to create order from chaotic pathological end results of multiple superimposed processes. When illnesses, injuries, and complications are limited in number, clinical pathological correlations are more readily available as, for example, in uncomplicated pulmonary contusion [2]. The problems arise in the patient with multiple injuries and illnesses with prolonged diverse therapy, multiplicity of surgical procedures, and complications of other organ system impairment. Martin, Soloway, and Simmons [34] studied pulmonary pathological findings in 100 patients who died of shock or trauma, or both, during the Vietnam conflict. All had been clinically observed and complete postmortem examinations were available. They list pulmonary findings, including edema, congestion, fat embolism, bronchopneumonia, hyaline membrane atelectasis, hemorrhage, thromboemboli, and so on. Their limited discussion notes that the 14 patients with observed hyaline membrane lungs included 4 in whom clinical respiratory distress preceded the development of bronchopneumonia, edema, renal failure, or the use of high concentrations of oxygen. Parenthetically it should be noted that the fat embolism syndrome [21] exists, but pathological findings of pulmonary fat emboli rarely result in the syndrome. Such emboli in the absence of the syndrome may add to the burden of pulmonary insufficiency from other causation [27].

Lindquist, Rammer, and Saldeen [32] emphasized the problem of unexplained posttraumatic respiratory insufficiency and commented that the symptoms and morphological pulmonary changes were analogous to fat embolism. They searched for evidence of microembolism and fibrinolysis inhibition in posttraumatic postmortem material obtained in 28 cases of delayed automobile trauma at Upsala during the years 1964 to 1970. A progression of changes from early edema to later hyaline membrane and subsequent fibrosis were noted, as well as pneumonia and fat embolism. In 27 of the 28 a pattern of intravascular coagulation and fibrinolysis inhibition was noted. They interpret the fibrin within the vasculature to be microemboli from damaged areas of the body. Later Hill and colleagues [23] published a series of open lung biopsy findings during the early phase of acute respiratory insufficiency. They studied 42 patients, including 20 with trauma, 18 with pneumonia, 3 with nonpulmonary systemic sepsis, and 1 with paraquat poisoning. Large intravascular aggregation of fibrin was present in small amounts in two-thirds of these patients. Almost all had hyaline membranes and two-thirds had fibrinogen immunofluorescent material within alveoli. Twenty-

two had fibrosis. This appeared to be of prognostic importance since one-third without fibrosis survived while two-thirds with fibrosis did not. The trauma group (18 patients) had a more favorable survival rate, 39 percent, than the pneumonia group, 11 percent, but each had an equal incidence of fibrosis.

Blaisdell [6] summarized the sequential changes noted in the unexplained respiratory distress syndrome following trauma. Initially fibrin and platelet microemboli occur with later periarterial hemorrhages. After 12 to 24 hours severe congestion, alveolar septal hemorrhage, and edema are noted and the microemboli become less pronounced. At 72 hours alveolar hemorrhage is most pronounced, with some hyaline membranes being noted. After 72 hours hyaline membranes become quite prominent and are predominant at 3 to 5 days, at which time superimposed bronchopneumonia is prominent. At 10 to 14 days, if the patient survives, organization with subsequent fibrosis is noted. Blaisdell concludes that "pulmonary microembolism does cause the respiratory distress syndrome seen in traumatic shock and many other types of critical illness" [6].

Some clues as to the behavior of circulating platelets when exposed to irritants may be evident from the report of Wiedeman, Tuma, and Mayrovitz [66]. This study, applied to intra-arterial injections of parenteral or oral barbiturate preparations in the experimental bat model, revealed the sequential pathological effects of platelet mechanical blockage of arteriolar branch openings and the subsequent loss of lymphatic and venous vasomotion that would be expected to aggravate edema tendencies by virtue of lymphatic and venous insufficiency.

The pathological findings of Blaisdell [6] tend to correlate with the clinical observations of Zapol and Snider [69] that pulmonary hypertension may be demonstrated in severe acute respiratory failure. In postmortem studies of patients with severe acute respiratory failure Zapol and co-workers [68] have demonstrated progressive disintegration of microvasculature and have further demonstrated an increase in collagen content in patients with acute respiratory distress syndrome [70].

Of additional interest is a clinical study of two young adults who survived hanging episodes and subsequent respiratory distress syndrome characterized by respiratory distress, severe hypoxemia, and right-to-left shunting. One patient's pulmonary problem was complicated by aspiration of vomitus [16].

Pardy and Dudley [43] present a masterful hypothesis supported by a collective review of the literature in which an attempt is made to bring order and understanding to the problem of posttraumatic and postsepsis pulmonary insufficiency. They hypothesize that portal system materials injurious to lungs—endotoxins, bacteria, and others—are normally kept in check by the reticuloendothelial system of the liver, the Kupfer cells, which represent 80 percent of the body's reticuloendothelial system. With severe shock the intestinal mucosa line of defense is weakened, thus increasing the portal content of noxious substances. With liver injury, frequently occurring concomitant with nonpenetrating chest injury, the liver barrier is breached. The lung, containing only 1 percent of the reticuloendothelial system and that efficient mainly for airway contamination, is now vulnerable to an accumulation of material from the portal system, which may play a significant role in the pathogenesis of the acute respiratory distress syndrome picture. From a functional and morphological correlative standpoint this hypothesis is attractive and merits more investigation.

Pulmonary edema is common to many disease and injury states investigated by medical examiners. A particularly dramatic form is the profuse pulmonary edema associated with deaths following acute, intravenous "street" heroin abuse. To some this has been a great mystery postulated as allergy [22]. To me this represents simply the superimposition of several mechanisms. One is the dying asphyxial state when respirations are centrally depressed by the circulating blood morphinans. Under these circumstances the heart continues to beat (slow heart stoppage) and circulation lacks the assistance of respiratory excursions. Delayed heart stoppage has been well documented in cases of sudden respiratory cessation for well over a century [5]. Central nervous system hypoxia-induced pulmonary edema may also play a role [13]. In addition in these patients a bolus of filth, particulate matter, and miscellaneous chemicals, opiates, barbiturates, tranquilizers, quinine, and so on enter a lung whose reticuloendothelial system may already be overloaded by previous abuses. It is common to find granulomata, mineral matter, cellulose, and starch entrapped in the lungs and elsewhere from previous intravenous injections [64]. The result is features

that are similar in respects to the pathological findings described in early phases of the acute respiratory distress syndrome, with the exception that edema is more pronounced.

The complexity of superimposed direct and indirect trauma upon the lungs, aspiration, sepsis, and therapeutic intervention results in great difficulties in retrospective postmortem reconstruction of events. Injuries received during emergency cardiopulmonary resuscitation may merge with other injury [57]. Obviously well-documented clinical observations are a necessity for a dynamic clinicopathological correlation. An excellent example of such complexity is a clinicopathological correlation from the Massachusetts General Hospital [35]. A 23-year-old patient seriously injured in an automobile accident subsequently had two lung biopsies, but he died after 22 days of intense hospital study. Noteworthy in the clinical history was the lack of an attempt to ascertain from rescue and scene investigative personnel the immediate postcrash position of the victim and any observations pertaining to apparent aspiration of blood or gastric content, or problems associated with the patient's extrication from the wrecked vehicle. Wright and Harris [67] pinpoint the necessity for such scene-investigative information from a series of patients with postural asphyxia in whom neck flexion restricted the airway during the immediate postcrash situation or during rescue transport. Such hypoxic positions and other significant, immediate postcrash observations should be of great value to clinicians concerned with subsequent problems of diagnosis and treatment.

The inhalation of fumes likewise adds to the complexity of diagnosis and treatment. Most common is cigarette smoke, which may be expected to account for a significant depression of bronchial-clearing ability and also to result in increased levels of carbon monoxide in the blood. It is commonly accepted that up to 10 percent of carbon monoxide saturation of hemoglobin may be explained by cigarette smoking, but it is possible, in heavy chain smokers, to observe twice this concentration. This is an additional burden upon respiratory function in the traumatized patient. More severe smoke inhalation may be expected when there has been postcrash fire, with or without other physical injury. Genovesi and colleagues [18] document mild to moderately severe hypoxemia in 19 firemen exposed to smoke from burning polyvinylchloride plastic in which the mean

PaO$_2$ was 64 mm Hg at 2 to 10 hours after exposure. Fortunately no chronic effects could be documented 1 month later [61]. Clinical study of pyrolytic noxious compounds is in its infancy and only recently has serious consideration been given to this problem [40].

DROWNING

Drowning, in company with other forms of trauma, is most frequently associated with motor vehicle entry into waterways. The pathophysiology is complex due to variabilities of age, preexisting disease, chemical impairment, resuscitative attempts, composition of the watery environment, and, quite significantly, the variable amounts of water that may have been inhaled. In many victims the amount of water inhaled may be very little, due to protective reflex laryngospasm and resultant breathholding. However, even a small amount of water, as little as 1 ml per pound of body weight, has been shown to result in prolonged arterial hypoxemia under experimental conditions [38, 39].

The final common pathway of drowning is hypoxia, whether the water is fresh or seawater. Fresh water destroys surfactant, with a resulting decrease in compliance along with an alveolar cell membrane increase in permeability. This results in pulmonary edema and increased hypoxia. Seawater has less surfactant effect, but, being hypertonic, it results in more intra-alveolar edema and even hemoconcentration, depending on the amount aspirated. With fresh water there may be hemodilution. Although electrolyte changes have been theoretically involved in the resulting clinical picture, this has not been substantiated in the detailed and excellent clinical and laboratory studies of Modell [37].

Near-drowning, or postimmersion syndrome, is a medical emergency necessitating the utmost in respiratory care therapy. The treatment has been well detailed by Modell [37]. The target organs are either the lungs or the brain. With aspiration of little water and minimal pneumonitis, lack of recovery may be due to hypoxic brain effects, the patient remaining neurologically depressed after rescue. On the other hand, the postrescue clinical picture may be that of loss of pulmonary function, even though consciousness has returned. Persistent hypoxemia and increasingly poor response to oxygen therapy results. The pathological end result is a pneumonitis characterized by copious fibrinous alveolar exudate, hyaline membranes, and hemorrhages. All this represents the summation of aspirated water effect, vomit aspiration, oxygen toxicity, and bacterial invasion.

Aspiration of the fuel-contaminated water, following automobile or aircraft submersion, may add to the risk of pulmonary complications. The effect can be subtle and might escape detection unless adequate observation is maintained. For example, the helicopter used for the transportation of President Nixon lost power and crashed into the sea on approach to Grand Cay, Bahamas, on the evening of May 26, 1973. The president was not aboard but seven Secret Service agent passengers and three crew members were. The craft capsized, commenced to sink, and trapped the passengers in a partially flooded JP-4 fuel-contaminated compartment. Six were rescued by the crew who had escaped through a hatch. The seventh passenger had drowned. Four survivors had skin "burns" from the solvent action of fuel, and 3 had temporarily clouded sensorium from fume inhalation. All were flown to a military hospital for observation and released the next day, apparently well. A few days later, at the instigation of the physician in charge of the human factors aspect of crash investigation, the survivors had follow-up chest roentgenograms. One had evidence of an unsuspected pneumonia, most likely on the basis of minimal fuel inhalation.

Hypothermia, as a complication of the drowning process, is important in colder climates. Death from hypothermia may be rapid, occurring in as little as 45 minutes for an adult in water of 1.5°C [56]. With children the large ratio of surface area to body mass increases the cooling rate. When interior body temperature drops to below 30°C, consciousness diminishes and cardiac dysrhythmias may result [14].

NOTIFICATION OF MEDICAL EXAMINER—A LEGAL MATTER

In the event that the victim of an injury dies because of the injury or its complications, regardless of the duration of incapacity and regardless of where the injury occurred in the first place, attending physicians have a legal obligation to notify the medical examiner or coroner, depending on the system in that particular jurisdiction. The law usually provides a penalty for failure to comply with these requirements, a potential source of embarrassment for the busy practitioner who might consider it beneath his dignity to carry out such a task. In those jurisdictions with better systems of medicolegal death investigations, the body is removed to the central morgue for identification, photography, postmortem examination, toxicological study if needed, and correlation of findings with circumstances. On the other hand, the attending physician may find himself in a backward, poorly serviced jurisdiction where he alone is left to certify the cause of death. In such an event he must follow the format clearly outlined on the death certificate and should use terms that can be coded according to the International Classification of Diseases [63]. Noncausative terms such as *cardiac arrest, congestive heart failure, ventricular fibrillation* or nonqualified *bronchopneumonia* or *pulmonary embolism* should be avoided. Rather, the terminology should include the primary causative disease or agent of injury. If a patient dies of hemorrhage associated with carcinoma of the lung, the certificate should read, for example, "pulmonary hemorrhage due to bronchogenic carcinoma of the lung." In the event of an injury, an example might be "laceration of heart and lung due to gunshot wound of chest" or "pulmonary thromboembolism due to multiple fractures of ribs, spine, and pelvis."

In summary, it should be reiterated that a large jurisdiction adequately represented by a well staffed medicolegal death-investigative agency, hopefully affiliated with schools of medicine and law, is in the position of providing a central data bank from which the physician can derive data to enable better care of injured patients. The community can draw upon this same source for the basic facts needed to cope with problems of transportation, overcrowding, crime, accidents, and many other aspects of public health and social problems.

REFERENCES

1. Adelson L: The Pathology of Homicide (A Vade Mecum for Pathologist, Prosecutor and Defense Counsel). Springfield, Ill, Thomas, 1974, Chap. V
2. Alfano GS, Hale HW: Pulmonary contusion. J Trauma 5:647, 1965
3. Amato JJ, Billy LJ, Gruber RP, et al: Vascular injuries, an experimental study of high and low velocity missile wounds. Arch Surg 101:167, 1970
4. Ashbaugh DG, Peters GN, Halgrimson CG, et al: Chest trauma, analysis of 685 patients. Arch Surg 95:546, 1967
5. Atlee WL: Report of a series of experiments made by the Medical Faculty of Lancaster, upon the body of Henry Cobler Mosselman, executed in the jail yard of Lancaster County, Pa., on the 20th of December, 1839. Am J Med Sci 51:2–34, 1840
6. Blaisdell FW: Pathophysiology of the respiratory distress syndrome. Arch Surg 108:44, 1974
7. Bloch B, Meir J: Isolated traumatic tears of the interventricular septum. J Forensic Sci 9:81, 1977
8. Briggs JN, Germann TD: Traumatic perforations of the esophagus. Surg Clin North Am 48:1297, 1968
9. Caseby NG, Porter MF: Blast injuries to the lungs: Clinical presentation, management and course. Injury 8:1, 1977
10. Charters AC III, Charters AC: Wounding mechanism of very high velocity projectiles. J Trauma 16:464, 1976
11. Committee on Public Works: 1968 Alcohol and Highway Safety Report. 90th Congress, 2nd session. Washington, DC, US Government Printing Office, 1968
12. DeMuth WE: High velocity bullet wounds of the thorax. Am J Surg 115:616, 1968
13. Ducker TB, Simmons RL, Anderson RW: Increased intracranial pressure and pulmonary edema. 3: The effect of increased intracranial pressure on the cardiovascular hemodynamics of chimpanzees. J Neurosurg 29:475, 1968
14. Editorial: Immersion and drowning in children. Br Med J 2:146, 1977
15. Fine PR, Stafford MA, Miller JM III, et al: Gunshot wounds of the spinal cord: A survey of literature and epidemiologic study of 48 lesions in Alabama. Ala J Med 13:173, 1976
16. Fischman CM, Goldstein MS, Gardner LB: Suicidal hanging, an association with the adult respiratory distress syndrome. Chest 71:225, 1977
17. Friedman M: The coronary thrombus, its origin and fate. Hum Pathol 2:81, 1971
18. Genovesi MG, Tashkin DP, Chopra S, et al: Transient hypoxemia in firemen following inhalation of smoke. Chest 71:441, 1977
19. Greendyke RM: Traumatic rupture of the aorta, special reference to automobile accidents. JAMA 195:527, 1966
20. Griffiths DK, Hayes HRM, Gloyns PF, et al: Car occupant fatalities and the effects of future safety legislation. In Proceedings of the 20th Stapp Car Crash Conference. Warrendale, Penn, Society of Automotive Engineers, 1976, p. 383

21. Gurd AR, Wilson RI: The fat embolism syndrome. J Bone Joint Surg [Br] 56:408, 1974

22. Helpern M: Fatalities from narcotic addiction in New York City. Incidence, circumstances, and pathologic findings. Hum Pathol 3:13, 1972

23. Hill JD, Ratliff JL, Parrott JCW, et al: Pulmonary pathology in acute respiratory insufficiency: Lung biopsy as a diagnostic tool. J Thorac Cardiovasc Surg 71:64, 1976

24. Honkanen R, Ottelin J: Blood alcohol levels in injury victims at the emergency station of a rural central hospital. Ann Chir Gynaecol Fenn 65:282, 1976

25. Honkanen R, Visuri T: Blood alcohol levels in a series of injured patients with special reference to accident and type of injury. Ann Chir Gynaecol Fenn 65:287, 1976

26. Huller T, Bazini Y: Blast injuries of the chest and abdomen. Arch Surg 100:24, 1970

27. Kallos T: Impaired arterial oxygenation associated with use of bone cement in the femoral shaft. Anesthesiology 42:210, 1975

28. Kihlberg JK: Multiplicity of injury in automobile accidents. Impact Injury and Crash Protection. Edited by ES Gurdjian et al. Springfield, Ill, Thomas, 1970, Chap. 1

29. Kirsh MM, Orringer MB, Behrendt DM, et al: Management of tracheobronchial disruption secondary to nonpenetrating trauma. (Collective review.) Ann Thorac Surg 22:93, 1976

30. Knight B: The dynamics of stab wounds. J Forensic Sci 6:249, 1975

31. Kulowski J: Crash Injuries: the Integrated Medical Aspects of Automobile Injuries and Deaths (Preface). Springfield, Ill, Thomas, 1960

32. Lindquist O, Rammer L, Saldeen T: Pulmonary insufficiency, microembolism and fibrinolysis inhibition in post-traumatic autopsy material. Acta Chir Scand 138:545, 1972

33. Macklin MT, Macklin CC: Malignant interstitial emphysema of the lungs and mediastinum as an important occult complication in many respiratory diseases and other conditions: An interpretation of the clinical literature in the light of laboratory experiment. (Review.) Medicine 23:281, 1944

34. Martin AM, Soloway HB, Simmons RL: Pathologic anatomy of the lungs following shock and trauma. J Trauma 8:687, 1968

35. Massachusetts General Hospital: Case 22–1977. N Engl J Med 296:1279, 1977

36. Mattila S: Rupture and successful repair of the heart following blunt chest injury. Ann Chir Gynaecol Fenn 65:145, 1976

37. Modell JH: The Pathophysiology and Treatment of Drowning and Near Drowning. Springfield, Ill, Thomas, 1971

38. Modell JH, Moya F: Effects of volume of aspirated fluid during chlorinated fresh water drowning. Anesthesiology 27:662, 1966

39. Modell JH, Moya F, Newby EJ, et al: Effects of fluid volume in seawater drowning. Ann Int Med 67:68, 1967

40. National Research Council: Physiological and Toxicological Aspects of Combustion Products: International Symposium. Washington, DC, National Academy of Sciences, 1976

41. Oparah SS, Mandal AK: Penetrating stab wounds of the chest: Experience with 200 consecutive cases. J Trauma 16:868, 1976

42. Oren A, Bar-Shlomo B, Stern S: Acute coronary occlusion following blunt injury to the chest in the absence of coronary atherosclerosis. Am Heart J 92:501, 1976

43. Pardy BJ, Dudley HAF: Post-traumatic pulmonary insufficiency. (Review.) Surg Gynecol Obstet 144:259, 1977

44. Robbins DH, Melvin JW, Stalnaker RL: The prediction of thoracic impact injuries. In Proceedings of the 20th Stapp Car Crash Conference. Warrendale, Penn, Society of Automotive Engineers, 1976, p. 699

45. Rybeck B: Missile wounding and hemodynamic effects of energy absorption. (Thesis and review.) Acta Chir Scand (suppl. 450), 1974

46. Saunders CR, Doty DB: Myocardial contusion. (Review.) Surg Gynecol Obstet 144:595, 1977

47. Sevitt S: Fatal road accidents in Birmingham, times of death and their causes. Injury 4:281, 1973

48. Sevitt S: Traumatic ruptures of the aorta: A clinico-pathological study. Injury 8:159, 1977

49. Sevitt S: The mechanisms of traumatic rupture of the thoracic aorta. Br J Surg 64:166, 1977

50. Shatsky SA, Alter WA III, Evans DE, et al: Traumatic distortions of the primate head and chest: Correlation of biomechanical, radiological and pathological data. In Proceedings of the 18th Stapp Car Crash Conference. Warrendale, Penn, Society of Automotive Engineers, 1974, p. 378

51. Sims JK, Ebisu RJ, Wong RKM, et al: Automobile accident occupant injuries. (Review.) JACEP 5:796, 1976

52. Smith JM III, Grover FL, Marcos JJ, et al: Blunt traumatic rupture of the atria. J Thorac Cardiovasc Surg 71:617, 1976

53. Spees EK, Strevey TE, Geiger JP, et al: Persistent traumatic lung cavities resulting from medium- and high-velocity missiles. Ann Thorac Surg 4:133, 1967

54. Spenler CW, Benfield JR: Esophageal disruption from blunt and penetrating external trauma. Arch Surg 111:663, 1976

55. Spitz WU, Wilhelm RM: Stud gun injuries. J Forensic Med 17:5, 1970
56. Spitz WU: Drowning. In Medicolegal Investigation of Death Guidelines for the Application of Pathology to Crime Investigation. Springfield, Ill, Thomas, 1973, Chap XIII
57. Stephenson HE: Cardiac Complications (Chap. 57), and Complications to Other Organs and Systems in Cardiac Resuscitation (Chap. 58). In Cardiac Arrest and Resuscitation (4th ed.). St. Louis, Mosby, 1974
58. Stephenson LW, Workman RB, Aldrete JS, et al: Bullet emboli to the pulmonary artery: A report of 2 patients and review of the literature. Ann Thorac Surg 21:333, 1976
59. Stoppa R, Ossart JL, Henry X, et al: Thoracic and abdominal injuries in multiple trauma. Int Surg 62:8, 1970
60. Sugg WL, Rea WJ, Ecker RR, et al: Penetrating wounds of the heart, an analysis of 459 cases. J Thorac Cardiovasc Surg 56:531, 1968
61. Tashkin DP, Genovesi MG, Chopra S, et al: Respiratory status of Los Angeles firemen. One-month follow-up after inhalation of dense smoke. Chest 71:445, 1977
62. Turney SZ, Attar S, Ayella R, et al: Traumatic rupture of the aorta. A five year experience. J Thorac Cardiovasc Surg 72:727, 1976
63. U.S. Department of Health, Education, and Welfare: Eighth Revision of International Classification of Disease. Washington, DC, US

Public Health Service Publication No. 1693. Vol. 1.
64. Wetli CV, Davis JH, Blackbourne BD: Narcotic addiction in Dade County, Florida. An analysis of 100 consecutive cases. Arch Pathol 93:330, 1972
65. Whelan P, Ackroyd CE: Seat belts: A study of their use by the victims of road traffic accidents. Injury 8:269, 1977
66. Wiedeman MP, Tuma RF, Mayrovitz HN: In vivo microscopic observations of intra-arterial injections of barbiturates. J Surg Res 22:97, 1977
67. Wright RK, Harris LS: Auto fatalities by postural asphyxia. Proceedings of the 18th Conference of the American Association of Automotive Medicine, 1974, pp. 104–107
68. Zapol WM, Kobayashi K, Snider MT, et al: Vascular obstruction causes pulmonary hypertension in severe acute respiratory failure. Chest 71:306, 1977
69. Zapol WM, Snider MT: Pulmonary hypertension in severe acute respiratory failure. N Engl J Med 296:476, 1977
70. Zapol WM, Trelstad R, Coffey J, et al: Total lung collagen content (TLC) rapidly increases during adult respiratory distress syndrome (ARDS). Am Rev Resp Dis (Suppl.) 115:183, 1977
71. Ziperman HH, Cromack JR, Clark JM: Air bags and seatbelts in injury amelioration. J Trauma 16:686, 1976

INDEX